HEARING
CONSERVATION

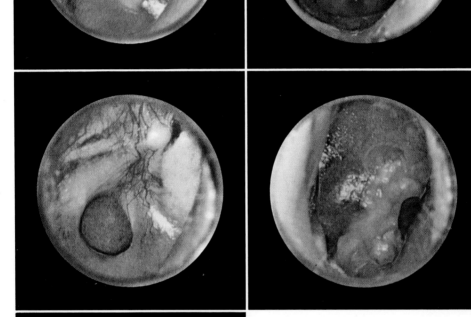

Plate 1. Normal eardrum. Plate 2. Large inferior central type perforation with inflammation of medial wall of middle ear. Plate 3. Postero-inferior perforation which has healed with thin atrophic scar. Remaining pars tensa is thickened and heavily scarred anteriorly. Very prominent corda tympany. This type scar is frequently misinterpreted as an open perforation. Plate 4. Cholesteatoma-growth in the middle ear. Eardrum is gone. Plate 5. Chronic otitis media, adhesive. The entire posterior quadrant of the drum is so deeply retracted that there appears to be a perforation of the drum. The yellow-brown color of the drum is due to presence of serous fluid in the middle ear. (40 dB hearing loss) (Note: Plate 1-5 photos by R. Buckingham)

RF291
S29

HEARING
CONSERVATION

By

JOSEPH SATALOFF, M.D., D.Sc.

Professor of Otology
Thomas Jefferson University
Philadelphia, Pennsylvania
Scientific Member
United States Department of Labor's Standards Advisory
Committee on Noise

and

PAUL MICHAEL, Ph.D.

Professor of Environmental Acoustics
Director of the Environmental Acoustics Laboratory
The Pennsylvania State University
State College, Pennsylvania

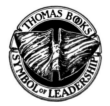

CHARLES C THOMAS · PUBLISHER
Springfield · Illinois · U.S.A.

NO LONGER THE PROPERTY
OF THE
UNIVERSITY OF R. I. LIBRARY

Published and Distributed Throughout the World by

CHARLES C THOMAS • PUBLISHER

Bannerstone House

301-327 East Lawrence Avenue, Springfield, Illinois, U.S.A.

This book is protected by copyright. No part of it
may be reproduced in any manner without written
permission from the publisher.

© *1973, by* CHARLES C THOMAS • PUBLISHER

ISBN 0-398-02822-2

Library of Congress Catalog Card Number: 73-200

*With THOMAS BOOKS careful attention is given to all details of
manufacturing and design. It is the Publisher's desire to present books that are
satisfactory as to their physical qualities and artistic possibilities and
appropriate for their particular use. THOMAS BOOKS will be true to those
laws of quality that assure a good name and good will.*

Printed in the United States of America

C-1

34368

INTRODUCTION

THE INCREASE in industrial noise and a greater appreciation of deafness in general has focused attention upon occupational deafness during recent years. The federal government and many state governments have shown their concern by passing rules and regulations to prevent occupational deafness.

Noisy industries face many challenging problems in the development of effective hearing conservation programs which will comply with current rules and regulations. To cope with these problems there is needed:

1. A complete understanding and a clear perspective of all aspects of occupational deafness as it relates to employees and management.
2. The ability to measure and evaluate noise exposures.
3. The ability to perform meaningful hearing tests.
4. An understanding of noise reduction procedures.

This book is intended to cover all of these vital topics on a level that will be useful for engineers, executives, hearing testers, industrial hygienists, nurses, otologists, physicians, and safety personnel. No previous experience in the field is required to understand the material presented.

The book provides a basic and practical overview of the physics of sound, how we hear, and the causes of deafness, which are needed to understand the problem of occupational deafness. In addition, it provides basic and practical instruction in hearing measurement, noise measurement, noise control, and other factors needed in the development of effective hearing conservation programs. Extra-auditory effects of noise are covered from the point of view of community reaction.

The authors express their gratitude to many colleagues and friends, especially the faculty at Colby College and Penn State University whose sustained interest and encouragement have made this book possible. We are particularly indebted to the following persons for their direct and indirect assistance in the preparations of this book: Eddie Anderson, Chester Arnold, Lawrence Ballou, Edward Bartlett, Duane L. Block, D. Bolka, T. B. Bonney, Howard Bunn, Ross Coles, Aram Glorig, R. E. Gosztonyi, Vaughn Hill, Harold Imbus, E. Irvin, Roger Maas, R. M. Marrazzo, Calvin Michaels, K. M. Morse, Anne Murphy, Robert Sataloff, Floyd Van Atta, John Zapp, L. G. Doerfler, Alexander Cohen and C. W. Nixon.

The authors express their appreciation to the J. B. Lippincott Company, Philadelphia, for permitting them to extract freely from Dr. Sataloff's book, *Hearing Loss.*

Mr. Lawrence Vassallo warrants special appreciation for his major contribution in the chapters on hearing testing and for his careful editing of the manuscript. To our secretaries, Paula Francia, Mary Jane Grooms, and Mrs. D. L. Tindal and others we are indebted for their tireless efforts.

JOSEPH SATALOFF
PAUL L. MICHAEL

CONTENTS

HEARING
CONSERVATION

Chapter I

THE IMPORTANCE OF
GOOD HEARING

PREVENTING HEARING LOSS due to excessive noise exposure and reducing annoyance from environmental noise have become major issues in America. The federal government evidenced its serious concern by passing the Walsh-Healey Regulation in May 1969 and then the Occupational Safety and Health Act in April 1971. These specify that 90 decibels (dB) on the "A" scale of the noise level meter is the point at which industry must begin hearing conservation if employees are exposed to high decibel noises all day for many years. The Occupational Safety and Health Act makes the noise regulations in Walsh-Healey applicable to all American industry. The Department of Labor is conducting an active program of inspection to encourage compliance with these regulations.

Many states (such as New York, Wisconsin, California, Missouri, Maryland and Maine) have recognized the importance of hearing loss and have passed special legislation for compensating employees suffering from deafness due to occupational noise. Some states, like California, and even the City of Philadelphia have passed regulations limiting the amount of noise exposure permitted in industry. New York, advanced in this area of study, established a regulation of the noise transmission characteristics of walls, ceilings and floors in apartment houses. Most major cities have noise ordinances applying to sirens, horn-blowing and the use of amplifiers in the streets. It is apparent from the countless scientific and lay publications on noise and its deleterious effects, and from the increasing regulations, legislation and compensation activity, that industry and government must take positive measures to correct the problem. The urgent necessity to comply with the federal regulations is of prime importance. Only by instituting effective hearing conservation programs can industries prevent occupational hearing loss. Providing compensation for a permanent and incurable hearing loss that is caused by noise is not an acceptable or satisfactory solution. Emphasis must be placed on prevention rather than on compensation for if the former succeeds the latter is eliminated. Occupational hearing loss is one of the most solvable issues in American public health. It *is* possible in years to come to prevent over 95 percent of all cases of occupational deafness due to excessive noise exposures that now affect many millions of workers. The growing emphasis on environmental pollution will undoubtedly focus even more attention upon noise during the coming decade. Legislation, regulation, and compensation will become major issues and cannot be overlooked in considering the many solutions to occupational deafness and excessive environmental noise. The legal and economic aspects of occupational hearing loss are discussed in Chapter 9.

Physicians, nurses, hygienists, safety engineers and executives must be aware of the economic and legal aspects of occupational hearing loss, but by far the most compelling and moving reasons for our interest in this important problem are the medical and humane aspects. There are millions of people in this country with substantial hearing impairments because they work in noisy jobs, and inadequate measures have been taken to quiet the noise or to establish effective ear protection programs. There are, in addition, millions of people with hearing losses due to causes other than noise exposure that are curable and not enough has been done to help them. In industry there are probably more people with occupational hearing loss than there are with all other occupational diseases combined, such as silicosis, emphysema, radium poisoning, lead poisoning, etc. Of even greater importance is the growing awareness that no physical handicap can have so many and so serious repercussions on the personalities of people as can a hearing loss. Many employees, because of their high frequency nerve deafness become unable to distinguish speech especially in groups or in noisy environments. Most of them do not go to movies, theatres, or churches, or purchase radios or television as freely as the normal population. This type of hearing loss is poorly compensated, if at all, by hearing aids. Consequently many of these people are excluded by their handicap from any type of advancement that requires them to participate in educational meetings or conversations in groups and they are deprived of normal enjoyments, becoming outcasts to some degree and occasionally even misfits. Interestingly enough, some of the worst effects on the personality are associated with hearing deficits which seem mild on a numerical or percentage basis and this is because the quality of hearing suffers more than the quantity, and the quality is sometimes hard to measure. Hearing is a phenomenon that utilizes the pathway between the ears and the brain and is an essential part of human response. In any discussion of hearing it is necessary to think of the person as a whole and not merely as a pair of ears. This is because the whole person is affected if he is frustrated in a promotion, education, recreation or self-fulfillment. To add to all of this, a further reason why occupational hearing loss is of such crucial importance is that the type of nerve deafness produced by exposure to excessive noise is irreversible and incurable.

We are becoming increasingly aware that occupational hearing loss is a serious threat to the well-being of our industrial population, especially skilled labor. Industry is obligated to preserve its greatest asset; the good health of its employees.

The Relationship Between Hearing and Speech

To understand the basis for the personality changes and communication handicaps that hearing loss may produce, it is necessary to recall the relationship between hearing and speech. The ear is sensitive to a certain range of sound frequencies and obviously speech falls within that range. Speech can be divided into two types of sounds: vowels and consonants. Roughly speaking, the vowels fall into the frequencies below 1,500 cycles per second (cps) or Hertz (Hz) and consonants above 1,500 Hz. The vowels are relatively powerful sounds, whereas consonants are weak and quite often are not pronounced clearly. Sometimes consonants are even dropped entirely in everyday speech.

Vowels give power to speech, that is, they signify that someone is speaking, but by themselves they give very little information about what the speaker is saying. To give specific meaning to words, consonants are interspersed among the vowels. Thus it can be roughly stated that vowels indicate someone is saying something, whereas consonants help the listener to distinguish *what* the speaker is saying. This ability to distinguish words is called "discrimination."

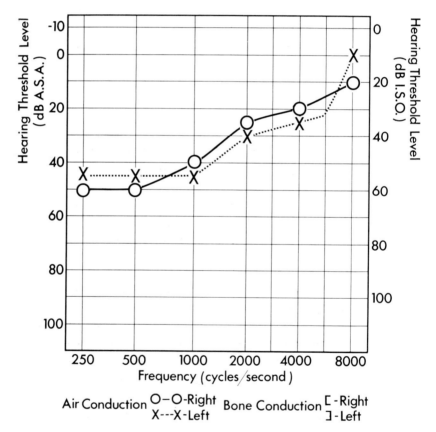

Figure 1. Audiogram showing a hearing loss chiefly in the lower frequencies and due to infection in the middle ears.

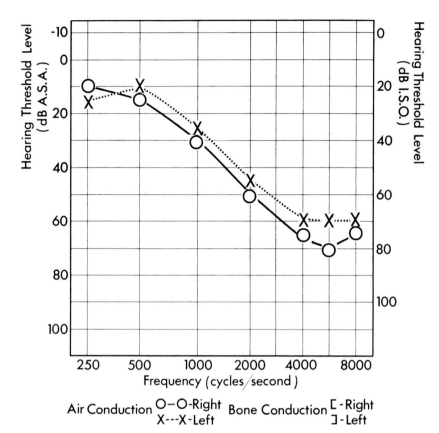

Figure 2. Audiogram showing a hearing loss chiefly in the high frequencies and due to nerve deafness resulting from congenital and hereditary factors.

To show the difference between hearing trouble merely for loudness as opposed to reduced discrimination let us examine the audiogram of a person whose hearing loss is in the low register, not due to noise exposure but resulting, let's say, from ear infection (Fig. 1). Such an individual would have difficulty hearing speech unless it was quite loud. His difficulty lies in the low tones, and so he cannot hear vowels. He would not be able to hear a soft voice, but if the voice was raised he would understand it clearly. His principal need is one of loudness or amplification, therefore a hearing aid would serve him well.

On the other hand, the person whose audiogram is portrayed

in Figure 2 has a high tone loss with almost normal hearing in the low register. This person hears vowels almost normally but has difficulty in hearing and distinguishing between consonants. If addressed in a loud voice, this person might find it disturbing since the raised voice would emphasize the missing consonants only slightly, while increasing the loudness of the vowels to an intolerable degree. The individual's chief problem is not so much hearing as understanding what he hears. He hears the vowels and knows someone is speaking; but he cannot distinguish between some of the consonants, and so he has to guess at what is being said. Such a person would want the speaker to enunciate more clearly and especially to pronounce the consonants more distinctively, rather than to speak in a loud voice.

Hearing loss of the latter type is found commonly in presbycusis (old age deafness), occupational deafness, and in certain types of congenital deafness and other causes.

The handicap imposed by deafness may vary from very little to a crushing burden. There are many causes of deafness not connected with excessive noise, and persons with hearing loss are so numerous that it would not be possible to avoid hiring employees so affected since they include thousands of gifted and high qualified workers. Management people should therefore have some comprehension of how workers are affected by various kinds of hearing loss, and bear in mind that nonindustrial hearing loss can have industrial deafness superimposed on it.

Reactions to Hearing Loss

The manner in which people react to hearing loss varies considerably. Some may try to minimize or to hide their defect. One such person, to keep up with a conversation, makes strenuous listening efforts and fills in hearing gaps by guessing, while carefully concealing his frustration by acting particularly pleasant and affable. His effort to "save face" leads to numerous embarrassing situations, becomes fatiguing and leads to nervousness, irritability and instability. He sits on the edge of his chair and leans forward to hear better. From the strain of listening his brow becomes wrinkled and his face serious and strained. Toward evening he is worn out from his efforts to hide and to deny his handicap. The sense of humor in which he once took great pride falters in a losing effort to maintain a pretense of normalcy, and makes way for a desperate show of sham amiability and a grim smile.

Some people react to hearing loss, particularly that of slow and insidious onset, by becoming withdrawn and losing interest in their environment. This, the most common type of reaction, is reflected in an avoidance of social contacts and in a preoccupation with the subject's own misfortunes. He shuns his friends and makes excuses to avoid social contacts that might cause his handicap to become more apparent to friends and to himself.

Economic and Family Aspects

This reaction may be seen in a businessman who has to sit at board meetings and planning or training meetings for salesmen and executives. The hearing-handicapped person soon realizes that he cannot keep up with what is going on, though his mental ability may still be as good as ever. Rather than tolerate criticism and suspicious remarks reflecting on his alertness and proper interest in business, he may resign his responsibilities and step down to a position less worthy of his potential. In one instance a successful executive, after years of effort and hard work had at last been rewarded with a vice-presidency of his firm. He found, however, that he was getting little enjoyment out of his new position because of his weariness at the end of the day from straining to hear what was said during business hours. He found that more and more often he was asking people to repeat what they said and, worst of all, in conferences and business meetings he was missing important parts of conversations, sometimes improvising answers to questions that he had not clearly heard so that his answers were proving embarrassing. He was extremely reluctant to admit to himself that it was his hearing which was causing his difficulty.

When a salesman becomes hard-of-hearing, his business usually suffers, and his ambitions frequently are suppressed or completely surrendered.

A hearing impairment may cause no handicap to a chipper or a riveter while he is at work. His deafness may even seem to be an advantage, since the noise of his work is not as loud to him as it is to his fellow workers with normal hearing. Because there is little or no verbal communication in most jobs that produce intense noise, a hearing loss will not be made apparent by inability to understand complicated verbal directions in a noisy environment. However, when such a workman returns to his family at night or goes on vacation, the situation assumes a completely different perspective. He has trouble understanding what his wife is saying, especially if he is reading the paper, and his wife is talking while attending noisy chores in the kitchen. This kind of situation frequently leads at first to a mild dispute and later to a serious family tension.

The wife accuses the husband of inattention which he denies, while he complains in rebuttal that she mumbles. Actually, he eventually does become inattentive when he realizes how frustrating and fatiguing it is to strain to hear. When the same individual tries to attend meetings, visit with friends, or go to church services and finds he cannot hear what is going on, or is laughed at for giving an answer unrelated to the subject under discussion he soon, but very reluctantly, realizes that something is wrong with him. He stops going to places where he feels pilloried by his handicap. He stops going to the movies, the theatre, the concert, for the voices and the music are not only far away but frequently distorted. Little by little his whole family life may be undermined, and a cloud overhangs his future and that of his dependents.

He may have been taking evening courses to improve his education and qualify for advancement, and finds he misses large portions of the lectures. Afterwards he tries to make up by asking fellow students to share their notes. Finally, he may become a "drop-out," though gifted with a brilliant mind. He finds the road to advancement barred, his natural ambitions frustrated, and a lifetime of mediocrity facing him. No wonder he becomes resentful of his fate, and critical of acquaintances who make light of his handicap.

The Plight of the Aged Deaf

Hearing losses in older persons, whether from causes associated with aging or owing to other sensori-neural (nerve deafness) causes, are often quite profound. All too often the unfortunate oldster begins to believe that his inability to hear and to understand a conversation, particularly when several people are talking at once, is due to deterioration of his brain. This belief generally is forced on him by his family and friends, who disregard him in group conversations and assume the attitude that he does not understand what is going on anyhow, so why include him in the conversation? Occasionally, he will overhear a remark or notice a gesture signifying that he is getting old and slowing down. Such talk and such attitudes further undermine the old person's already weakened self-confidence and hasten the personality changes so common in deafness, and more particularly in the aged deaf.

Effect of Mild Hearing Losses

Strangely enough, some of the most profound personality changes and communication handicaps occur in people who have comparatively mild hearing losses. This effect is particularly evident in *otosclerosis*. It is seen also in occupational deafness of moderate degree and in that accompanied by distortion of hearing and *tinnitus* (ear noises). Often such an individual is constantly disturbed not only by noises in his ears (the artificial tinny sound of music, the loud blur of amplified sound, and certain voices) but even more by the haunting fear that he will not be able to understand what someone is going to say to him. On some occasions he may hear and understand very well and at other times he cannot make out what is being said.

People with borderline losses tend to hide their handicap and to deny it even to themselves. They conceal their deafness just as they try to conceal their hearing aids if they can be induced to use them. The feelings of uncertainty and insecurity that result from so-called borderline hearing loss may lay the foundation for profound changes in a subject's personality structure. They lead to irritability and suspicion. Since he catches only stray

24368

words of a nearby conversation, an individual may come to feel that others are talking about him in a contemptuous and derogatory manner. This makes him feel resentful and tends to bring out in him latent neurotic tendencies for which he might otherwise have compensated successfully.

Effect of Profound Hearing Losses

In general, people with profound hearing losses are somewhat easier to help than the borderline cases, since the severely deafened are more ready to admit that they have a handicap. Of course the major handicaps of persons with severe losses concern communication as well as some personality problems. Often these individuals cannot hear warning signals, such as a fire bell or a siren. They cannot maintain a job on engines which require the use of hearing to detect flaws in operation. This is particularly true in persons working with airplanes, diesel engines and other types of machinery. Another important handicap in the more severe losses is the inability to tell the direction from which a sound is coming. This difficulty is particularly prominent when the deafness exists in only one ear, or when the hearing loss in one ear is much worse than in the other, because two ears with reasonably normal hearing are needed to localize the source and the direction of sound.

Another interesting aspect of profound hearing loss is that after a time the person so handicapped tends to speak less clearly. His speech deteriorates, he begins to slur his "s's," and his voice becomes rigid and somewhat monotonous. This frequently happens when a person can no longer hear his own voice. He cannot hear himself speak so he raises his voice, often to the point of shouting. After a while he may find this still unsatisfactory, and then he loses interest in his ability to speak clearly, and he will not even realize that his speech is deteriorating. The reason is that one of the important functions of the ear is to serve as a monitor for speech. Hearing his own voice tells a person whether it is loud enough but not too loud, and also whether he is modulating and pronouncing his words correctly. With the loss of this important monitoring system in nerve deafness, speech and voice deterioration often occur.

Effect on Social Contacts

Unlike the blind and the crippled, the deafened have no outward signs of disability, and strangers are prone to confuse imperfect hearing with imperfect intelligence. This and similar attitudes hurt the feelings of the hard-of-hearing person and make for a strained relationship between speaker and listener. As a result, the hard-of-hearing person frequently limits his social contacts, and this often leads to moods of frustration, insecurity, and even aggression.

The hard-of-hearing person misses the small talk about him. He does not get the flavor of a conversation so much enriched by side-remarks and innuendoes. This eventually makes him feel shut off from the normal-hearing world around him and makes him a prey to discouragement and hopelessness. Until a person loses some hearing, he can scarcely realize how important it is to hear the small background sounds around him, and to what extent these sounds help him to feel alive, and how their absence makes life seem rather dull. Imagine missing the sounds of rustling leaves, footsteps, keys in doors, motors running and the thousands of other little sounds that make human beings feel that they "belong."

A Personal Tragedy With Progressive Aspects

When people become aware, if only to a small degree, of the possible effects of hearing loss, they wonder how a money value can be placed on such a handicap. Although the compensation aspects of occupational deafness demand standardized values on hearing losses, from the medical and social aspects a permanent hearing loss is a personal tragedy to each individual. Furthermore, the handicapping effects of hearing loss are often progressive. They are changing even as this book is being written. With the development of new media for sound communication, an individual's hearing comes to assume ever greater importance. For example, a hearing loss today is far more handicapping than it was before television, radio and the telephone began to play such major roles in education, leisure and the business world. Today the inability to understand on a telephone is indeed a major handicap for the vast majority of people. The loss of even high tones, alone, to a professional or an amateur musician or even to a high-fidelity fan can be a serious handicap. The hearing loss of tomorrow will affect a different handicap from the hearing loss of today.

RECOMMENDED READING

Ballantyne, John: *Deafness,* 2nd Edition, Williams and Wilkins, Baltimore, 1970.

Bender, Ruth E.: *The Conquest of Deafness,* Case Western Reserve University, Cleveland.

DeCarlo, Louis: *The Deaf,* Prentice-Hall, Inc., Englewood Cliffs, 1964.

Griffith, Jerry: Persons With Hearing Loss, Thomas, Springfield, 1969.

Mykebust, H. R.: *The Psychology of Deafness,* Grune and Stratton, New York, 1964.

O'Neill, John J.: *The Hard of Hearing,* Prentice-Hall, Englewood Cliffs, 1964.

VanItallie, Phillip H.: *How to Live With a Hearing Handicap,* Eriksson, New York, 1963.

Wallenfels, Herman G.: *Hearing Aids for Nerve Deafness,* Thomas, Springfield, 1971.

Chapter 2

HOW WE HEAR

THE EAR IS ONE of the most complex and intriguing organs known to science and it is necessary to understand, at least in a general way, how this delicate and intricate mechanism works in order to appreciate conservation of hearing. Its extreme sensitivity allows it to experience a sensation of hearing even when the sound stimulus has less energy in it than a fly might create when it lands on your hand. Such a very weak stimulus might only be vibrating the eardrum about a hydrogen molecule in diameter and yet be strong enough to transmit a sensation of hearing to the brain.

On the other extreme the ear is so sturdy it can withstand the intense sound pressure of explosions and noises of enormous energy output. It is almost inconceivable that so minute an amount of energy as is created in the mouth and larynx of a speaker has been able to transmit to our brain all the information and education we have acquired through our sense of hearing since birth. This is accomplished initially by a code of information that is placed in the bundle of energy created by our mouth and vocal cords. This energy produces sound waves in the air and eventually results in a pattern of impulses which travels along the auditory nerve to the brain where a concept of information is created, depending upon the coding in the original energy bundle. The hearing pathway is in essence a series of transducers that modify the stimulus so that it can be handled appropriately by the brain. Each part of the hearing mechanism has some role in handling the energy, and very frequently by testing for the specific function of each part of the hearing mechanism we can establish which part of the ear has been damaged. This is the basis for giving certain types of hearing tests. For instance, the chief function of the outer and middle ear is amplification. Should damage occur here the problem would involve loudness. The principal operation of the inner ear is the analysis of sound energy, and if the cochlea is damaged the resulting difficulty is not so much in loudness as in discrimination or in distinguishing speech sounds.

Sensitivity of the Human Ear

In young children the human ear is sensitive to sound waves vibrating at frequencies as low as 16 Hz and as high as 16,000 Hz or 20,000 Hz. As we grow older the upper limit of sensitivity decreases, so that many adults are not able to hear above 12,000 Hz, and it is not uncommon for individuals to be unable to hear tones at frequencies above 8,000 or 10,000 Hz. But the human ear will not hear any of these frequencies, despite the ear's sensitivity to them, unless they are loud enough.

Generally, the adult ear is most sensitive in the frequency range between 1,000 and 3,000 Hz, as shown in Figure 3. In this middle frequency range it takes less sound energy for tones to reach the threshold of hearing than it does for those tones above 3,000 Hz and those below 1,000.

In the very low frequency range it is difficult to distinguish between hearing and feeling. If these low tones are of sufficient intensity, they activate our sense of touch and since the sound waves stimulate the vibratory sense endings in our skin we can actually feel the sound. This can be demonstrated by taking a vibrating tuning fork of 128 or 64 Hz and placing it on your shin bone. The sensation of feeling the tone will be experienced readily. If a similar fork were placed on the mastoid bone to test bone conduction, the patient could readily misinterpret feeling for hearing.

Above 20,000 Hz we enter the ultrasonic range, which is inaudible to the human ear. The ear of the dog, for example, is sensitive to these higher frequencies, so that a dog responds to the so-called inaudible dog whistle whose frequency is above 20,000 Hz. The ears of bats are also sensitive to high frequencies, and their direction of flight is guided by their use of ultra-

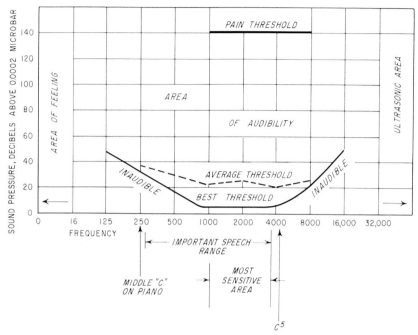

Figure 3. Graph showing area of audibility and sensitivity of the human ear. The best threshold (solid line) separates the audible from the inaudible sounds. This level is generally the reference level for sound-level meters. The average threshold of hearing (dashed line) lies considerably above the best threshold and is the reference level used in audiometers under ASA 1951. The new ANSI reference level lies much closer to the best threshold line. The ear is most sensitive between 1,000 and 3,000 Hz. The sound pressures are measured in the ear under the receiver of an audiometer. (With modifications from H. Davis, Hearing and Deafness, Rinehard Books, Inc., New York)

sonic frequencies in a manner closely paralleling the principle of radar.

The human ear is not sensitive to frequencies in the ultrasonic range and therefore is not likely to be notably damaged by sound waves in these frequencies, especially since it is difficult to generate high intensities in the ultrasonic frequencies.

Anatomy of the Ear

Figure 4 shows a cross-section of the human ear, which anatomically may be divided into three parts known as the outer, mid-

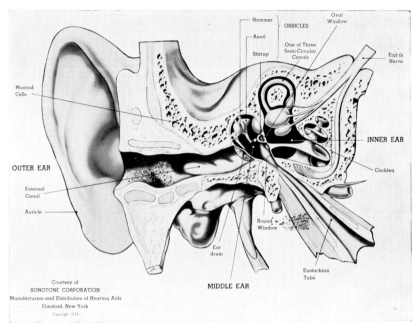

Figure 4. Diagrammatic cross section of the ear. The semicircular canals are concerned with maintaining balance. (Sonotone Corporation)

dle, and inner ears. The *outer ear* is that part which is readily visible and which extends, via the external auditory canal, 1⅛ inches to the eardrum (tympanic membrane). On the other side of the eardrum begins the area we call the *middle ear,* the air-filled cavity whose boundaries are the eardrum on the outer side and the oval window, into which the footplate of the stapes (stirrup) fits, on the inner side. The ossicular chain of three small bones, and the opening for the Eustachian tube are in the middle ear. On the other side of the oval window is the *inner ear,* deeply imbedded in the skull, which consists of a very complicated maze of chambers and tunnels within a small ebony-like bone known as the cochlea. The inner ear is filled with a clear fluid in which are membranous tunnels conforming to the bony tunnels. On the floor of one of these membranous tunnels is the amazing Organ of Corti (Fig. 5).

Now let us see how these three areas function when audible

sound waves are produced. As the sound waves are carried through the air and reach the outer ear they are collected into the external ear canal and directed toward the *eardrum,* and cause this sensitive membrane to vibrate in the range of several thousand times per second.

The eardrum (about 85 mm^2) (see Plate 1) is smaller than a dime, is semitransparent, and consists of three distinct layers: the outer layer, which is the extension of the skin covering the

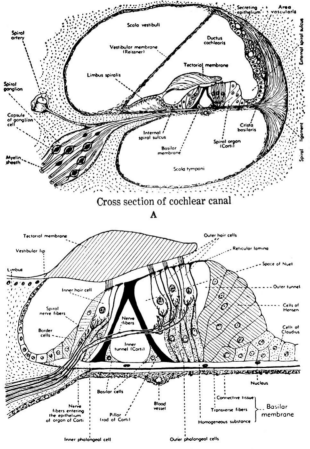

Figure 5. A cross section of the organ of Corti. Low magnification above and higher magnification below. The outer and inner hair cells are most important, since they are primarily damaged in noise deafness. (After Rasmussen, Outlines of Neuro-Anatomy, William C. Brown Co., Dubuque, Iowa)

external ear canal; the inner layer, which faces the middle ear and consists of a mucous membrane continuous with the membrane lining the middle ear; and between these two the middle layer, consisting of fibrous tissue encompassing the network of blood vessels and nerves that supply the eardrum. Despite the thinness of these layers the eardrum is very strongly attached at its edges to the bone.

The eardrum vibrations are transmitted through the middle ear area chiefly by means of a series of three small bones known as the *ossicular chain* (Fig. 4). The first is the malleus (hammer), which is firmly attached to the inner side of the eardrum. The eardrum embraces the handle of the malleus so tightly that it is difficult for it to be separated even by a surgeon. The smallest movements of the eardrum are thus immediately and intimately perceived by the malleus, and transmitted along the chain. The second is the *incus* (anvil), so named because it actually resembles a small anvil. The third is the *stapes* (stirrup), so named because of its resemblance to a stirrup on the side of a saddle.

Attached to the malleus and stapes are two small muscles which by reflexly contracting, serve as protection against very loud sounds and thus prevent too forceful movements of the bones of the ossicular chain. While these muscles may provide some early protection from continuous noise, especially at low frequencies, they have limited protection effect in screening sudden noises because the reflex action of the muscles may not be sufficiently rapid.

The stapes has a small footplate that fits exactly into the *oval window* and is attached to this oval window by an elastic membrane. As vibrations are received by the stapes along the chain from the eardrum, the footplate moves in and out of the oval window in a very complex manner.

The oval window is actually an opening in the solid bony wall of the *cochlea,* which constitutes the area we call the inner ear. The cochlea is a bony coil of about $2\frac{3}{4}$ turns filled with clear fluid and somewhat resembling a seashell. As the footplate of the stapes moves inward the fluid within the cochlea receives alternate positive and negative pressure at an extremely rapid rate.

The bony chamber of the cochlea has only one other outlet (known as the round window), which is also closed by an elastic membrane. The action of the stapedial footplate causes waves to form in the inner ear fluid (perilymph).

The coil of the cochlea is divided lengthwise into two compartments. The division is partially made by an incomplete bony shelf which somewhat resembles a circular stairway, and is completed by means of a firmly attached flexible membrane known as the *basilar membrane*. Upon this basilar membrane lies a tube-like structure which follows the turns of the cochlea and is known as the *scala media*. Inside the entire length of the scala media is the very sensitive mechanism of hearing called the Organ of Corti which, incredible as it may seem, contains between 20,000 and 30,000 minute sensory cells, from which very fine hairs extend. On top of these *hair cells* is a fine gelatinous membrane known as the tectorial membrane.

The hair cells respond selectively according to the frequencies of the sound the ear is transmitting. Fluid waves produced by tones of high frequency stimulate the hair cells at the lower or basal end of the cochlea (the large end of the seashell). Those produced by low frequencies chiefly (but not solely) stimulate hair cells towards the upper end (the pointed end of the seashell).

As the fluid waves, put in motion by the stapedial footplate at the oval window of the cochlea, selectively stimulate the hair cells, the nerves at the base of the hair cells gather together the impulses thus generated into a sort of cable that carries them along the eighth nerve and into the various sections of the brain. When the impulses reach the cortex of the brain, the sensation of hearing is experienced.

This is a brief and very simplified account of the hearing process, which is in fact a most complex operation. It will be noted from the above description that the complex sounds such as speech, which are not pure tones, are taken into the ear, broken down into pure tones somewhere in the inner ear and nervous system, and conducted along the nerve cable as nerve impulses (not sound) until they reach the brain. In the brain these nerve impulses, which are thought to consist of electrical and chemical phenomena, are integrated, interpreted, and perceived as meaningful speech.

This remarkable ability of the ear to analyze and break down speech sounds into their fundamental frequencies is still the wonder of researchers. When one considers that the many thousands of hair cells in the Organ of Corti, within the cochlea, are contained in an area smaller than that of an ordinary fingernail, the complexity of this organ is readily seen. It has been said, and with considerable justification that more surprising than why the ear sometimes does not function well, is why it does not have functional disorders much more frequently than it does. It is fortunate that the hearing mechanism is no more sensitive than it is, otherwise we might be forced to listen constantly to the vibrations of the molecules in the air around us.

Another remarkable feature in the functioning of the ear is the role the ossicular chain plays in preventing loss of sound wave energy when the waves reach the fluid of the cochlea. Everyone at one time or another has observed that if a swimmer's head is submerged, he has difficulty in hearing sounds from above the surface of the water because airborne sound waves are reflected from the surface and do not penetrate the water with their full energy. It seems reasonable to assume that a similar loss in energy would occur when the sound waves, after being airborne to the eardrum and ossicular chain, enter the fluid of the cochlea. Such is not the case inside the ear, however, for one of the important functions of the ossicular chain is to conduct the sound waves to the fluid without significant loss of energy. This it does essentially by matching the impedance of the sound waves in the air to that of the sound waves in the fluid. If for any reason the ossicular chain is disrupted behind the eardrum, a loss of about 60 decibels in hearing is experienced.

The Eustachian Tube

Earlier it was noted that the middle ear contains the opening for the *Eustachian tube*. As shown in Figure 6 it is a small tube (36 mm) leading from the middle ear and opening into the back of the nose and throat, and so constructed with a valve-like action that it is easy for air to pass from the middle ear to the

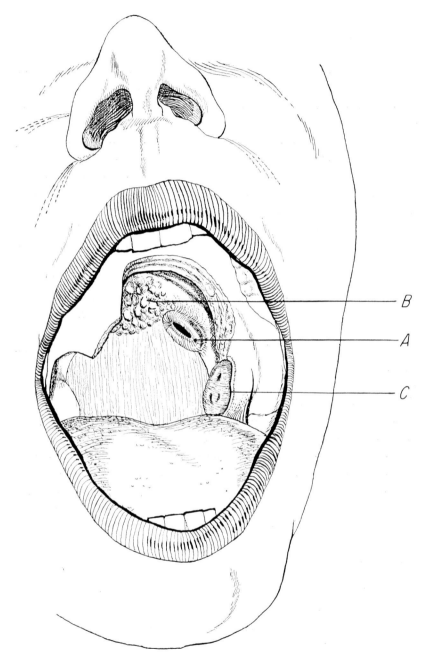

Figure 6. (A) The Eustachian tube opening in the back of the throat behind the soft palate that has been partly removed; (B) adenoids; (C) tonsils.

nasopharynx, but somewhat more difficult for air to return to the middle ear.

We are familiar with the popping sound in the ears that can be produced by pinching the nose and swallowing. Such action forces air into the middle ear and bulges the eardrum outward. In order to hear properly it is important that atmospheric pressure be equal on both sides of the eardrum at all times. If this is not the case, the eardrum cannot accurately detect and transmit the sound waves which impinge upon it. We keep this pressure equalized in normal ears by the action of swallowing, which opens the Eustachian tube and permits air in the nasopharynx to go up to the middle ear and equalize the pressure on the inner side of the eardrum with that on the outer side. We have all experienced the sensation of pressure in the ears when a rapid descent is made in an elevator, and recall how swallowing permits equalization of the air pressure on both sides of the eardrum. When swelling or infection occurs inside the Eustachian tube, the difficulties of equalizing pressure through the nasopharynx to the middle ear are magnified and certain abnormal conditions may result, some of which are discussed in the following chapter describing the causes of deafness.

Special Features of the Ear

One of the many extraordinary properties of the hearing mechanism is that it enables us to localize the source of sound. For instance, if a warning signal such as a horn should sound we would suddenly tense and turn in the direction of the source of the noise. This is important for protection from any danger which is not visible. Unless we have fairly good hearing in both ears, our ability to localize sound can be impeded. The most common cause of one-sided total deafness, which interferes with the localization of sound, is mumps. Mumps has a peculiar tendency to destroy the hearing in one ear without affecting the balance mechanism or the hearing in the opposite ear.

Another interesting aspect of our hearing is that it acts as a feedback mechanism. Through our sense of hearing we are able to determine how loud or soft our voices should be. For instance, in a loud factory or classroom we raise our voices to be heard, while in a very quiet room we have a tendency to speak more softly. If we are unable to hear the background noises we are unable to monitor our voices well. We hear our own voices by two mechanisms: airborne through the outer ear, or through the bone conduction system of our head. If an individual has a severe nerve deafness in both ears he has a tendency to speak loudly in order to hear himself the better. If, on the other hand, the nerve mechanism is intact but the middle ear is damaged causing a substantial degree of hearing loss, an individual has a tendency to speak softly. He believes he is speaking much louder than he actually is, and consequently lowers his voice. This is especially characteristic when otosclerosis is the cause of hearing loss.

Most of us fail to appreciate that our hearing is connected with more parts of our body than any of the other senses. For instance, it is connected with our entire muscular system, as is demonstrated merely by saying "boo" behind an individual; all of his muscles immediately tense and his head turns toward the source of the sound; even his pupils change size. The hearing mechanism is also connected with the blood vascular system. This also is easy to demonstrate since an individual will blush when an obscene word is used in mixed company. This blushing is the result of faster heart action and dilation of the peripheral blood vessels. Just the opposite effect can be produced by presenting bad news to an individual. This can result in his turning pale or even passing out because of the indirect effects on the blood vascular system. It is even more difficult to realize that the hearing mechanism is connected with the intestinal tract, especially the stomach. It very frequently controls the hydrochloric acid flow and gastric juice in the stomach. For instance, it is not difficult to make some people's gastric acidity overactive by merely saying such words as "income tax" or "mother-in-law." It would appear that the source of aggravation that may result in ulcer formation comes principally through our sense of hearing, rather than through other senses. Our imagination also is intimately tied up with our sense of hearing.

These features of our hearing mechanism are presented to especially emphasize the fact that when an individual is hard of hearing practically all his body systems are affected.

RECOMMENDED READING

Davis, Hallowell and Silverman, S. Richard: *Hearing and Deafness,* 3rd Edition, 1970.

Hawkins, Joseph E., Jr.: Hearing, *Annual Review of Physiology,* Vol. 26, 1964.

Littler, T. S.: *The Physics of the Ear,* Pergamon Press, New York, 1965.

Chapter 3

COMMON CAUSES OF CONDUCTIVE HEARING LOSS AND TREATMENT

FROM A STRICTLY MEDICAL viewpoint the term "deafness" describes any loss in hearing, regardless of degree or whether the loss is in one or more frequencies. In most instances the word "deaf" is used to characterize a person with a very profound hearing loss and the phrases "hearing loss" and "hard of hearing" indicate a comparatively mild hearing loss; such distinction is not made here, however, and throughout this book the terms "deafness" and "hearing loss" are used interchangeably. The term "hearing impairment," however, has acquired a specific meaning and will be used to refer to a hearing loss in which the average hearing level in the three frequencies 500, 1,000, and 2,000 Hz is greater than 15 dB (ASA reference levels or 26 dB ANSI reference levels).

Normal Hygiene of the Ear

The normal formation of wax in the ear canal is protective and is essential in keeping the skin of the canal soft and moist. Sometimes small pieces of wax may dry up and cause itching in the ear. In older people particularly wax glands may stop working or produce a peculiar type of wax that is so dry it serves no beneficial purpose. This dryness causes an annoying itching in the ear canal and many people either through lack of self-control, unconsciously, or perhaps in their sleep, vigorously scratch their

27

ear canals. Match sticks, hair pins, bobby pins, toothpicks and finger nails are probably the most frequent instruments used.

Since the skin of the ear canal is very thin and fragile, it is easily broken; as a result harmless germs that are normally present on the surface of the skin get inside and under the skin, become harmful, and produce infection. This in turn causes swelling of the canal, discharge, and further damage to the glands present in the skin. Such an ear requires medical attention. A satisfactory method of managing excess ear wax or mild itching of the ear is to take a toothpick with a small piece of cotton wrapped tightly around it and very gently try to get the wax out of the ear canal without pressing on the canal itself. Since most ear canals are very narrow and become narrower as they near the eardrum, the use of a large piece of cotton on an applicator is unsatisfactory because its use only serves to impact the wax deeper into the canal. Such impacted plugs of wax cause deafness.

People who are nervous or under excessive tension develop the habit of picking in their ear canals with any available object. Such action often has a deep emotional and sexual interpretation (recall the sensation one gets when a member of the opposite sex blows or "tongues" the ear canal). The final result of picking in the ear canal can be a persistent ear canal infection. In such cases the doctor's treatment is usually of little lasting value because some patients take a subconscious pleasure in surreptitiously scratching the ear canal, even to the extent of drawing blood and causing pain. For these cases it is essential not only to prescribe medication for the ears but also to give positive suggestions and explanations.

Forceful nose blowing should also be avoided, particularly when one has a cold. Wiping the runny nose with a tissue and blowing very gently will prevent forcing infected mucus from the nose through the Eustachian tube into the middle ear.

Protecting the ears of employees who work in dusty and dirty plants can be achieved by the use of either ear plugs or muffs.

Special precaution should be taken by women to avoid getting hair shampoo or spray into their ear canals, otherwise infection can result.

CONDUCTIVE DEAFNESS (DAMAGE IN THE MIDDLE OR OUTER EAR) CAUSES OF HEARING LOSS IN OUTER CANAL

Wax in the Ear

Impacted ear wax is a common cause of hearing loss. It occurs more frequently in persons whose ear canals are narrow and hairy, and is especially common in industry where employees work in a dirty or dusty environment. Wax must completely block the ear canal before deafness results. Even a pinpoint opening in the wax is enough to permit sound to get through and allow normal hearing. In the act of scratching an itching ear the finger may close the pinpoint opening and sudden hearing loss will occur.

Wax glands are present only in the skin covering the outer part of the ear canal. When wax is found deeper in the canal towards the eardrum it usually has been pushed there by a finger or a cotton applicator. Some ear canals are so narrow and tortuous that instead of the wax falling out normally in a self-cleaning way, it accumulates and plugs up the canal and causes hearing loss. Many individuals have large amounts of hair in their ear canals, and they readily accumulate impacted wax because it becomes enmeshed in the hairs and is prevented from falling out.

When wax is pushed into the ear canal and presses on the eardrum it may, on rare occasions, cause ear noises and even dizziness. Both of these symptoms completely disappear when the wax is removed.

It is a common error in industry to have a nurse or physician look in the ear, see a large amount of wax and assure the patient that this hearing loss is due to the wax and that the hearing will return when the wax is removed. Wax, even when impacted, produces a comparatively mild degree of hearing loss, and even when wax is present there may be underlying deafness due to other causes in the middle ear or even in the nerve of hearing. Caution should be exercised in making a diagnosis merely on the basis of seeing wax in an ear.

Removing impacted wax can be time consuming and difficult. Whenever possible it is advisable to refer an employee to his own physician for the removal of wax. If it becomes necessary to remove wax from the ear at the industrial medical clinic, irrigation of the canal with water should be avoided, if possible. The simplest method to suit the situation should be used to remove the wax. Dried and firm wax plugs can be removed best in one mass by gently easing them out with a fine forceps or dull curette (scoop). Gentleness, patience, and excellent lighting must be used. The forceps or scoop should touch only the wax and not the skin of the canal since the skin is thin and tender and can be easily irritated to the point of pain and bleeding. If the wax is soft it can be wiped out with a very thin cotton probe. If irrigation is necessary the employee should always be asked before irrigation whether he has or has had a perforated eardrum. If the answer is yes he should be referred to his own ear doctor, since irrigation of the ear canal with water may cause a flare-up in an old ear infection. Irrigation should be done with water at body temperature in order to avoid causing dizziness. The stream of water should be directed toward the edge of the wax so that the water can get behind the wax and force it out. After irrigation, the canal should be dried carefully with a piece of cotton.

Harsh chemicals, irritants, and medications that are supposed to soften wax when placed in the ear canal should be avoided, since they can irritate the tender skin and cause external ear infection. Water should not be used in the ear canal when infection of the skin of the outer canal is present.

Infections of the Outer Ear Canal

A common cause of temporary hearing loss, accompanied by pain and discomfort, is infection of the skin of the outer canal with blocking due to debris and swelling. This is especially common in the summertime when swimming is popular, and in occupations such as textile and foundry work where there is much humidity and high temperature. The most frequent cause is getting water into the ear during swimming, or from excessive washing or irrigation of the ear canal. Injury to the skin of the canal can also be caused by picking with sharp instruments, such as bobby pins and pencils, to remove cerumen (wax). With the increased use of certain earplugs we are also seeing more ear infections. When earplugs are wetted with saliva, over-sized or forced in, the very delicate skin of the ear canal may be damaged. Occasionally hair sprays and certain chemicals used in industry may cause a skin infection. This may be due to toxicity in the chemical or due to an allergy. Many general skin diseases, such as eczema, can cause infection of the outer ear canal.

Pain is usually associated with outer canal infections and it is therefore generally essential to treat the condition with gentleness. The pain in the ear is generally aggravated by chewing or swallowing, or by touching the outer part of the ear. This is in contrast to infection in the middle ear, where there is no pain on moving the outer ear or on chewing. If there is a discharge in the outer ear and it has a very stringy mucoid appearance such as is found being discharged from the nose during a cold, it indicates there is a hole in the eardrum and that the discharge is coming from the middle ear. This should not be misdiagnosed as outer ear infection.

Using strong chemicals and overtreatment for external otitis should be carefully avoided. Strong medicines frequently aggravate the condition and prolong it when it might have otherwise cleared up. One of the best treatments for external otitis which industry can use safely is to insert snugly into the swollen ear canal a cotton wick soaked with Burow's solution diluted 1:10: this changes the acidity or pH in the ear canal and prevents certain pathologic organisms from growing while the ear is healing. The wick should be kept in place for about 24 to 48 hours, and continually wetted with the same Burow's solution. If this does not cure the infection then the patient should be referred to an ear specialist for further treatment. Always be sure that the employee has pulled out the ear wick after 24 to 48 hours.

The Eardrum
Ruptured Eardrum

We speak of an eardrum being ruptured when it is suddenly penetrated by a foreign body, like a piece of metal, or by an explosion or slap across the ear. Otherwise, a hole in the eardrum is called a perforation rather than a rupture. Usually a rupture is more irregular and is not immediately accompanied by signs of inflammation.

Most ruptures of the eardrum caused by penetrating objects, occur in the posterior portion of the drum because of the curve of the external canal and the slope of the eardrum. Ruptures caused by sudden and intense pressure change, such as a blow to the side of the head or an explosion, are found more frequently in the anterior part of the drum, though occasionally in the pars flaccida or upper part.

Whenever an explosion occurs in the proximity of the patient, in addition to a complete examination for other injuries, it is advisable to examine the eardrums for rupture, in order that proper therapy may be started immediately.

The single treatment for ruptured eardrums is systemic antibiotics. Nose blowing should be avoided and, above all, there should be no unnecessary probing in the canal. The introduction of medications into the canal should be avoided to prevent entry of infection into the middle ear. In most instances, the rupture heals spontaneously, if infection is prevented. If healing does not occur, it may be necessary to encourage healing by cauterizing the edges of the ruptured eardrum or by performing a myringoplasty at some future date. The hearing loss may be as much as 60 dB if the rupture was due to a force severe enough to impair the ossicular chain, but usually the hearing loss is less than 30 dB and involves all frequencies.

Spark in the External Ear Canal

Unfortunately, getting a spark into the external ear canal is not a rare experience in industry, where employees are welding, grinding, chipping, or burning. The spark hits the eardrum with devasting effect. Usually the entire drum is cleanly destroyed, leaving just the handle of the malleus hanging down. Little or no infection accompanies this very painful and traumatic accident. The hearing loss can be as much as 50 dB in all frequencies. As in cases of ruptured eardrum, probing the canal and forceful nose blowing should be avoided. The eardrum does not regenerate by itself when such a large amount of it is destroyed. It is essential to graft a new eardrum.

The technique for grafting a new eardrum is now comparatively simple, as far as the patient is concerned. Using a piece of the patient's vein or skin or fascia, the material is placed around the edges of the excoriated eardrum perforation and in most instances the perforation closes. For several years the author has been using frozen heart valves from autopsy material, and has found them extraordinarily successful for closing perforations and for making entire new eardrums. In the near future it will even be possible to graft in entire eardrums and ossicular bones taken from autopsy material.

Most ruptured eardrums in industry are completely preventable. It is essential to protect individuals, not only with safety glasses but also with ear protectors when they work in industrial areas where free sparks are produced. The use of insert protectors is probably the most suitable means of protection. Absorbent cotton in the ears is of minimal help and provides inadequate protection.

Foreign Body in the Ear Canal

Hearing loss and fullness in the ear are often the only symptoms produced by a foreign body in the ear canal. It is surprising how long a piece of absorbent cotton or other foreign matter can remain in an ear canal without the patient being aware of its presence. It is only when this foreign body becomes impacted with wax or swollen with moisture that fullness and hearing loss ensue, and medical attention is sought. The hearing loss is due to the occlusion of the canal; it is usually very mild and usually greater in the lower frequencies.

The variety of foreign bodies removed from ear canals ranges from rubber erasers and pieces of slag to peas. Usually these cause enough ear discomfort to attract attention before hearing loss becomes prominent, but not always. Caution must always be observed when attempting to remove a foreign body from the ear canal. Usually, special grasping instruments are essential, depending upon the nature of the foreign body. General anesthesia may be advisable, unless the foreign body is obviously simple to

grasp and remove in one painless maneuver. It is easy to under-
estimate the difficulty in removing a foreign body, and to run into unexpected problems; excessive preparation is better than too
little.

Causes of Hearing Loss in the Middle Ear

Acute Otitis Media

Acute otitis media is an ear infection of comparatively short
duration, in contrast with chronic otitis media which persists continuously for many months or years. If an acute otitis media
clears up and, because of a persistent anterior perforation in the
eardrum, flares up again in a matter of months, this should be
considered a recurrent otitis media and not a chronic one.

The common causes of acute otitis media are upper respiratory
infections, sinusitis, hypertrophied adenoids, allergies, and improper nose blowing and sneezing. It is notable that all of these
causes are external to the ear itself. The otitis media is secondary
to a condition prevailing elsewhere in the body, and many of the
causative infections are influenced or precipitated by environmental conditions.

Thus irritant gases, vapors, or particular matter in the air may
cause irritation and inflammation of the nasopharynx, which
makes it more susceptible to invasion by ubiquitous pathogenic
bacteria. Prolonged exposure to chilling climatic conditions and
nutritionally inadequate diets may also contribute to a lowering
of the resistance to infection.

Many patients with anterior perforations whose ears have been
dry for months, or even years, may get water in them, or blow
their noses improperly during head cold, and in this way reinfect
the ear. In such cases the otorrhea (ear discharge) is usually
stringy and mucoid, and comes from the area of the Eustachian
tube.

To prevent otitis media, patients should be cautioned to re-
frain from improper nose blowing and sneezing. Too forceful
blowing while pinching both nares causes build-up of pressure
in the nasopharynx. This pressure may force small amounts of
infected mucus through the Eustachian tube into the ear with resultant otitis media.

While excellent results have been achieved with medication in preventing otitis media, some cases still become chronic. One of the principal causes for this is failure to use adequate doses of antibiotics. In many cases of middle ear infection, a much higher blood level of antibiotic is necessary than is generally recognized; the reason being that the infection has become walled off and can be reached only by very high blood levels of medications. If adequate antibiotics are prescribed to most patients with otitis media in the early stage, it can be cleared up before severe pain and disability develop. Early treatment can prevent discomfort and loss of work time for employees. If an employee reports to the medical department at a time when his eardrum is bulging a myringotomy is advisable, and relief will be immediate. The use of intensive antibiotics, along with oral decongestants and nose sprays is an effective measure against otitis media.

Chronic Otitis Media

When infection persists continuously in the middle ear for long periods of time, it is called chronic otitis media, and is a frequent cause of hearing impairment. The mechanism varies. There is invariably a perforation in the eardrum. In most cases the hole is in the back or top portion of the drum. Occasionally, the entire drum is eroded, and much of the middle ear is visible through the otoscope. The more severe hearing losses are due to erosion of some part of the ossicular chain. The most common ossicular defect is erosion of the long end of the incus, so that it does not contact the head of the stapes. Occasionally, the handle of the malleus and even the stapedial crura are eroded. In some ears the entire incus has been found to be destroyed. Scarlet fever and measles are notorious causes of severe erosion of the ossicles and the eardrum.

Another cause of hearing loss in chronic otitis media is discharge in the middle ear. This naturally adds a mass which impedes transmission of sound waves. Strangely enough, a patient may say he hears much less after the ear is cleared of discharge, and the audiogram often will substantiate this complaint. One explanation for this is that the discharge blocks sound waves bound for the round window niche, and thereby permits some semblance of normal phase difference for sound waves transmissions entering the inner ear. Sound waves in normal ears selectively enter the oval window rather than the round window, because of their direct transmission through the ossicular chain. When the drum is missing, and the ossicular chain is not functioning properly, sound waves occasionally directly strike both the round and the oval windows almost simultaneously, so that the waves may in part prevent the necessary movement of fluid in the inner ear. This causes hearing loss. A discharge in the mid-

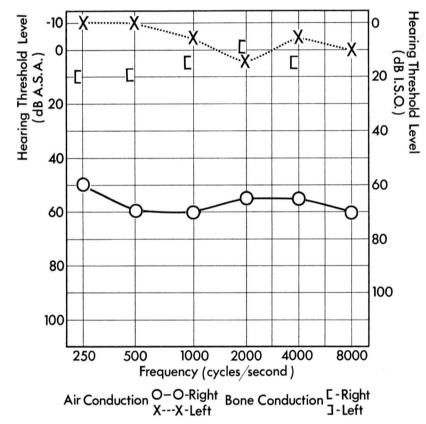

Figure 7. This audiogram shows the hearing of a 45-year-old woman whose left ear has been draining for many years. Examination showed absence of visible ossicles and a cholesteatoma with chronic infection in the ear and mastoid area. A radical mastoid operation was performed and the present audiogram shows her hearing level.

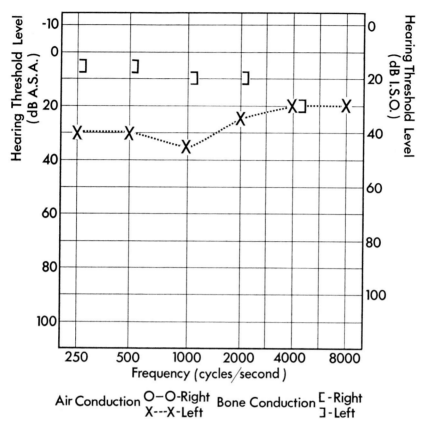

Air Conduction O–O-Right   Bone Conduction ⸢-Right
                 X---X-Left   ⸥-Left

Figure 8. *History:* The patient whose hearing is shown in this audiogram had a discharging left ear for many years. X-ray study showed a cholesteatoma. *Otologic:* Large posterior marginal perforation. The ossicular chain was not disrupted; otherwise, the hearing loss would have exceeded 50 dB. Ossicular continuity was confirmed at surgery. *Audiologic:* Pure tone thresholds in the left ear revealed a mild air conduction loss with a gradually decreasing air-bone gap at the higher frequencies. Right ear masked. *Classification:* Conductive. *Diagnosis:* Cholesteatoma with marginal perforation.

dle ear may sometimes prevent this effect by blocking sound waves that otherwise would reach the round window niche. Thus the patient's hearing may be better when his ear is moist. The same mechanism sometimes is used purposely to improve hearing in ears that are free of infection.

However, these considerations should not lead a physician to

disregard discharge in the hope of maintaining hearing, for infection can result in serious complications. There are many satisfactory methods to restore hearing after an infection has been
controlled. When a posterosuperior perforation is found in the
eardrum with a putrid discharge, it generally means that mas-
toiditis is present. If the infection is allowed to continue, it may
cause a number of complications, including erosion of the ossicles and severe hearing loss. A cholesteatoma (collection of
skin and infection) may form that could erode the semicircular
canals and the facial nerve, and even produce a brain abscess.

It is important, therefore, to cure a chronic middle ear infection as rapidly as possible. Unfortunately, systemic antibiotics do
not often succeed in clearing up chronic otitis media, because the
chronically diseased mastoid cells in the middle ear have such a
poor blood supply. Consequently, it is necessary to treat the ear
locally, and occasionally surgery must be performed when local
therapy has been unsuccessful, and complications threaten.

Figures 7 and 8 illustrate several audiometric patterns that can
occur in chronic otitis media.

Aerotitis Media

The condition known as aerotitis media has been associated
with work in caissons, with deep water diving, and with air travel.
The condition is now associated most frequently with rapid descent in an airplane.

If changes in atmospheric pressure occur, equalization of pressure between the middle ear and the external ear occurs through
the Eustachian tube, but if congestion exists in the Eustachian
tube, equalization of pressure between the middle ear and the
outer ear does not occur. When the atmospheric pressure increases rapidly, as in the descent of an airplane, and the Eustachian tube is blocked, the pressure on the outside of the eardrum
exceeds that on the inside and the eardrum is pushed inward towards the middle ear and the promontory in the middle ear. This
causes sudden pain, fullness, and hearing loss. If the atmospheric
pressure decreases rapidly, as in the rapid ascent of an airplane
or of a diver, and the Eustachian tube is blocked, the higher
pressure in the middle ear pushes the eardrum outward, result-

ing in tinnitus, vertigo, and slight hearing loss. In the event of a sudden decompression, as in deep scuba diving, an air embolus can occur in the inner ear as well as elsewhere in the body.

Aerotitis media is best prevented by avoiding rapid changes in pressure on the part of those suffering from congestion of the Eustachian tubes because of upper respiratory infection or allergy. If such pressure changes cannot be avoided, the preventive use of oral decongestants and nasal sprays or inhalants may produce a temporary decongestion of the Eustachian tube and facilitate equalization of pressure between the middle ear and the outer ear.

If aerotitis media has occurred, vigorous chewing movements may induce a temporary opening of the Eustachian tubes and bring relief. If the patient is seen soon after the symptoms develop, he can be relieved immediately by a myringotomy followed by politzerization (forcing air up the Eustachian tube). In all cases, hearing should return to normal when the eardrum is restored to its customary position.

Retracted Eardrum

The Eustachian tube plays a vital role in maintaining equal pressure on both sides of the eardrum. Each time we swallow, the tube has a tendency to open and allow air to pass into the middle ear. When we have head colds, allergy attacks, infections in the back of the nose and throat, or when the lining of the tube becomes inflamed and swollen, the tube closes so that no air can get into the middle ear. In such a situation the air normally present in the middle ear becomes locked in, some of it becomes absorbed by the lining of the middle ear, and the pressure in the middle ear is thus reduced. This makes the pressure inside the middle ear lower than the pressure on the outside in the external canal and results in the eardrum being gradually pushed inward by the extra pressure from the outside. The otologist refers to this type of an eardrum as a *retracted eardrum,* that is, it is retracted into the middle ear. Sometimes it can be pressed so far into the middle ear that it touches the bony area of the cochlea itself, almost completely obliterating the area of the middle ear.

Obviously such an abnormal process reduces the efficiency of the eardrum and ossicular chain in transmitting sound to the inner ear. It is noteworthy, however, that the appearance of the eardrum, particularly the amount of retraction, is no indication of the amount of hearing impairment resulting from the damage in the middle ear.

Some eardrums are so completely retracted that the whole incus can be observed clearly to be wrapped in the eardrum, and yet the hearing is practically normal. On the other hand a slight amount of retraction may produce a fair degree of hearing loss. The amount of hearing loss present is mostly determined by the site and type of damage in the ossicular chain and this cannot be evaluated by appearance alone.

THE EUSTACHIAN TUBE AND HEARING LOSS

No part of the auditory system has been incriminated more wrongly and mistreated more often than the Eustachian tube. At the present time there should be no reasonable excuse for blaming or mistreating the Eustachian tube when actually the cause of the hearing loss lies elsewhere.

Malfunction of the Eustachian tube causes only conductive hearing loss. If nerve deafness is present the Eustachian tube should not be the target for treatment, even though politzerization or tubal inflation may give the patient a subjective sense of well-being and an apparent hearing improvement for a few moments. Such treatment often delays the patient's actual auditory rehabilitation.

In general, simple blockage of the Eustachian tube causes only a comparatively mild hearing loss not exceeding 25 dB; and most of the time much less. The loss is greater in the lower frequencies than in the higher. The most common causes are acute upper respiratory infections and allergies of the nose, in which the Eustachian tube becomes boggy and obstructed due to congestion and inflammation. This condition makes the ears feel full and the individual appears to be slightly hard of hearing. If the obstruction in the tube persists, the air in the middle ear is absorbed by the mucosal lining, and the eardrum becomes slightly retracted; thus the hearing loss is aggravated, so that it may reach a measurable level of about 25 dB. If fluid forms in the middle ear, there may be an even greater level of hearing loss, but in this case the loss is often greater in the higher frequencies. This frequency change is due to the addition of the fluid mass to the contents of the middle ear. When there is fluid in the middle ear the bone conduction also may be slightly reduced, and this may suggest a false diagnosis of sensorineural hearing loss. Removal of the fluid however, restores both air and bone conduction to normal.

There are exceptions to these generalizations. When the tube has been closed for many months or years, the drum may become retracted so completely that it becomes "plastered" to the promontory, a condition which causes a hearing loss of about 40 dB; or if the fluid is thick and gelatinous, the loss may exceed 40 dB. In general, however, the Eustachian tube obstruction *per se* causes only a mild loss in hearing. The loss increases only when complications arise in the middle ear, such as the presence of a fluid mass and retraction of the drum. Therefore, it is safe to conclude that with rare exception, if the hearing loss exceeds 25 dB and the eardrum and middle ear appear to be practically normal, the fault does not lie in the Eustachian tube. The cause is more likely to be found in the ossicular chain and especially in the stapes.

One of the signs of Eustachian tube obstruction is observed during politzerizing. The air may go up the Eustachian tube quite well and distend the eardrum, but instead of the eardrum returning immediately to its normal position, as it does in a person with normal tubal aeration, it stays slightly puffed out and returns slowly.

Secretory Otitis Media

For unknown reasons an abnormal accumulation of fluid may occur in the middle ear, usually straw-colored but sometimes mucoid or gel-like in consistency. This is called secretory otitis media. In most cases the Eustachian tube may be patent and the tube is not the primary reason for the abnormal collection of fluid in the middle ear. The fluid can be removed readily by myringotomy and politzerization (forcing air up the Eustachian tube). However, the fluid occasionally continues to accumulate in spite of numerous myringotomies and varied treatments, and hearing loss occurs, usually to a greater degree in the higher tones. Secretory otitis may be present in one or both ears, and is found in babies as well as in adults.

Quite often the condition suddenly stops spontaneously, and the treatment used at that particular time is likely to get the credit, but this conclusion proves to be unjustified in the long run. In some cases the secretion continues to form and causes a perforation in the eardrum. When this occurs, the findings resemble those seen in chronic otitis media, but the discharge is free of infectious elements; as a matter of fact, the discharge generally is almost sterile, and attempts to culture bacteria and viruses from the fluid have been unsuccessful. Figure 9 shows the type of hearing loss characteristically present in this condition.

Otosclerosis

In otosclerosis there is a gradual fixation of the stapes footplate in the oval window because of boney changes in the stapes footplate and the cochlear bone. The cause is unknown but heredity is the most prominent factor. The hearing gradually diminishes as the footplate becomes more fixed. The only treatment for this condition is surgery, chiefly in the form of stapedectomy where the stapes is removed and replaced with an artificial prosthesis that is attached to the incus.

Because of the high prevalance of otosclerosis in our population it is essential to diagnose this condition in industry, so that employees can be advised to seek expert attention to restore their hearing. There is no causal relation between industrial noise and otosclerosis.

When conductive hearing loss is present in an adult, and the eardrum and the middle ear appear to be normal through the otoscope, the most likely diagnosis is otosclerosis. There are other possible causes, but they are comparatively uncommon. Actually, the name "otosclerosis" is misleading for it is really not a sclerotic process; it is more like a vascularization in the bone with formation of spongy bone. Such changes have been reported nowhere in the body except in the bony labyrinth.

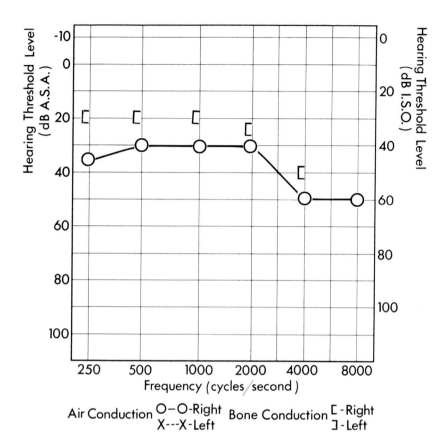

Figure 9. *History:* 24-year-old patient who sustained a head injury causing right middle ear to be filled with blood. *Otologic:* Tympanic membrane was intact but was deep red in color due to blood on the middle ear. The eardrum did not move well with air pressure. Resolution occurred spontaneously without myringotomy. *Audiologic:* Pure-tone thresholds in the right ear revealed a mild air conduction loss with reduced bone conduction (left ear masked). Note the greater loss in the high frequencies and the reduced bone thresholds because of the fluid in the middle ear. Hearing returned to normal at all frequencies after spontaneous resolution. *Classification:* Conductive; damage in middle ear. *Diagnosis:* Post-traumatic hemotympanum.

Clinical Otosclerosis

There are more people with otosclerosis than there are patients who seek medical advice for their hearing loss in order to receive the benefit of diagnosis. For instance, it has been shown that otosclerosis is found at autopsy in the ears of many individuals who in life gave no evidence of hearing impairment. This happens when otosclerotic changes affect areas of the bony labyrinth and cochlea, other than the oval window. It is only when the oval window and the stapes are involved that hearing loss develops, and then it is called clinical otosclerosis. For the purposes of this book we shall call it simply otosclerosis, because the condition does not concern us clinically until hearing impairment develops. Fixation of the stapes may occur over a period of many months or even years. Figure 10 shows a serial audiogram of a patient with otosclerosis whose hearing level has been followed repeatedly for years as her hearing loss progressed.

Extent of Hearing Loss

In some cases the hearing loss stops progressing after reaching only a very mild level. We do not know why this occurs. More frequently the hearing deteriorates until it stabilizes at about 50 to 60 dB. The hearing deficiency classically starts in the lower frequencies and gradually progresses to the high ones. Eventually, all frequencies are involved. In numerous patients the high tones continue to deteriorate even more than the low frequencies due to superimposed sensorineural deafness.

Characteristic Features

There are many intriguing and challenging features about otosclerosis. It is far more common in females than in males, and it is generally first noted around the age of 18. Quite often the hearing loss is accompanied by a most annoying buzzing tinnitus; both symptoms usually are aggravated by pregnancy. The tinnitus commonly subsides over a period of many years.

Psychological Aspects

Of particular interest is the strange psychological complex almost invariably present in otosclerotic patients. Most of them be-

JOSEPH SATALOFF, M. D.
1721 PINE STREET   PHILADELPHIA, PA. 19103

HEARING RECORD

NAME _____ AGE _____

AIR CONDUCTION

			RIGHT							LEFT						
DATE	Exam.	LEFT MASK	250	500	1000	2000	4000	8000	RIGHT MASK	250	500	1000	2000	4000	8000	AUD.
6/1955			35	35	30	20	10	5		35	40	30	20	5	5	
4/1956			45	40	40	20	10	10		40	40	30	20	10	10	
6/1957			50	50	50	25	15	15		40	45	35	20	15	15	
4/1959			55	55	50	40	20	25		45	45	40	35	30	25	
4/1962			60	55	50	50	40	35		50	55	50	45	45	40	
2/1964			60	55	55	60	65	50		55	55	55	55	60	45	

BONE CONDUCTION

			RIGHT							LEFT					
DATE	Exam.	LEFT MASK	250	500	1000	2000	4000		RIGHT MASK	250	500	1000	2000	4000	AUD.
6/1955			0	0	0	5	5			0	0	0	5	5	
4/1959			0	5	5	10	15			0	5	10	10	15	
2/1964			0	10	20	25	30			0	10	25	20	35	

SPEECH RECEPTION — DISCRIMINATION

DATE	RIGHT	LEFT MASK	LEFT	RIGHT MASK	FREE FIELD	MIC.	DATE	% SCORE	TEST LEVEL	LIST	LEFT MASK	% SCORE	TEST LEVEL	LIST	RIGHT MASK	EXAM.
6/1955	30		35					100	70			100	75			

HIGH FREQUENCY THRESHOLDS

	RIGHT							LEFT					
DATE	4000	8000	10000	12000	14000	LEFT MASK	RIGHT MASK	4000	8000	10000	12000	14000	

RIGHT		WEBER	LEFT		HEARING AID			
RINNE	SCHWABACH		RINNE	SCHWABACH	DATE	MAKE		MODEL
					RECEIVER	GAIN		EXAM.
					EAR	DISCRIM.		COUNC.

REMARKS

Figure 10. This serial audiogram shows the manner in which hearing can deteriorate with time in an individual who has otosclerosis.

come suspicious and feel people are talking about them. Many become introspective and have marked personality changes. They creep into their own shells. Some try to appear to be lighthearted and even humorous, but the attempt lacks conviction. Perhaps these symptoms are related to the gradual onset of the otosclerosis.

It has been suggested, without any proof, that otosclerosis is a psychosomatic disease. Certainly, the psychological aspects of otosclerosis are of paramount importance. One of the vital reasons for trying to restore hearing early with surgery, is to head off adverse personality changes.

Familial Aspects

Otosclerosis is familial to some extent. It often is found in several people in the same family. On the other hand, many patients with otosclerosis deny any hearing loss in their families for as many generations as they may recall. It is not possible to predict on genetic principles who in a family will exhibit clinical otosclerosis but on theoretical grounds marriages between members of two families in both of which there are clear-cut cases of otosclerosis seem to be inadvisable. Nevertheless, the risk does not warrant an extreme position, and one should not stand in the way of a man and woman who wish to marry after they have been made aware of the facts. None of their offspring may develop a hearing loss. Certainly there is no justification for a therapeutic abortion in a pregnant woman with otosclerosis merely because her hearing loss might be aggravated during pregnancy. Some older textbooks took a contrary view, but such a stand is unwarranted in the light of the present knowledge of otosclerosis.

Effects of Excellent Bone Conduction

A prominent feature in otosclerosis is that the patient speaks in a very soft and modulated voice. As previously pointed out, this is easily explained by the fact that these patients have excellent bone conduction. They may also complain that their hearing gets worse when they chew crunchy foods like celery. This, too, is related to excellent bone conduction, which causes the crunching noise to interfere with hearing conversation.

Differentiation

During pure tone audiometry, patients with otosclerosis often are uncertain whether or not they really hear the tone when they are being tested at threshold. In contrast, patients with sensori-neural deafness are sure when they hear and when they do not.

In spite of the classic symptoms that otosclerotic patients present, many cases are still misdiagnosed as catarrhal deafness, allergic deafness, adhesive deafness or deafness due to Eustachian tube blockage. Whenever a patient with normal otoscopic findings has conductive hearing loss exceeding 30 dB in the speech frequencies, the cause is in all likelihood otosclerosis or ossicular defect, even though there may be a marked allergic history and changes in the nose, or slight retraction of the eardrum, or even a demonstrably blocked Eustachian tube. Few if any causes other than otosclerosis, produce progressive conductive hearing losses of more than 30 dB accompanied by tinnitus and a familial history.

Variable Progression in the Hearing Loss of Each Ear

Otosclerosis sometimes does occur unilaterally, with normal hearing in the other ear. The progression of hearing loss in each ear, when otosclerosis is present in both ears, may differ widely, so that most of the time a patient states that the hearing is better in one ear than in the other. This difference may change, however and the patient often says, "My left ear used to be the better ear, but the hearing in that ear has decreased so much that the right ear is now the better one." This subjective experience, corroborated by hearing tests, may determine which ear should be operated upon when an attempt is made to restore hearing by stapes surgery.

Other Types

The most characteristic type of otosclerosis has been described but there are many other types that the otologist can almost clas-

Hearing Conservation

JOSEPH SATALOFF, M. D.
1721 PINE STREET   PHILADELPHIA, PA. 19103

HEARING RECORD

NAME _____   AGE _____

AIR CONDUCTION

DATE	Exam.	LEFT MASK	250	500	1000	2000	4000	8000	RIGHT MASK	250	500	1000	2000	4000	8000	AUD.
					RIGHT								LEFT			
9/17/56			90	95	85	90	NR	NR		85	NR	NR	NR	NR	NR	
10/31/56			Right stapes mobilization													
1/31/57			45	50	45	75	65	65								
2/10/57										Left stapes mobilization						
2/18/57										60	70	70	70	75	NR	

BONE CONDUCTION

DATE	Exam.	LEFT MASK	250	500	1000	2000	4000		RIGHT MASK	250	500	1000	2000	4000	AUD.
					RIGHT								LEFT		
9/17/56			40	30	40	50	55			15	35	35	50	45	

SPEECH RECEPTION

DATE	RIGHT	LEFT MASK	LEFT	RIGHT MASK	FREE FIELD	MIC.
2/18/57	58		86			

DISCRIMINATION

DATE	% SCORE	TEST LEVEL	LIST	LEFT MASK	% SCORE	TEST LEVEL	LIST	RIGHT MASK	EXAM.
		RIGHT				LEFT			
	44	88			68	98			

HIGH FREQUENCY THRESHOLDS

DATE	4000	8000	10000	12000	14000	LEFT MASK	RIGHT MASK	4000	8000	10000	12000	14000	
			RIGHT							LEFT			

RIGHT		WEBER		LEFT		HEARING AID		
RINNE	SCHWABACH		RINNE		SCHWABACH	DATE	MAKE	MODEL
						RECEIVER	GAIN	EXAM.
						EAR	DISCRIM.	COUNC.

REMARKS

Figure 11. Severe type of otosclerosis with secondary nerve involvement. In some of these patients the hearing can be improved with stapes surgery.

sify mentally. One is the so-called "malignant type," which is most disturbing. It may occur in young patients and is characterized by a rapidly progressing hearing loss which often reaches serious proportions in 1 or 2 years, and is accompanied by diminished bone conduction as a result of sensorineural involvement. Frequently these cases are not seen until the sensorineural damage is already so pronounced that the otosclerotic origin is largely obscured, and surgery is of doubtful value.

As yet the relationship between otosclerosis and sensorineural deafness is not known, but the latter is a frequent companion of otosclerosis. For this reason some otologic surgeons advise doing stapes surgery as early as possible in otosclerosis, to obviate not only any adverse psychological changes but perhaps to forestall sensorineural damage.

Another type of otosclerosis is characterized by the audiogram in Figure 11. This is hardly recognizable as otosclerosis, and yet the patient has all the classic history and symptoms, that the hearing loss is greater than 60 dB, and sensorineural deafness is also present. This is definitely otosclerosis, and the hearing can be improved by surgery, as shown in the audiogram. It is also to be noted that the absence of any response to audiometric testing does not mean necessarily that the ear is "dead." It means merely that the threshold is beyond the limits of the audiometer. Another unusual but severe type of otosclerosis occurs when there is obstruction, not only of the oval window but also of the round window. Here again the bone conduction is reduced severely, along with the air conduction loss.

The cases of otosclerosis just described that have a sensorineural component in addition to the conductive loss, are considered "mixed hearing impairment."

Correction of Conductive Deafness

Thus far the cause of deafness described are those that damage the outer or middle ear, and prevent sound waves from reaching the inner ear. This type of hearing loss is called conductive deafness, and there is no damage to the inner ear or auditory nerve. Most authorities agree that the maximum air conduction hearing loss that can result from a conductive deafness is about 60 dB. Any deafness greater than this suggests the presence of sensorineural deafness, either exclusively or superimposed upon a conductive hearing loss. An otologist classifies a hearing loss as either conductive or sensorineural because he needs to localize the area in the auditory pathway that has been damaged, in order to establish the cause and possible cure.

Fortunately, most cases of conductive hearing loss are subject to cure through expert otological attention. The most dramatic otologic therapy now available is for otosclerosis where the stapes footplate is fixed in the oval window. A surgical procedure under local anesthesia makes it possible to lift up the eardrum, remove the fixed stapes bone, and replace it with an artificial prosthesis made from a piece of Teflon or Gelfoam wire. The eardrum is replaced without requiring sutures or leaving any visible scar. In the majority of cases, the surgery has resulted in the restoration of hearing to thousands of hard-of-hearing people with otosclerosis.

A new field of reconstructive middle ear surgery has been developed for people who have had chronic ear infections, with destruction of the eardrum and even of the ossicular chain of bones. With the use of artificial or even natural bones taken from autopsy material, it is possible to reconstruct the eardrum and ossicles and thereby restore hearing in many cases. It is advisable however, that all infection be cleared up before this type of reconstructive surgery is performed.

Chapter 4

COMMON CAUSES OF NERVE DEAFNESS AND TREATMENT

W HEN A HEARING LOSS results from damage in the inner ear (cochlea) or in the auditory nerve proper, we classify such deafness as being sensorineural—more commonly called neural or nerve deafness. (The obsolete term "perceptive" was used earlier for this type of loss.)

Nerve deafness is one of the most challenging problems confronting physicians. Not only are there many millions of people with this type of loss (particularly industrial workers and older citizens) but perhaps more important, the hearing loss generally is incurable and can affect the personality adversely and create many psychological problems. Unfortunately our knowledge about nerve deafness is inadequate. In some cases we are unable to establish the precise cause of the nerve deafness, but we can generally localize the precise site of the damage in the neural pathway and thereby deduce the cause of the hearing loss. By doing this we are able to provide a prognosis, such as the degree of hearing loss we can expect in the years to come, and we can also eliminate unnecessary treatment, especially surgery that might be misdirected to the middle ear. There is no logical reason for example, to treat the Eustachian tube, or perform a stapes operation, or remove adenoids and tonsils when the diagnosis is nerve deafness.

Sensorineural hearing loss can occur suddenly or gradually, and in one or both ears. Causes of sudden deafness in both ears are (1) meningitis, (2) infections, (3) drugs, (4) functional deafness, (5) multiple sclerosis and (6) unknown causes. Causes of one-sided sudden deafness are (1) mumps and other viruses, (2) direct head injury, (3) acoustic trauma, and (4) vascular disorders. Causes of gradual hearing loss in one or both ears include (1) presbycusis, (2) occupational noise, (3) heredity, (4) otosclerosis, (5) neuritis, (6) vestibular disorders, and (7) unknown causes. A brief description of some of these causes of sensorineural deafness is included to enable the reader to recognize the

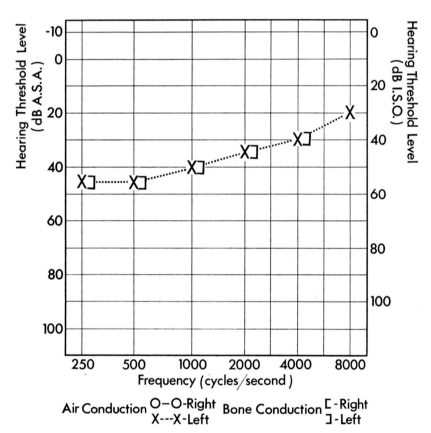

Figure 12. *History:* 37-year-old male with recurrent sudden attacks of rotary vertigo accompanied by nausea, vomiting and an ocean-roaring tinnitus in the left ear. Between attacks the patient reports fullness and deafness, aggravated during attacks. Patient is annoyed by loud noise in the left ear, and voices sound fuzzy and unclear. *Otologic:* Normal. *Audiologic:* Moderate

many problems that must be considered before narrowing down the diagnosis in any specific patient.

Meniere's Disease

There is increasing interest in a condition called "Meniere's disease" which is characterized by recurring attacks of dizziness, deafness and tinnitus. The attacks of dizziness may last only a few minutes or last for a day or more, and they can recur frequently or disappear for a number of years. Some patients can predict the onset of the dizziness by a rather full feeling in the ear that is involved. In over 90 percent of the cases the disease occurs in only one ear. The dizziness is often so severe that the patient cannot remain standing. He sees the room spinning around him or feels himself rotating which causes nausea and vomiting. At the same time he hears a loud roaring noise in his ear or head, as if the ocean were creating a storm inside. If one looks at the patient's eyes at the time of this attack, he will see a rapid back and forth movement of the eye balls from side to side or round and round. This is called nystagmus, and may last as long as the dizziness lasts. In the early stages of the condition the hearing worsens during the attack and the patient may be hard of hear-

---

hearing loss with no air-bone gap. Left ear discrimination: 60%. Binaural loudness balance studies show complete recruitment in the left ear:

1,000 Hz	
R	L
0	40
10	45
20	50
30	55
40	55
50	60
60	65
70	70

During the loudness balance test the patient reported that the tone in the left ear was not as clear as the tone in the good ear. This is diplacusis and is an important symptom in inner ear pathology. The patient also has a lowered threshold of discomfort. There was no abnormal tone decay. *Classification:* Sensory impairment. *Diagnosis:* Meniere's disease.

ing for a week or two after the dizziness subsides; but then the hearing often returns to normal and stays normal until the next attack. If the attacks occur frequently, there may be a permanent loss in hearing (Fig. 12). Some patients have a permanent loss of hearing even after the first attack. It is common for this condition to desist spontaneously; that is, to disappear for a number of years.

The real damage occurs in the inner ear. While we are not completely certain of the precise cause of the disease, we do know there is an abnormality in the endolymphatic fluid of the inner ear with damage to the hair cells and eventually to the nerve fibers supplying them. There is some question as to the likely role of viruses or allergy in this condition. Emotional tension is also considered as a possible cause. Most patients with Meniere's disease seem to be under considerable emotional strain, and there is a strong impression among physicians that dizzy attacks are less frequent if the patient learns to relax.

The deafness in Meniere's disease has very characteristic features: (1) the hearing fluctuates widely, and may even return to normal between attacks, (2) there is distortion in hearing; voices may sound tinny, hollow, or fuzzy in the ear which has the Meniere's condition, (3) the same pitch may sound different in the normal ear than it does in the ear with Meniere's disease; the pitch in the bad ear usually sounds higher than it does in the good ear (this is called diplacusis), (4) loud voices and noises ordinarily well tolerated by the normal ear produce discomfort and even pain in the affected ear; this is known as a reduced threshold of discomfort for hearing, (5) there are very clear-cut endpoints during audiometric testing; this means the subject answers very promptly when given a very weak tone and does not seem hesitant about the continuance or discontinuance of the tone as is ordinarily expected in normal ears or ears having conductive deafness, and (6) the hearing loss that occurs is sensorineural and usually the low notes are involved more than the high ones. At present we have no specific cure for Meniere's disease but symptomatic treatment with medicine is generally successful.

Deafness Due to Injury to the Head

Severe head injuries can cause sensorineural deafness in one or both ears. Usually there is accompanying dizziness. Many times the X-ray shows a fracture in the skull bone which houses the delicate ear mechanism. Sometimes there is also associated weakness of the face, due to injury to the nerve that supplies the face. Often there is bleeding in the ear canal.

There are really two types of deafness that result from head injury. One is a conductive deafness due to damage in the middle ear and the other is sensorineural deafness. In the conductive type the deafness is due to the presence of blood in the middle ear and external canal, and sometimes a disruption of the ossicular chain. Generally there is also a rupture in the eardrum. As the blood is absorbed, however, the hearing usually returns to its original level, and the eardrum heals. Occasionally the damage is such that the conductive deafness is permanent, but being conductive the maximum degree of hearing loss is usually around 60 dB; hence, if the individual is spoken to loudly enough in the damaged ear, he not only can hear well but can understand what is being said. New types of surgery can sometimes restore much of the hearing loss.

Sensorineural deafness due to severe head trauma can be associated with a so-called transverse fracture of the temporal bone, which causes a complete destruction of the hearing and balance mechanism on the affected side. The deafness is usually permanent, and is accompanied by severe dizziness and vomiting which can last for several days. The dizziness gradually subsides over a period of several weeks, but unsteadiness and swaying towards the affected side may last for several months. There are some cases of transverse fracture of the ear bone in which the hearing loss is incomplete, but this is not the common type.

It is also possible to have hearing damage without there actually being a fracture in the temporal bone. Such an injury usually results from a blow to the back or side of the head, but the blow generally must be severe enough to cause at least some loss of consciousness. Hearing loss due to such an injury is the same as that which results from exposure to noise. The most severe damage to the hearing in both instances occurs at around 4,000 Hz and its neighboring frequencies. Unlike injury resulting from exposure to noise, however, injury resulting from a severe blow to the head is also accompanied by dizziness, which generally is aggravated by changes in position of the head, such as sudden turning or bending. Another interesting aspect of injury to the head is the fact that not only may deafness occur on the side which sustained a fracture of the temporal bone, but there may also be a mild hearing loss on the opposite side due to a concussion in the inner ear. The initial damage that results from the injury is to the organ of Corti and its hair cells, and any nerve damage is usually secondary to this.

Mumps Deafness

Mumps is the most common cause of severe one-sided deafness. The deafness is sudden in onset, and comes on without pain or ear discomfort. Frequently, the deafness goes unnoticed for many days or even years after its onset. A patient may state he has noticed only recently the sudden onset of deafness in his right ear, for example, and have no idea of its cause. A careful investigation may reveal that while the patient is now grown, the deafness in his right ear actually has been present since an attack of mumps during childhood. The fact that he used the telephone at his left ear and wrote with his right hand all these years, prevented him from recognizing that he had always been getting along with only one ear. The reason he noticed this suddenly is that he recently switched the telephone receiver to the right ear, then jumped to the obvious conclusion that the deafness has just occurred in the right ear.

Deafness due to mumps generally causes complete loss of hearing in one ear by destroying the inner ear without affecting the balance mechanism. We do not have any cure. If any hearing does remain in the affected ear, this amount of hearing persists and does not get progressively worse (Fig. 13).

Congenital Deafness

The term "congenital deafness" merely indicates that deafness was present at birth. It neither indicates the cause of the deaf-

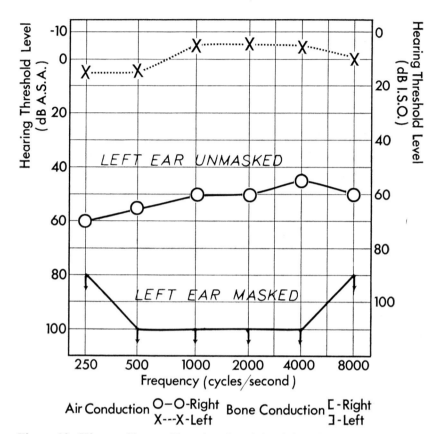

Air Conduction O–O-Right Bone Conduction ⊏ -Right
X---X-Left   ⊐ -Left

Figure 13. *History:* 33-year-old male who claimed his right ear went deaf after he hit his head on a pole protruding from a building. There was no head wound or unconsciousness. He denied having vertigo or tinnitus. *Otologic:* Normal with normal caloric responses. *Audiologic:* No response in the right ear with the left ear masked. *Classification:* Unilateral sensorineural deafness. *Diagnosis:* Mumps deafness. Established by further detailed history. *Comment:* So severe a unilateral deafness with normal labyrinthine responses is not produced by such a head injury.

ness nor suggests a possible cure. In the past most cases of congenital deafness were attributed to heredity or birth injury, but we are gradually discovering other causes.

There are two important causes of congenital nerve deafness, one resulting from Rh incompatability with cerebral palsy, and one resulting from the mother's having had German measles during her first three months of pregnancy.

Congenital Deafness Due to Rh Incompatability

There is a certain factor carried in our red blood cells which is called the Rh factor. About 85 percent of the population is Rh positive, and about 15 percent is Rh negative. Nothing abnormal occurs in a Rh negative person unless Rh positive blood is introduced into his bloodstream. This introduction can generally occur in two ways: through a blood transfusion, or through the placenta in a pregnant mother. When an Rh negative mother has an Rh positive child, the mixture of these blood factors sometimes causes the mother to develop antibodies against the

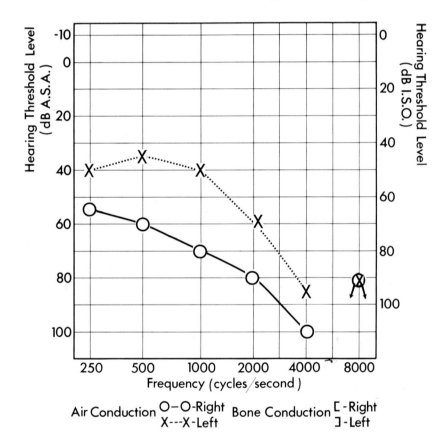

Figure 14. Audiogram of a 12-year-old boy who had marked jaundice shortly after birth and whose parents had a blood Rh incompatability.

Rh positive blood of the child. Since it takes some time for these antibodies to develop, the first child is seldom affected by them. On the next pregnancy, however, it can happen that the antibodies present in the mother's blood go through the placenta and affect the child by causing damage to the child's blood cells. From this may result a certain type of destruction of the blood cells, called erythroblastosis. This can cause severe jaundice (yellowing of the skin) and many other harmful affects. We find that a fair percentage of children with athetoid cerebral palsy have congenital hearing loss as the result of this Rh disparity.

It has been established that children who have deafness due to Rh incompatability show the following characteristics: the hearing loss is the same in both ears, and is usually worse in the high frequencies than it is in the lower ones; the loss is present at birth and there is frequently an accompanying speech difficulty, particularly in pronouncing the letter "S"; there is reduced bone conduction; and, foremost, the hearing loss is non-progressive in that it does not get any worse as the years go on (nor does it get better) (Fig. 14).

Congenital Deafness Due to German Measles in Pregnancy

Until recently the disease called German Measles has been considered a very mild one, which almost never resulted in any serious complications. This view has been drastically changed. A fuller understanding has revealed serious effects that German Measles can have upon the unborn infant when the disease affects the mother during the first three or four months of pregnancy. German Measles during early pregnancy can cause such a serious condition that young girls should be vaccinated against it. Exposure to the virus of German Measles, and perhaps other viruses, during early pregnancy may cause not only deafness but also deformities of the body such as defects in the heart, blindness, and mental disorders.

Hearing and Amplification

Whenever a patient who uses a hearing aid complains that his hearing is getting much worse in the aided ear, we should suspect

amplification as a possible cause if the loss is sensorineural. In
such instances, the hearing aid should be removed and the hearing watched to see if it returns to its original level. It may be necessary for the patient to use the aid in his other ear, and if this
ear shows the same sensitivity to amplification a less powerful
type of hearing aid might be indicated.

Neuritis of the Auditory Nerve and Systemic Diseases

Neuritis of the auditory nerve may follow such systemic infections as scarlet fever, typhoid fever, and other infectious diseases that produce high fevers. The hearing loss may be noted
immediately, but the onset is generally progressive over a period
of days or weeks. The type of neuritis more commonly encountered in present day practice would, perhaps, be more aptly classified under "unknown etiology." There is an insidious development of sensorineural deafness very similar to presbycusis, but
occurring at a much earlier age and attributed to such causes as
anoxia, anemia, nonspecific viruses, vague labyrinthitis of uncertain origin, and other conditions that are as yet poorly understood.

Meningitis

The sudden profound irreversible bilateral deafness caused by
meningitis makes this disease of great and singular concern to all
physicians. Since the damage is irreversible, every effort must be
exerted to prevent meningitis or to treat it vigorously and early
to obviate such complications. Occasionally a small amount of
hearing remains and a powerful hearing aid is then of some value but only to hear sounds, not to recognize speech. Tinnitus is
rarely present and rotary vertigo is usually of short duration. Imbalance, particularly in a dark room, is common because of
labyrinthine instability. Caloric studies, except in rare cases, reveal absent or poor vestibular function.

Acute Infections

Systemic infections, such as scarlet fever, typhoid fever, measles, and tuberculosis may occasionally cause bilateral sensorineural hearing impairment. In the past, syphilis has been blamed

for many cases of deafness that were actually due to other causes. At present syphilis is a rare cause of deafness, but in some cases it can cause sudden bilateral hearing loss that is not amenable to treatment. It is important to bear in mind that although a patient may have positive serological findings for syphilis along with sensorineural deafness, there may not be a causal relationship. The incidence of sensorineural deafness is so high that undoubtedly some people so affected have syphilis without any relation between the two. Scarlet fever, however, still causes a moderate degree of sensorineural deafness, usually accompanied by bilateral acute and later chronic otitis media.

Functional Deafness

Some cases of bilateral deafness are due to emotional disturbances, and while there is no real damage to the sensorineural mechanism the clinical findings so strongly resemble organic disease that it is discussed in greater detail in Chapter 7.

Ototoxic Drugs

With the increasing use of drugs that damage hearing it is important to inquire from every patient with sensorineural hearing loss what kind of drugs he has taken, particularly in relation to the onset of deafness. The most important offenders have been dihydrostreptomycin, neomycin, and kanamycin when used systemically and without proper precautions. Sudden deafness from these drugs occurs principally in the presence of impaired kidney function. It may also occur, however, from overdosage.

Multiple Sclerosis

Multiple sclerosis is a rare cause of deafness but it has been reported as a cause of sudden bilateral hearing loss. Usually the deafness fluctuates and hearing may return to normal even after a very severe depression. The precise mechanism of this loss has not yet been established.

Acoustic Trauma

In order to differentiate between sudden hearing loss, due to accidental brief exposure to intense noise, and gradual hearing loss, caused by prolonged exposure over many months and years, we restrict the term acoustic trauma to the former and call the latter occupational hearing loss.

In acoustic trauma the patient is usually exposed to a very intense noise of short duration such as an explosion or a rifle shot. This causes immediate hearing loss accompanied by fullness and ringing in the ear. If the cause is an explosion, there may also be a rupture of the eardrum and disruption of the ossicular chain. If this occurs, a conductive hearing loss is immediately caused without much serious nerve damage developing because the middle ear defect now serves as a protection for the inner ear.

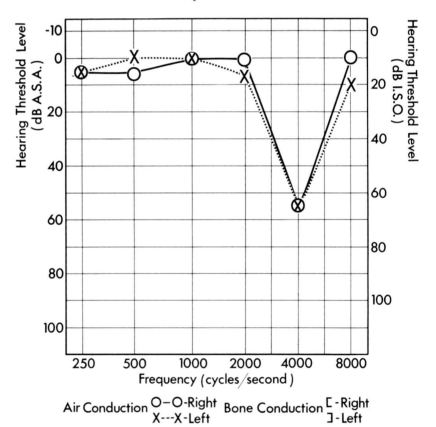

Figure 15. Audiogram showing a 4,000 Hz dip (C[5]) resulting from hair cell damage in the inner ear due to explosion of a firecracker very close to the ears.

Following acoustic trauma to the inner ear, the patient usually notes that his fullness and ringing tinnitus subside and his hearing improves. Generally the hearing returns to normal. Most of us have been exposed to gunfire at one time or another and have experienced some temporary hearing loss and had our hearing return to normal. In some cases, however, a degree of permanent hearing loss remains. The amount of loss depends on the intensity and duration of the noise, and the sensitivity of the ear. Usually the permanent loss is very mild and consists only of a high tone dip around 3,000 to 6,000 Hz. If the noise is very intense and the ear is particularly sensitive, the loss may be greater and involve a broader range of frequencies. The milder cases of hearing loss involve only one ear, usually the one closer to the gun or the source of the noise. If the noise is very intense and the hearing loss moderate, then both ears are usually affected to an almost identical degree or perhaps one slightly more so than the other. It is hardly possible (as a result of exposure to intense noise) to have a nerve deafness in one ear greater than 60 dB in all frequencies, with normal hearing in the other ear. This has important medicolegal aspects.

Because there is practically always some degree of temporary hearing loss or fatigue in acoustic trauma, the amount of permanent damage cannot be established until some time after the exposure. In the interim the individual must be free of other exposure to intense noise that might aggravate the hearing loss. The audiometric patterns in acoustic trauma are similar to those in noise-induced hearing loss, but the history is different and probably the manner in which the permanent hearing loss is produced is also different (Fig. 15).

Viruses

Herpes zoster, or shingles, is also known to cause sudden unilateral deafness of a severe degree. The author has seen one case of total loss of hearing that returned to normal in a few days. The patient had a typical picture of shingles on his face.

Many cases of sudden unilateral deafness that are now attributed to blood vessel spasm or rupture, may prove due to virus infections (Fig. 16).

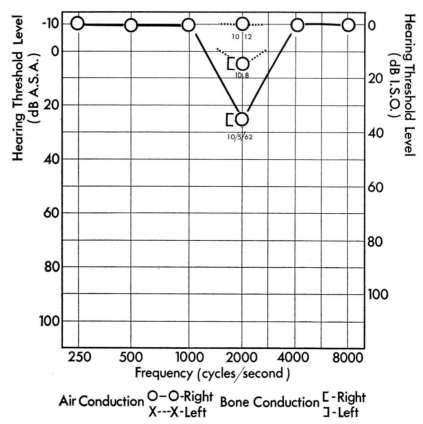

Air Conduction O—O-Right Bone Conduction ⊏-Right
              X---X-Left   ⊐-Left

Figure 16. *History:* 2 days following the onset of an upper respiratory infection this 25-year-old male complained of a ringing tinnitus in his right ear. *Otologic:* Normal. *Audiological:* All thresholds normal except for a dip at 2,000 Hz in the right ear. Complete recruitment was present at 2,000 Hz but not at 1,000 or 3,000 Hz. The tinnitus matched the frequency of a 2,000 Hz tone. No abnormal tone decay at 2,000 Hz. *Classification:* Sensory impairment. *Diagnosis:* Viral infection of the right inner ear.

Viruses are a common cause of high frequency hearing loss commonly attributed to vascular problems.

Vascular Disorders

The role of blood vessel spasm, thrombosis, embolism, and rupture as causes of hearing loss is still not clear. It is common and logical to attribute a progressive sensorineural deafness in an older person to arteriosclerosis or thrombosis. Such an explanation, however, has not been confirmed by histopathologic studies. While we continue to blame terminal blood vessels in the ear for many causes of hearing loss, we do not have proof that this is so. Other logical causes should also be considered.

The roles of hypertension and hypotension in deafness are also not clear. In the author's experience, hypertension is rarely, in itself, the cause of either insidious or sudden hearing loss. Hypotension on the other hand seems to be vaguely associated with progressive high tone sensorineural deafness in some patients. Usually recurrent attacks of imbalance are also present in these patients. Hypotension may predispose to sudden losses in hearing, but here again convincing proof is lacking.

Presbycusis

The most common cause of sensorineural deafness is presbycusis, the gradual reduction in hearing with advancing age. The hearing loss takes place in a well-defined manner. It occurs gradually over a period of years, with the very highest frequencies affected first and the lower ones gradually following. Both ears are affected at about the same rate, but sometimes the loss in one ear may progress faster than in the other. Whenever an older patient is encountered who has a hearing loss much greater in one ear than in the other, a diagnosis of presbycusis should not be made without reservation, for in all likelihood some other cause is present.

Actually, the process of presbycusis starts quite early in life. Children can hear up to about 20,000 Hz. But many adults can hear only up to 14,000, 12,000, or 10,000 Hz. With advancing years the ability to hear the higher frequencies becomes less acute, and by the age of 70 most people do not hear frequencies above 6,000 Hz. Since human beings make very little use of frequencies above 8,000 Hz, they do not become aware of any loss in hearing until the frequencies well below 8,000 Hz are affected. These frequencies begin to be affected around age 50. The rate at which presbycusis advances, and the degree to which the individual becomes affected varies widely. To some extent heredity plays a role, for early or premature presbycusis often is found in several members of the same family.

There may be a rare form of early presbycusis in which the inner ear structures may be affected in such a manner that only the frequencies between 2,000 and 6,000 Hz become involved, before there are any changes in the higher ranges. This is not a common condition but when it occurs, deafness does not progress to a marked degree before the higher frequencies also become involved. It should be noted that this picture closely resembles that of the hearing loss caused by intense noise exposure.

A Typical Case and Average Values

Figure 17 shows the typical manner in which presbycusis de-

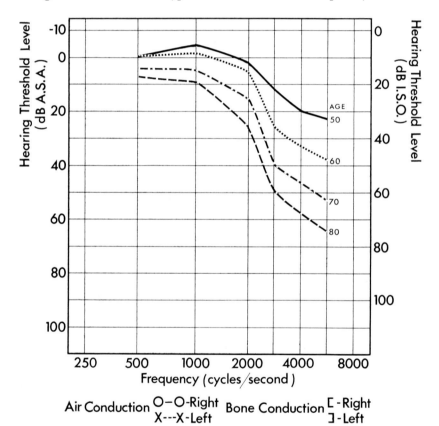

Air Conduction O–O-Right   Bone Conduction ⊏-Right
                X---X-Left   ⊐-Left

Figure 17. Presbycusis in a male patient. This shows the gradual deterioration of hearing with age. The 8,000 Hz threshold was always worse than the 4,000 Hz threshold.

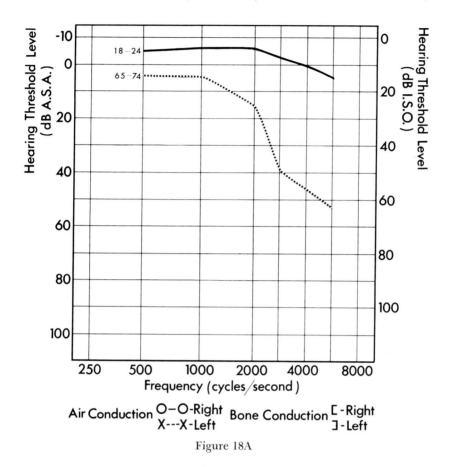

Figure 18A

velops in one individual. This is a longitudinal study, since the same man has been examined for about 20 years. In all presbycusis cases in which frequencies of 6,000 and 8,000 Hz are impaired, there is always a greater loss in the higher frequencies (10,000 and 12,000 Hz). It is possible to find middle-aged people with substantial presbycusis, whereas some quite elderly people may be found who have very little hearing loss for pure tone thresholds. Presbycusis should not be confused with hereditary progressive nerve deafness, which starting at a much earlier age and becoming quite severe, is undoubtedly inherited. Figure 18 shows the average hearing loss in each frequency that can be ex-

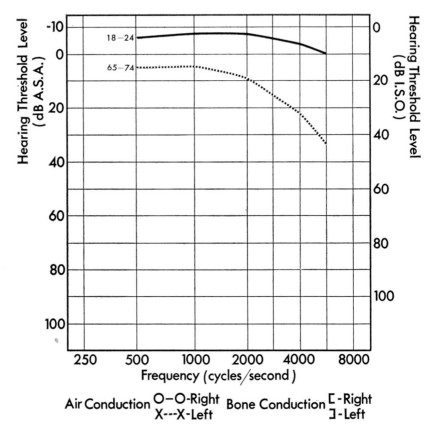

Figure 18B

Figure 18. (A-B) These composite curves show the manner in which presbycusis develops in the better ear of the average male population (A), and of
the average female population (B). (From Hearing Levels of Adults by
Age and Sex, U. S. Dept. HEW, Series 11, No. 11, 1965)

pected with aging, in the general population. These are average
values to be used for statistical purposes; they do not hold necessarily for specific individuals.

It is helpful at this point to emphasize one distinction between
presbycusis and noise-induced hearing loss. If the highest frequencies are at a more normal hearing level than the lower ones,

the cause is not likely to be presbycusis, except rarely in the unusual type of mild epithelial damage.

RECOMMENDED READINGS

Ballantyne, John: *Deafness,* 2nd Edition, Williams and Wilkins, Baltimore, 1970.

Davis, Hallowell and Silverman, S. Richard: *Hearing and Deafness,* 3rd Edition, 1970.

Sataloff, Joseph: *Hearing Loss,* Lippincott, 1966.

Chapter 5

NOISE INDUCED HEARING LOSS

OCCUPATIONAL HEARING LOSS is the gradual deafness caused by many months and years of exposure to very loud noise produced in industry. The following industrial environments produce sufficient noise to impair hearing: boilermaking, weaving, aircraft maintenance, blacksmithing, chipping, riveting, blasting, machine manufacturing, gunfiring, metal working, and numerous others utilizing large presses, high pressure steam, large wood saws, and heavy hammering, such as are used in steel and iron works, and many others.

There are actually two types of hearing loss produced by exposure to intense noise. One is temporary hearing loss such as is experienced after exposure to very loud jet noise. This loss gradually subsides and hearing returns to normal. In contrast, permanent hearing loss may follow prolonged exposure to intense noise. The latter type is referred to as occupational hearing loss. The relationship between temporary hearing loss, commonly abbreviated TTS (temporary threshold shift), and permanent hearing loss (PTS) is not yet clearly established. However, such a relationship serves as a useful guide in the conservation of hearing, but helps establish criteria for guidance purposes only. In particular, caution should be exercised in drawing any conclusion concerning an individual's susceptibility to permanent deafness from his temporary hearing loss characteristics.

Acoustic Trauma

If a hearing loss is produced by a noise, such as an accidental

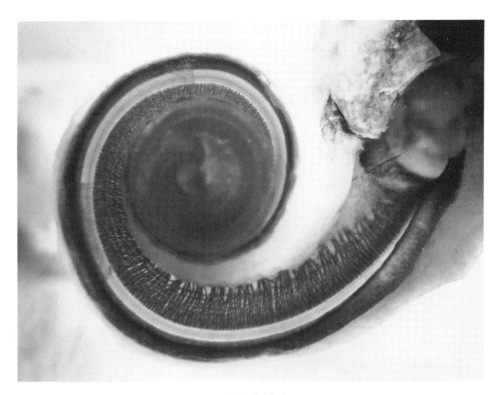

FIGURE 19 A

Figure 19 A. Anterolateral view of the left cochlea from a 17-year-old female car accident victim. Most of the vestibular portion of the membranous wall of the cochlea, Reissner's membrane, and the tectorial membrane have been removed for surface preparations. At 12 o'clock, a part of Reissner's membrane is still in situ, and at 9 o'clock, a portion of the spiral ligament is arching over the scala vestibuli. OW oval window; RW round window niche; H helicotreme; SL spiral ligament; OC organ of Corti. N network of radial and spiral myelinated nerve fibres in the osseous lamina. Paraformaldehyde 6 hours post mortem, OsO_4.

Figure 19 B. The left cochlea from a 76-year-old male cancer patient with hypertension and generalized arteriosclerosis. Note the patchy degeneration of Corti's organ in the lower basal turn and the nerve degeneration. Paraformaldehyde 11 hours post mortem, OsO_4.

(These are reprinted with the kind permission of Lars-Göran, M.D., Kresge Hearing Research Institute, University of Michigan, Ann Arbor, Michigan)

Figure 19 C. The right cochlea from a 59-year-old male patient who had worked in noisy surroundings and had been an enthusiastic hunter. There is a total loss of hair cells and nerve fibres in the middle of the basal turn. Note in the upper basal turn the presence of nerve fibres in an area where no organ of Corti remains. Paraformaldehyde 8 hours post mortem, OsO_4.

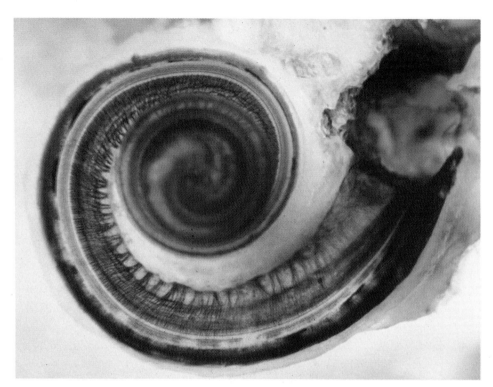

FIGURE 19 B

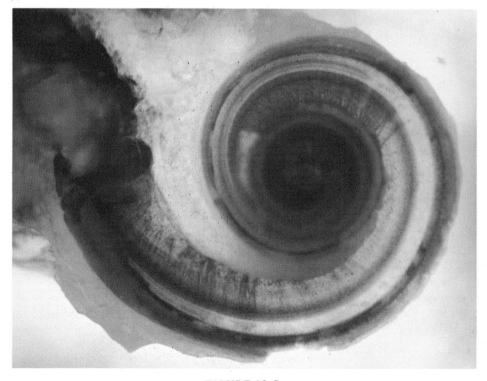

FIGURE 19 C

explosion, it is called "acoustic trauma," and is considered an occupational accident.

Inner Ear Damage from Noise

Environmental noise damages the organ of Corti in the cochlea of the inner ear (not the middle ear). Sound-induced motion of the fluid in the cochlea induces shearing and bending movements in the organ of Corti which, in turn, result in electrical stimuli to the auditory nerve. Prolonged and excessive noise injures and finally destroys the hair cells, and thus disrupts the sound transmission mechanism (Fig. 19). The damage generally occurs first to hair cells associated with the perception of frequencies higher than 2,000 Hz and below 8,000 Hz and thus does not interfere markedly with the reception of everyday speech. In its earliest stage prolonged exposure to intense noise may affect only the outer hair cells of the organ of Corti and reduce a slight dip at about 4,000 Hz. Actually, the hearing loss affects a range from 3,000 to 6,000 Hz, but measurements do not always cover this frequency spectrum. As the exposure to noise continues, inner hair cells also become affected and the hearing impairment increases. The supporting cells in the cochlea also may become damaged, and subsequently the nerve fibers themselves become affected. As exposure continues over many years the damage spreads to higher and lower frequencies (2,000, 1,000 and 500 Hz), and loss for the hearing of speech becomes apparent.

From the social point of view, the preservation of hearing for speech is of greatest importance; and in general, workman's compensation laws permit payment only for hearing loss in the speech frequencies (500, 1,000 and 2,000 Hz). The fact that initial noise-induced hearing loss generally occurs at frequencies above 2,000 Hz provides a powerful tool for the detection of the condition and for preventive action before the loss spreads to the speech-hearing frequencies.

The pure tone air conduction audiogram, if taken properly, provides an accurate map of hearing acuity for a range of selected frequencies. The frequencies monitored by audiometry should cover the range 500 to 8,000 Hz. Early noise-induced hearing loss is usually centered about 4,000 Hz, and thus is detected as a 4,000 Hz (or thereabouts) dip or notch. A deepening and spreading of this notch, as exposure to damaging noise continues may be predictive of eventual loss in the speech hearing frequencies and should trigger the initiation of a hearing conservation program.

Figure 20 shows a composite audiogram of the manner in which hearing thresholds become progressively worse in most cases of occupational hearing loss. Not all cases of high tone hearing loss affecting the frequencies mentioned are due to exposure to intense noise. Many other causes produce the same effects and patterns upon the hearing. Therefore, a careful otologic ex-

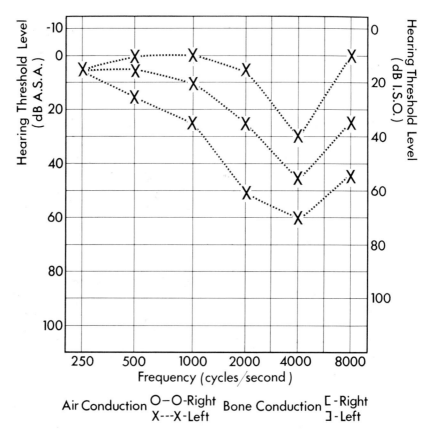

Figure 20. Series of audiometric curves showing a "classic" progressive loss that may be found in employees with excessive noise exposure.

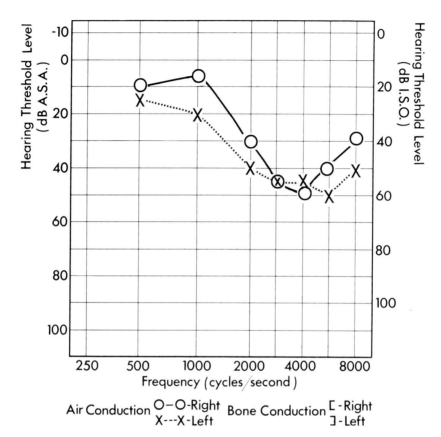

Figure 21. Audiometric threshold of a 59-year-old man showing the severe nerve deafness that can ensue in the high frequencies from many years of exposure to 101 dB in a plant.

amination and hearing evaluation are essential to an accurate individual diagnosis.

Figure 15 demonstrates the more common type of permanent hearing loss resulting from exposure to intense noise, such as small arms gunfire. This mild loss has little handicapping effect in communication and usually goes unnoticed by the subject. Figure 21 shows the gradual hearing loss that may ultimately result from extensive exposure in a metal plant for instance. An interesting example of hearing loss caused by noise is shown in Fig-

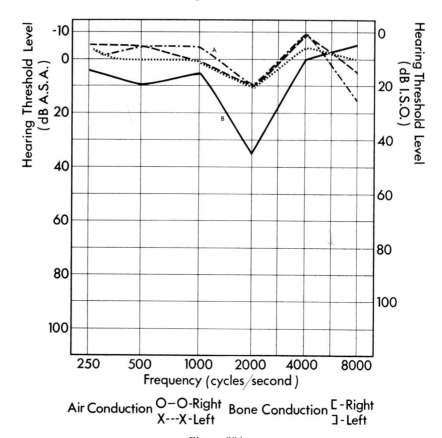

Figure 22A

ures 22 A & B. In this case the employee was wearing ear protectors but they failed to give adequate protection. Still another example is seen in Figure 23, in which an employee was exposed to a reciprocating engine for about 30 minutes. This employee also wore ear protectors (of another type) which were obviously ineffective. The examples also demonstrate the importance of proper hearing protection.

Temporary Hearing Loss (TTS)

The degree of TTS depends to a great extent upon the intensity and duration of the noise exposure, in addition to the spectral configuration. The degree of TTS and the rate of recovery from

TTS vary greatly among individuals, but seem to be about the same in both ears in the same individual. There is considerable difference of opinion as to how long it takes for TTS to disappear after long exposure to intense noise. The estimates vary from several days to several months, but as yet we have no well-controlled study to establish the facts. Figure 22 describes an interesting case of TTS occurring principally in the speech fre-

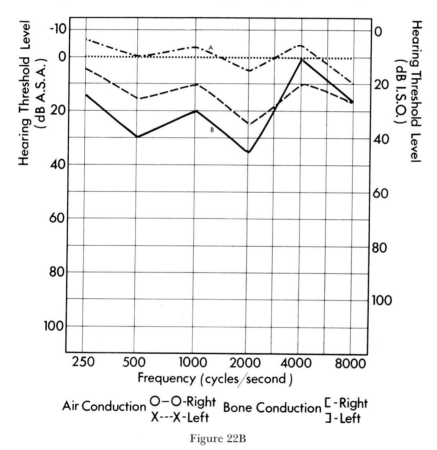

Air Conduction O–O-Right   Bone Conduction ⊏-Right
              X---X-Left   ⊐-Left

Figure 22B

Figure 22. (Note: 2 Figs.—right and left ear) Legend: ------ before exposure, ———— 15 min. after exposure, — — — 24 hours after exposure, —··—48 hours after exposure. Subject was exposed to intense noise of a certain type of jet engine for a long period. The hearing loss (B) returned to its original level (A) after 2 days of rest. During this period the subject experienced ringing tinnitus and much distortion with reduced discrimination.

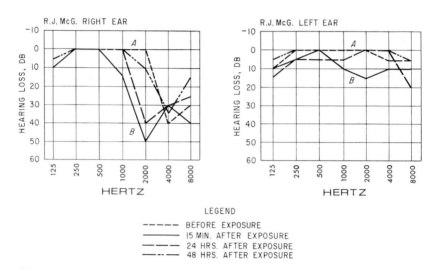

Figure. 23. Temporary hearing loss curves produced after exposure to a reciprocating engine. Curve A shows hearing before exposure and Curve B the subsequent loss in hearing of about 50 dB in the right ear.

quencies and demonstrates the exception that noise may not always involve the higher frequencies first. Certain types of noise, such as that produced by a paper machine, can involve 2,000 and 1,000 Hz, and with greater intensity 4,000 and 6,000 Hz. It would appear logical to relate temporary and permanent hearing loss, and to assume that individuals who sustain a temporary hearing loss everyday eventually sustain a permanent hearing loss. However, there is no satisfactory proof for this in the individual worker. In many instances workers who have sustained some degree of temporary hearing loss for years experience a return of hearing which remains normal after continued years of exposure. We also know that we are unable to predict the sensitivity of an individual to intense noise by determining his temporary threshold shift characteristics, such as magnitude and rate of growth or return to normal. Until more valid information is available it is safer to consider the relations between TTS and PTS unresolved at this time.

Factors in Making a Diagnosis.

Distinguishing Noise-induced Sensorineural Deafness

How does one go about making a diagnosis of sensorineural deafness due to prolonged exposure to intense noise and how does one distinguish its cause from other possible causes, especially presbycusis. In the former the early audiometric pattern is a dip at about 4,000 Hz with better hearing in the higher frequencies. Testing at 8,000 Hz shows fairly good residual hearing in early occupational deafness. In presbycusis the highest frequencies almost invariably are more depressed than the lower ones. Furthermore, complete and continuous recruitment is present in early cases of occupational deafness but not in presbycusis. In addition, a diagnosis of occupational deafness requires a proven history of many months' exposure to a damaging noise level. It is not always possible to distinguish more advanced cases of occupational deafness from cases of presbycusis. Age, too, must be given consideration in making a distinction.

If the patient hears much better at 8,000 Hz than at lower frequency levels, the principal cause of hearing loss is probably exposure to intense noise rather than aging. The presence of complete recruitment also favors a diagnosis of noise induced deafness, provided the patient has worked in a very noisy area. The subject's age is an important diagnostic criterion, since a marked hearing loss in a young man would not be expected without other corroborating evidence of hereditary nerve deafness, ototoxic drugs, Meniere's disease, etc. Another point of distinction is that occupational deafness does not seem to progress when noise exposure stops, whereas presbycusis generally progresses, though very slowly. Of course it may take many months or years to make a comparison.

Very High Frequencies in Occupational Hearing Loss

Studies with very high frequency testing of noise-exposed and non-noise-exposed personnel indicate that noise apparently has severe deleterious effect, not only in the well-known areas of

4,000 and 6,000 Hz, but also in high frequency areas above 8,000 Hz. The slopes of the high frequency curves for both groups parallel each other, but thresholds of the noise-exposed group are significantly poorer by approximately 20 dB at 10,000, 12,000 and 14,000 Hz. Preliminary studies on subjects with presbycusis suggest much less retention of perception for higher frequencies. If this continues to be borne out, we may then be able to differentiate between normal decline of threshold sensitivity with age, noise-induced loss and sensorineural deafness due to other causes.

Unilateral Deafness not Occupational Deafness

The likelihood that prolonged exposure to intense noise may be the cause of severe deafness in only one ear while the other ear remains practically normal is in conflict with available facts. Patients with unilateral total or subtotal deafness who work in noisy industries may claim that their deafness was produced by many years' exposure to intense noise. Since many physicians have heard of a link between noise and hearing loss, some are likely to assume such a connection. All evidence reported by competent investigators and extensive clinical practice agrees, however, that a severe sudden or even insidious hearing loss in one ear cannot result from prolonged exposure (for months or years) to intense industrial noise that is heard in both ears. Sudden acoustic trauma is a different story entirely.

If severe unilateral deafness develops over a period of several weeks, the probability of its being caused by prolonged exposure to intense industrial noise is almost negligible. Since both ears are almost equally sensitive in an individual, and industrial noise usually reaches both ears with equal intensity, it is unlikely that one ear could be seriously affected and the other not at all.

Effects of High Tone Hearing Loss in Industrial Deafness

The employee who develops industrial deafness has in the early stages a high tone hearing loss without involvement of the frequencies below 2,000 Hz. Consequently, he has little difficulty in hearing ordinary conversation, but he may on occasion have some difficulty in understanding poorly enunciated speech or whispers.

He may also have trouble hearing in the presence of much noise, because noise masks out some of the discriminating characteristics of the consonants and makes them even more difficult for him to distinguish. In addition, he may find it difficult to understand some voices projected by the telephone, television, records, movies or even radio, because the reproduction of voices through amplification system often reduces their clarity.

The word "deafness" when commonly used to refer to industrial or occupational hearing loss may be somewhat misleading when applied to its early phases since to most of us the word implies obvious difficulty in the hearing of speech. Actually, the difficulty lies not so much in hearing speech as in understanding it. Hence, unless one specifically looks for this lack of consonant discrimination, he is likely to miss the diagnosis of industrial deafness in its early stages because the employee usually tries to compensate for his handicap.

As a result of these factors, many representatives of management innocently deny the presence of occupational deafness in their plants, since they can walk repeatedly through their noisy shops and converse satisfactorily with all the employees. Too frequently management fails to recognize that conversing in a noisy environment requires one to speak above the level of the noise, and the vocabulary used in these brief conversations is such that any employee may be able to carry on a kind of limited and stereotyped conversation even though he has a substantial deafness.

It is not until the hearing loss extends to the lower frequencies and becomes more profound in the higher ones that poor hearing as well as understanding of speech becomes a prominent symptom. By then the damage to hearing is severe, irreversible, and often seriously handicapping. Furthermore, it assumes medicolegal importance as grounds for compensation.

The major handicaps in the severe cases are in communication, and because this enters into every phase of personal and business life, the psychological ramifications can cause personality problems. Often these individuals cannot hear warning signals, such as fire alarms or telephone bells. If they should happen to be employed in engine or machinery repair work and are expected to detect the need for adjustment by listening to the sounds in the motor, they are handicapped and may lose their jobs.

Recruitment

A factor often present in industrial deafness is a reduction of the individual's ability to understand speech because of distortion resulting from recruitment. At a railroad station reverberations of the voice of a train announcer make the message difficult for everybody to understand and become completely unintelligible blurs to the person with sensorineural deafness. The louder the reverberations, the less he understands. Like letters written with ink on blotting paper, the sounds of "Coach S 231 on Track 9 on the Panama Limited" dissolve and diffuse to a throbbing roll of thunderous sound signifying nothing.

Persons with recruitment often ask an individual to speak a little louder, but when the individual raises his voice a trifle more than necessary they understand even less. Instead of helping such individuals to understand better, loudness actually may reduce discrimination. This symptom of distortion is in itself a major cause for annoyance. It is natural that people who do not hear clearly should become frustrated and irritable.

Biologic Hypersensitivity to Noise

The phrase "hypersensitivity to noise" is very misleading and is being abused. There is no acceptable proof that any individual is so hypersensitive to noise of comparatively low intensity (90 dBA) that he will sustain a hearing loss of more than roughly 20 dB in the speech frequencies (or 30 dB ANSI) after several years of exposure. If an individual sustains a substantial hearing loss in a comparatively short period of exposure to these low intensities, the cause for his hearing loss is not the noise, but some other factor. The term "hypersensitivity" should be restricted to the individual who sustains an abnormal degree of hearing loss as compared to most of his fellow employees in the same noise level when exposed to intensities of over 95 dBA.

Tinnitus

Tinnitus, or noise in the ear, is one of the most challenging symptoms in otology and medicine. It usually indicates some damage to the auditory pathway. It has been speculated that tinnitus may be the result of a continuous stream of discharges along the auditory nerve to the brain, due to abnormal irritation in the sensorineural pathway. Though no sound is reaching the ear, the spontaneous nerve discharge may cause the patient to experience a false sensation of sound. While this theory sounds logical, there is as yet no scientific proof of its validity.

One of the surprising features about tinnitus is that not everybody has it. After all, the cochlea is exquisitely sensitive to sounds and relatively loud sounds are being produced inside our own heads: the rushing of blood through our cranial arteries, the noises that muscles make in the head when we chew. That we rarely hear these body noises may be explained by the way the temporal bone is situated in the skull and by considering how deeply the cochlea is imbedded in the temporal bone. The architecture and acoustics of the head ordinarily prevent the transmission of these noises through the skull bones to the cochlea, and thus to our consciousness; yet, the cochlea is so built and situated that it normally can respond to very weak sounds carried by the air from outside the head. Only when there are certain changes in our vascular walls—perhaps caused by arteriosclerosis—or in our temporal bone structure does the ear pick up these internal noises. The patient may say he hears his own pulse beat as a result of a vascular disorder, and it may seem louder when the room is quiet or at night when he is trying to go to sleep. Pressing on various blood vessels in the neck rarely stops this type of tinnitus, unassociated with gross hearing loss.

While always troublesome, tinnitus may serve as an early warning of auditory injury. For example, a high-pitched ringing or hissing may be the first indication of impending cochlear damage from an ototoxic drug and a clear signal that the drug should be stopped or its dosage reduced. Generally, the tinnitus disappears and hearing loss may not result, though in some instances the head noises may persist for months or even years.

When an observer can independently hear or feel the cause of head noises that bother the patient, the tinnitus is called objective and is usually associated with certain vascular disorders and soft palate abnormalities. The vast majority of cases of tinnitus are subjective, that is, heard by the patient alone. Objective tinnitus is comparatively easy to detect and localize because it can either be heard with a stethoscope, or determined by special studies such as x-rays and angiography.

Description of Tinnitus May Aid Diagnosis

Because tinnitus, like pain, is subjective, it can be described by the patient only by comparing it to some familiar noise. The patient may say it sounds like the hissing of steam, the ringing of bells, the roar of the ocean, a running motor, buzzing, or a machine shop. Very often it is difficult for the patient to localize the noise in the ears. He may not even be able to tell from which ear it is coming, or it may sound as though it is in the center of the head. Some people even say the noises are not in their ears at all but inside the head. Quite frequently a patient claims that the noise is in one ear and not in the other, yet when by some surgical or medical procedure the noise is stopped in the ear in question, the patient notices the noise in the opposite ear. This means that the patient had the tinnitus in the ear in which it was louder but did not realize that it was also present in the opposite ear.

How the patient describes his tinnitus is often of diagnostic significance. For example, a low-pitched type of tinnitus is more common in otosclerosis and other forms of conductive deafness. Sounds like ringing bells and hissing are more usual in sensorineural deafness. The ocean roaring type of noise or a noise like that of a hollow seashell held to the ear is most often described in Meniere's disease.

Patients sometimes say their ear noises are so loud that they are unable to hear what is going on around them. They also claim that if the head noises would stop, they would be able to hear better. Unfortunately, this is not the case. It is possible to measure how loud these noises actually are. These measurements show that tinnitus is rarely louder than a very soft whisper, and it is actually the concomitant hearing loss that prevents patients from hearing or else a psychological disturbance rather than the masking effect of the tinnitus is at fault.

Tinnitus After Exposure to Occupational Noise

Ringing tinnitus is almost invariably experienced after an accident to the ear, such as a slap across the ear, or after close exposure to loud impact noise, such as the explosion of a firecracker or the firing of a gun. In most instances tinnitus is accompanied by a high tone hearing loss. Generally, the hearing loss and the tinnitus are temporary and subside in a few hours or in several days. If a permanent hearing loss persists due to damage in the inner ear, a ringing tinnitus may also be present for many years. This is especially common after gunfire target practice in the military.

Tinnitus in habitual exposure to everyday occupational noise is not common. It does occur in employees who are exposed to very high-pitched intense noise, such as pounding of metal upon metal in foundries, and occasionally following long exposure to intense air-jet noise. However, tinnitus in these cases is not disturbing enough to make individuals complain severely, as they would in otosclerosis or Meniere's disease.

RECOMMENDED READINGS

Davis, H., Morgan, C. T. and Hawkins, J. E. et al.: Temporary deafness following exposure to loud tones and noise, *Acta Otolaryngol [Suppl]* 88, 1950.

Davis, Hallowell and Silverman, S. Richard, eds.: *Hearing and Deafness,* New York, Holt, Rinehart & Winston, 1960.

Engstrom, H. and Ades, H. W.: Effect of high intensity noise on inner ear sensory epithelia, *Acta Otolaryngol [Suppl]* 158:219-29, 1960.

Glorig, Aram: *Noise and Your Ear,* New York, Grune and Stratton, 1958.

Igarashi, M., Schuknecht, H. F. and Myers, E. N.: Cochlear pathology in humans with stimulation deafness, *J Laryngol Otol* 78:115-23, 1964.

Lawrence, M. and Yantis, P. S.: Individual differences in functional recovery and structural repair following overstimulation of the guinea pig ear, *Ann Otol* 66:595-621, 1957.

Lurie, M. H., Davis, H. and Hawkins, J. E.: Acoustic trauma of the organ of corti in the guinea pig, *Laryngoscope, 54*:375-86, 1944.

Miller, J. D., Watson, C. S. and Covell, W. E.: Deafening effects of noise on the cat, *Acta Otolaryngol [Suppl] 176,* 1963.

Nakashima, T., Meiring, N. L. and Snow, J. B., Jr.: Cations in the endolymph of the guinea pig with noise-induced deafness, *Surg Forum 21*:489-91, 1970.

Perlman, H. B. and Kimura, R.: Cochlear blood flow in acoustic trauma, *Acta Otolaryngol 54*:99-110, 1962.

Ward, W. D.: Biochemical implications in auditory fatigue and noise-induced hearing loss, Paparella, M. M. (Ed.) *Biochemical Mechanisms In Hearing and Deafness,* Springfield, Thomas, 1970.

Chapter 6

EQUIPMENT AND ROOM
FOR HEARING TESTING

The Audiometer

A PURE-TONE AUDIOMETER is recommended for testing hearing in industry. An audiometer consists of (1) an electronic oscillator for generating the test tones, (2) a carefully controlled amplifier-attenuator network, and (3) earphones to introduce the test tones into the ear canal.

Every audiometer has a series of switches and controls to direct its operation. The on-and-off switch controls the electrical power supplied to the audiometer. A frequency selector dial designates the tone that is produced in the earphones. The level control determines the sound-pressure level of the tone produced under the earphones. Attenuators which are used in the level control circuitry are normally calibrated in 5-dB steps ranging from 0 to 110 dB, with the exception of the very low and high frequencies, for which the maximum usually is around 90 dB. For industrial purposes, readings should not be made between the 5-dB steps. An interrupter switch is used to turn the tone on and off. A "normally on-normally off" switch provides a choice for interrupter switch operation. At the "normally on" position, depressing the interrupter switch causes the test tone to go off, while at the "normally off" position, depressing the interrupter switch causes the tone to come on. For industrial purposes, the "normally off" position is recommended. Some instruments have other switches such as microphone, masking, bone conduction, etc., which are not useful for industrial testing. These controls should be turned to an off position during testing.

Two cords leading from the audiometer are attached to earphones which are held by a spring headband. Earphones are very fragile and should be handled with extreme caution, for their sensitivities can be easily changed by rough handling. The function of earphones is to convert electric current supplied from the audiometer into sound, which then impinges on the eardrum. A switch normally provided on the audiometer enables the operator to shift the sound from one earphone to another. The earphones are equipped with a rubber cushion that must be of a specified size and shape so that the volume of air that it encloses is the same as that provided when the instrument was calibrated (approximately 6 cc.).[1] The cushion cannot be replaced by a larger or smaller one for reasons of comfort without disturbing the calibration of the instrument.

A push-button cord also accompanies most audiometers so that the patient may signal his response by pressing the button. When the subject hears the tone, he presses the button, causing a light to appear on the instrument panelboard. This is an acceptable way of getting a response from the subject; however, many experienced testers prefer to rely on the patient's raising a finger or a hand.

Selecting an Audiometer

Although standard specifications for approved audiometers are established by the American National Standards Institute, audiometers differ in many features. These differences help determine which audiometer is best suited for an individual tester or for an individual purpose. For industrial testing, it is advisable for the audiometer to be as simple as possible since only air conduction testing is to be performed. Additional features such as masking, bone conduction, and others only serve to increase the cost of the audiometer and to complicate its use without making it either more efficient or more helpful to the program.

Some of the features which should be considered before purchasing an audiometer for industrial testing are:

1. The audiometer should not be complicated to operate. It should have all of the essentials for air conduction threshold measurements and as few complicating and intricate extras as possible.

2. It is advisable for the instrument to have test frequencies including 500, 1,000, 2,000, 3,000, 4,000, 6,000 and 8,000 Hz. The purchaser should not be influenced by such accessories as speech reception, masking, bone conduction, or loudness balance testing facilities, since these will be of little value in industrial testing.

3. The tone interrupter switch should be designed so that the tone can be turned on when the switch is pressed.

4. The instrument should have a headband that has adequate tension to hold the earphones securely against the ears. A standard headband will have adequate tension if there is about one-half inch between the inner surfaces of the earphone cushions then the headband is in a free unmounted condition.

5. The earphone cushion should be the standard MX-41/AR type.[1]

6. The general appearance and facility with which the frequencies can be selected and the attenuator dial moved are also factors important to consider.

7. The audiometer should be purchased from a company which will assure prompt attention in case repairs are needed and which has facilities for accurately calibrating any instrument that is returned for adjustment.

Audiometer Calibration

An audiometer's accuracy, or calibration, must be checked daily prior to using the instrument and upon completion of its use for the day. In addition, complete laboratory calibrations should be made periodically.

CAUSES FOR INACCURACY IN INSTRUMENTATION. An audiometer that is in calibration produces a specified test tone at the level and frequency shown on the dial settings. Further, it produces the test tone only in the earphone to which it is directed, and it produces this signal free from unwanted noises or tones. It is important to realize that a properly calibrated audiometer can lose its accuracy in time if mistreated or even by aging of components. The following is a list of factors that can affect the accuracy of an audiometer:

1. Rough handling of the instrument or earphones. Shipping an audiometer or dropping the earphones are two common causes for loss of instrument accuracy.

2. Heat can cause audiometer electronic component values to change and result in a loss of accuracy. Overheating may occur when the instrument is stored in a warm place such as in a closed car on a hot day, or when the power is left on while the instrument is covered by a dust cover.

3. Dust or dirt inside the audiometer can cause switches to become noisy, and, in some cases, cause poor electrical contact that will affect the instrument accuracy. Dust covers should be used to protect the instruments when not in use, and when the instrument case is cleaned, care must be taken to prevent dust and dirt from getting brushed into the case.

4. High humidity, salt air, and acid fumes may cause corrosion of electrical contacts that can cause noise or affect the instrument accuracy.

5. Normal aging of component parts can change an audiometer's response characteristics significantly. Thus, an audiometer can go out of calibration even if it has not been in use.

CALIBRATION PROCEDURE. If the change in an audiometer's operating characteristics is sudden and onsiderable in extent, it is usually obvious that the instrument should be serviced. However, if the change is slow, it may not be obvious, and poor measurements may result. If changes in instrument accuracy are not detected, measurements may be made over many weeks or months before a calibration check discloses the inaccuracy. These wasted measurements can be prevented by simple daily checks designed to detect changes in instrument operating characteristics and potential trouble spots.

The following tests and inspections should be made by the technician at the beginning of each day:

1. All control knobs on the audiometer should be checked to be sure that they are tight on their shafts and not misaligned.

2. Earphone cords should be straightened so that there are no sharp bends or knots. If the cord covers are worn or cracked, they should be replaced. A recalibration is not necessary when earphone cords are replaced.

3. Earphone cushions should be replaced if they are not resilient or if cracks, bubbles, or crevices develop. A recalibration should not be necessary when earphone cushions are replaced.

4. The audiometer calibration should be checked by measuring the hearing threshold at each test frequency of a normal-hearing person[2] whose hearing levels are well known. A persistent change of

10 dB or more in the hearing threshold at any test frequency for this person from one day to the next which cannot be explained by temporary threshold shifts due to colds, noise exposure, etc., indicates the need for an instrument recalibration.[3] A normal-hearing technician may serve as the test subject. These threshold levels should be recorded serially at the beginning and at the end of each day of testing in ink, with no erasures, if the records are to have legal significance. Any mistakes made in entries to these records should be crossed once with ink, initialed, and dated.

5. The linearity of the hearing level control should be checked with the tone control set on 2,000 cps by listening to the earphones while slowly increasing the hearing level from threshold. Each 5-dB step should produce a small but noticeable increase in level without changes in tone quality or audible extraneous noise.

6. Test the earphone cords electrically with the dials set at 2,000 cps and 60 dB by listening to the earphones while bending the cords along their length. Any scratching noise, intermittency, or change in test tone indicates a need for new cords.

7. Test the operation of the tone interrupter with dials set at 2,000 cps and 60 dB by listening to the earphones and operating the interrupter several times. No audible noise, such as clicks or scratches, nor changes in test tone quality should be heard when the interrupter switch is used.

8. Check extraneous noises from the case and the earphone not in use with the hearing level control set at 60 dB and the test earphone jack disconnected from the amplifier. No audible noise should be heard while wearing the earphones when the tone control is switched to each test tone.

9. Check the headband tension by observing the distance between the inner surfaces of the earphone cushions when it is held in a free unmounted condition. While at the center of its adjustment range, the distance between cushions should be about one-half inch. The band may be bent to reach this adjustment.

Audiometer Repairs

When an audiometer's accuracy is suspected, it should be serviced and calibrated by a qualified laboratory. Preferably, the instrument should be hand-carried to and from the laboratory because rough handling encountered in normal shipping procedures may change its operating characteristics after calibration.

There are no certified facilities for the calibration of audiometers, so it may be difficult to find competent laboratories nearby. Even the audiometer distributor may not be competent in servicing or calibration procedures. When a servicing and calibration facility is located, some understanding should be reached on the kind of calibration to be performed. Determine that hearing level accuracy will be checked for each test tone at each 5 dB interval throughout the operating range. For industrial applications, the range should cover hearing levels from 10 dB to 70 dB re ANSI S3.6-1969 and at least test tones of 500, 1,000, 2,000, 3,000, 4,000, 6,000 and 8,000 Hz. In addition to these tests, the several other specifications listed in the American National Standard Specifications for Audiometers should be included. These specifications include tolerance limits on attenuator linearity, test tone accuracy and purity, interrupter switch operation, masking noise, and the effects of power supply variations. It is always good practice to require a written report that includes all measurement data. A simple statement that the audiometer meets ANSI specifications should not be accepted without some evidence that all tests have been made.

In addition to the possible bad effects of shipping on instrument accuracy, the inconvenience of not having an instrument for several weeks makes shipping an instrument off for service very unsatisfactory. If the instrument must be shipped away for service or calibration, it may be advisable to have two instruments on hand. Another solution may be to borrow an instrument during the repair period. If a second instrument is used, its calibration must be carefully established and a note must be made on each audiogram stating the change of instruments.

Accuracy of the instrument should not be taken for granted following a factory adjustment, particularly after shipment. The instrument should always be checked subjectively as described in the above steps.

A factor that should not be overlooked when an instrument's accuracy is suspected is that the tester may not be using the instrument properly. For this reason, it is always wise to discuss the problem with some person who is very familiar with the operation of the instrument to determine if a simple solution is available.

Audiometer Specifications

Wide range, limited range, and narrow range audiometers are specified in the American National Standards Institute (ANSI) Specifications for Audiometers.[1] The wide range audiometer is "intended primarily for clinical and diagnostic purposes, or for the measurement of the hearing thresholds of children." The limited range audiometer is "intended for measuring the hearing threshold levels of adult populations such as those found in industry." The narrow range audiometer is "more restricted than a limited range audiometer in its ranges of frequency and sound-pressure levels."

The limited range audiometer which is of primary interest to industry is intended for air conduction threshold measurements with test tones provided at least at 500, 1,000, 2,000, 3,000, 4,000 and 6,000 Hz, with hearing levels from 10 dB to at least 70 dB referenced to the new ANSI S3.6-1969 threshold levels. Facilities for bone conduction measurements and masking may be omitted.

Other significant provisions which have been changed from the previous audiometer standard include:

1. The accuracy of sound-pressure levels shall be ± 3 dB at test frequencies from 250 to 3,000 Hz, ± 4 dB at 4,000 Hz, and ± 5 dB at all other test frequencies above or below this range.
2. The measured difference between two successive designations of hearing threshold level shall not differ from the dial-indicated difference by more than (1) three-tenths of the dial interval measured in decibels, or (2) 1 dB, whichever is larger.
3. The accuracy of test tone frequencies shall be ± 3 percent of the indicated frequency for discrete-frequency audiometers.
4. The sound-pressure level of any harmonic of the fundamental shall be at least 30 dB below the sound-pressure level of the fundamental.

Most manual and automatic audiometers used in hearing conservation programs are discrete-frequency types which are covered by the above specifications. Those few audiometers that supply test tones over a continuous frequency range shall meet the above specifications except that frequency accuracy shall be within 5 percent at all indicated test frequencies.

ASA-1951 vs. ANSI-1969 Reference Threshold Levels

The new American National Standards Specifications for Audiometers, S3.6-1969, which became effective September 1, 1970, are much more complete and specify closer tolerance limits than the ASA-1951 specifications that they replace.

The most significant change in the audiometer specifications, and one which caused much controversy over the 15 years while the new specifications were being written, is in the hearing threshold reference levels. The sound-pressure levels corresponding to the new threshold reference levels are lower (higher hearing sensitivity) than those in the old standard at all test frequencies, the changes ranging from 14 decibels at 500 hertz to 6 decibels at 4,000 hertz (see Table I). The new threshold levels simply provide new numbers for given sound-pressure levels produced under the earphones and obviously do not change the ear's ability to perceive sound. The Scope and Purpose section of the new specifications clearly states that the new threshold levels should not be interpreted as altering previously implied physical sound-pressure levels for specific purposes such as in laws and administrative rules and regulations relating to the impairment of hearing, to minimum requirements for employment, to audiometric screening levels in school systems, etc.

Hearing Test Rooms

It is essential that hearing threshold measurements be made in a room sufficiently quiet so that the ambient noise does not mask the test tones. In addition, the testing space must be free from

TABLE I

MAXIMUM ALLOWABLE BAND PRESSURE LEVELS FOR NO MASKING
ABOVE THE ANSI S3.6-1969 TEN-DECIBEL HEARING LEVELS

Audiometric test frequency (Hz)	125	250	500	1,000	2,000	3,000	4,000	6,000	8,000
Octave band frequency (Hz)	125	250	500	1,000	2,000	4,000	4,000	8,000	8,000
Sound pressure level in dB re 0.00002 N/m²	35	35	35	35	42	47	52	57	62

any activities that will prevent the person being tested from concentrating upon the test tone. Any available room that can be made quiet enough and free from distractions can be used for hearing tests; however, the most satisfactory and practical test space is often provided by a commercially available pre-fabricated test room.

Allowable Sound Levels in a Test Room. The ANSI S3.6-1969 specifications for audiometers sets the 10 dB hearing level as the lowest necessary for limited range or industrial audiometry. Measurements at and above the 10 dB hearing level should be possible with no significant masking effects if the background noise levels do not exceed the levels shown in Table I.

Some hearing conservation program directors may want to measure hearing thresholds down to the 0 dB hearing level (recommended for clinical audiometry) in order to obtain accurate data for those persons with very good hearing. The maximum test room noise levels for no masking at and above the ANSI S3.6-1969 0 dB hearing level would be 10 dB lower than the levels shown in Table I.

In addition to the noise level requirements given in Table I, subjective tests should be made inside the closed test booth on location to determine that no noises, such as talking and clicking of a woman's heels, are audible. Any audible noises in the test room will interfere with hearing threshold measurements so they must be eliminated. Such extraneous noises and, in particular, short impulse-type noises, may be heard even though the measured sound-pressure levels are below the limits given in Table I.

Factors in Selecting Pre-Fabricated Test Rooms. The noise reduction provided by a good pre-fabricated audiometric test booth should be adequate to permit limited range threshold measurements (at and above 10 dB hearing level) in most areas selected for hearing tests. However, it is recommended that the burden of on-location performance be placed on the supplier to be sure that the booth is erected properly. In any purchase agreement, there should be a guarantee that the booth will provide the required test environment when installed at the specified test site. An agreement of this kind will obviate any unexpected problems that might result from such factors as poor vibration isolation or faulty assembly procedures.

In addition to the attenuation characteristics and cost, pre-fabricated test rooms may differ in other features that should be considered. Size and appearance are important points. Will opening and closing the door result in wearing of contact material and require frequent replacement? Are the interior surfaces durable and easily cleaned? Is the door easily opened from the inside so that the subject will not feel "locked in"? The observation window must be located so that the seated tester can comfortably see the subject's arm or hand response through the window. A ventilation system should be provided for the test booth and the noise produced by the ventilation system must be below the limits specified above. Portability of the room is seldom an important factor because test rooms are rarely moved.

Modifying an Available Room for Audiometric Testing

The most reliable means of providing noise reduction is massive construction. A room with heavy masonry walls, floors, and ceilings will provide good noise isolation provided care is taken to prevent leakage paths.

Leakage. Small cracks that might be found around windows, doors, electrical fixtures, pipes, etc., provide significant leakage paths that may nullify the benefits of a good noise barrier. A hole 1.5 inch x 1.5 inch in a wall will transmit about the same amount of acoustical energy as 100 square feet of wall area that has a transmission loss of 40 dB. Wherever possible, all holes and cracks should be sealed permanently. Openings around an operating door or window should be closed by flexible gaskets.

Radiation. Leakage and re-radiation of noise can occur through thin or light sections such as single-pane windows and doors. If additional noise reduction is required, double doors or double-pane windows can be used to provide more reduction.

Vibration. Structure-borne vibration can be transmitted through heavy walls and re-radiated into the air of an enclosed space. If noise levels from structure-borne sources are high, a "room within a room" construction[4, 5] may be required and this work should be undertaken only by experienced acousticians.

Interior Absorption. Interior noise-absorbing materials have little effect on the amount of noise leaking into a room from the outside. However, some absorbent material is required to prevent noise reaching the interior of the room from outside, or from the subject, from building up. For rooms of moderate size, adequate absorption is provided by a carpet on the floor and full drapes on two walls. If conventional sound-absorbing treatment is used, it should be distributed between the ceiling and two adjoining walls for maximum effectiveness.[4, 5]

Ventilation. Two general principles are normally applied in the design of ventilation systems for hearing test rooms. One is to use long inlet and outlet ducts that are heavily lined with noise-absorbing material. The second is to use low air velocities that will minimize noise caused by turbulence. The amount of noise reduction resulting from the duct dimensions, thickness of absorption materials, and air velocity may be found in other literature[4-6] and in Chapter 14.

REFERENCES

1. American National Standard Specifications for Audiometers, S3.6-1969. American National Standards Institute, New York, N. Y. 10018.
2. Normal hearing is defined here to be more sensitive than 25 dB (hearing levels re ANSI S3.6-1969 at all test frequencies).
3. When a tester uses his own or other normal ears to determine the calibration of an audiometer, he is testing only the calibration at threshold, and assuming that the attenuators are working properly and producing accurate readings at above threshold levels. This assumption is not always justifiable, but, at present, it is the most practical and inexpensive means other than experience and contradictory findings to establish the accuracy of the instrument.
4. Harris, C. M.: *Handbook of Noise Control.* New York, McGraw-Hill, 1957.
5. Beranek, L. L.: *Noise Reduction.* New York, McGraw-Hill, 1960.
6. *Fan Engineering,* 6th edition, edited by Robert Jorgensen, Buffalo, N. Y., Buffalo Forge Company, 1961.

Chapter 7

HEARING TESTING

To obtain an accurate quantitative measurement of a person's ability to hear may seem reasonably simple, but in actual practice it is often very difficult. Many methods have been used, including listening to watch ticks, tuning forks, monochords, whistles and other devices.

The most reliable and accepted method of testing hearing acuity is to use a standard pure-tone audiometer. In order to perform satisfactory audiometry specialized training is necessary, and for industrial hearing testing certification is advisable and may soon be required.

Because the testing of hearing is a complex subject with new factors constantly developing, the hearing tester should be familiar with certain basic aspects of hearing and its measurement.

What Is Hearing?

In a general way we all know that hearing is a sensation produced by sound waves of certain frequencies and intensities which enter the ear. But how can we tell whether or not an individual hears?

For example, if a subject repeatedly responds correctly to questions that he receives exclusively through hearing, it is reasonably safe to conclude he hears. However, if the subject does not respond to a question or sound signal, are we safe in assuming he does not hear? Obviously not. The subject may hear but may not wish to respond, or may be unable to respond, or may not know how to respond. There may be many other reasons. The difficulty in deciding whether or not an individual hears can be illustrated by the common experience of attending a dull lecture and being able with relative ease, to shut out the speaker's voice by merely placing a mental block somewhere between our ears and our brain. The sound most certainly enters our ears, but it is not integrated into information. Can it be said in such a case that we hear the speaker?

It is not within the province of this book to consider the psychological complexities of hearing but they must be assessed during industrial hearing testing. For the purpose of making accurate hearing measurements a response from the listener must be obtainable. This response may take many forms, such as merely answering a question, repeating a phrase or word, raising a hand or finger, pressing a button, or nodding the head. Such responses are voluntary and require cooperation of the listener. He must *want* to raise his finger or to answer the question. While it is true certain sounds may involuntarily cause a person to blink his eyes or turn his head, this generally occurs only when the sound is loud and possibly unexpected.

It would be more satisfactory if our method of determining hearing could be truly objective, but unfortunately such methods are not yet available for general use.

The Response Mechanism

Since we are measuring hearing through the medium of a response, we must make the response an accurate indication of the actual hearing acuity. This can be accomplished best by adhering to the following principles:

1. Make the response mechanism as simple as possible. For example: Raising a finger is simpler than writing down information.
2. Try by positive suggestion and encouragement to condition the subject to respond each time he hears the sound signal.
3. Explain the method of response to the listener in a simple positive manner, and give a practical demonstration.
4. During the hearing testing, occasionally check the accuracy of the response by other than the usual means.
5. Give the slow subject sufficient time to respond after presenting the sound signal.

The experienced hearing tester often develops an intuitive feeling for the extent of accuracy of a subject's responses, and can usually modify the response in one manner or another to make the test more reliable and more efficient. For example, if a tester notes that the subject's finger continually moves up and down independently of the tone in his ear, the tester can ask the subject to raise his hand or answer yes when he hears the tone instead of using the small range of motion permitted in the finger response.

Test Material

Another basic problem in measuring hearing concerns itself with the type of material used to test the hearing. This material is presently of two main forms—(1) *Pure Tones,* and (2) *Speech.*

Pure Tones

For industrial programs only pure tones are used at present for hearing testing, and the commercial instrument used to produce these pure tones is called an audiometer. These pure tones are usually in octave or half-octave steps and cover the frequencies between 250 and 8,000 Hz (formerly known as cycles per second). Since everyday speech falls within this range, in a limited way it is possible to measure a person's ability to hear conversation by testing his hearing with pure tones.

There are certain advantages in testing hearing by means of pure tones rather than by complex tones, noise, speech sounds or discourse.

1. Pure-tone testing methods have been standardized, and there are available inexpensive commercial instruments with which to perform such tests.
2. The intensities and frequencies of pure tones can be more accurately measured than other types of sound signals on available commercial equipment.
3. The frequencies of the pure tones used for testing have their anatomical counterpart in the Organ of Corti, and the use of pure tones can indicate the degree and may even indicate the cause of any hearing loss present.
4. A defect of the peripheral hearing mechanism can be detected much earlier with pure-tone testing than with tests using speech.

This last is one of the best reasons for using pure tones in industrial hearing testing. The very early effects of intense noise upon hearing can be detected by careful observation of the threshold in the frequencies above 2,000 Hz, and proper protective measures can be taken. In occupational deafness, it is these higher frequencies that first show the effects of intense noise.

There are several methods of using pure tones to test hearing. The best and the one recommended for all industrial testing is the standard procedure for performing individual audiograms described in this chapter.

Occasionally, individual screening by means of pure tones is used, but this screening method is not recommended and should be used only when individual audiometry is not possible. In using the screening method the test is performed by setting the intensity at perhaps 20 dB and merely asking the individual to respond if he hears each of the test tones. If he hears them, he is passed; if not, he is recommended for individual threshold audiometry or perhaps even rejected for employment on the basis of such screening. Such screening audiometry, using above threshold levels, does not meet the rigid standards of testing required in cases of industrial deafness.

Another method is to do pure tone group screening in which many subjects are simultaneously given the tones and asked to fill out certain coded forms that establish whether or not the subject hears at the levels tested. This method is most useful when it is essential to test large numbers of personnel at the same time in the military, for example, or in instances when a plant might hire hundreds of employees in one or two days. Such a method of testing is not advisable in industrial hearing testing, but if it must be used, it is recommended that later, when the opportunity presents itself, all personnel so tested be rechecked by individual threshold audiometry.

Self-recording audiometry with either discreet or continuous tones is another method which has some value in industrial hearing testing. This is done by a special type of instrument which requires a tester, but not necessarily in constant attendance.

The sounds are presented to the subject in a specified manner and his response leaves a written record of his hearing acuity.

Speech

One of the disadvantages of testing hearing with pure tones is that the sounds we hear in everyday life are not pure tones but very complex speech sounds, and these speech sounds would seem logically to be the ideal material for testing hearing.

A reasonably accurate and practical measure of an individual's ability to hear and understand speech can be obtained by using two different tests. One test determines the threshold at which the individual can repeat about half of such materials as two-syllable words, sentences, or discourse. This threshold generally compares favorably with the average pure tone loss at 500, 1,000 and 2,000 Hz. The other test determines the individual's ability to discriminate the important sounds, principally the consonants. These tests are not performed in industry but should be done on all patients referred to an otologist for hearing studies.

These two tests are commonly known as (1) *The speech reception threshold* (SRT), and (2) *The discrimination test.*

The former determines the weakest intensity at which an individual can repeat about 50 percent of what he hears. The latter seeks to determine how well an individual can discriminate speech at intensities 30 to 40 dB above his SRT.

The speech reception threshold test uses words called "spondee" words. These words consist of two syllables equally accented, such as are listed in Figure 24.

Sentences and discourse can also be used for this purpose. The threshold is determined as the lowest intensity at which the sub-

SPONDEE LIST 2

1. ALTHOUGH	12. GRANDSON	23. NUTMEG	34. SUNDOWN
2. BEEHIVE	13. GREYHOUND	24. OUTSIDE	35. THEREFORE
3. BLACKOUT	14. HORSEHOE	25. PADLOCK	36. TOOTHBRUSH
4. CARGO	15. HOTDOG	26. PANCAKE	37. VAMPIRE
5. COOKBOOK	16. HOUSEWORK	27. PINBALL	38. WASHBOARD
6. DAYBREAK	17. ICEBERG	28. PLATFORM	39. WHIZZBANG
7. DOORMAT	18. JACKNIFE	29. PLAYMATE	40. WOODCHUCK
8. DUCKPONT	19. LIFEBOAT	30. SCARECROW	41. WORKSHOP
9. EARDRUM	20. MIDWAY	31. SCHOOLBOY	42. YARDSTICK
10. FAREWELL	21. MISHAP	32. SOYBEAN	
11. FOOTSTOOL	22. MUSHROOM	33. STARLIGHT	

Figure 24. Spondee Word List.

PB-50 LIST 14

1. AT	11. DEAD	21. ISLE	31. PRUDE	41. STUFF
2. BARN	12. DOUSE	22. KICK	32. PURGE	42. TELL
3. BUST	13. DUNG	23. LATHE	33. QUACK	43. TENT
4. CAR	14. FIFE	24. LIFE	34. RID	44. THY
5. CLIP	15. FOAM	25. ME	35. SHOOK	45. TRAY
6. COAX	16. GRATE	26. MUSS	36. SHRUG	46. VAGUE
7. CURVE	17. GROUP	27. NEWS	37. SING	47. VOTE
8. CUTE	18. HEAT	28. NICK	38. SLAB	48. WAG
9. DARN	19. HOWL	29. NOD	39. SMITE	49. WAIF
10. DASH	20. HUNK	30. OFT	40. SOIL	50. WRIST

Figure 25. Phonetically balanced word list.

ject can repeat approximately 50 percent of this material correctly. This test, like other speech tests, must be performed with accurately calibrated equipment specifically constructed for speech hearing testing.

In order to determine the discrimination score, which is to a great extent the ability of the ear to discriminate consonants, lists of phonetically balanced (PB) words (one syllable) are used. These discrimination tests are made not at the level of the previously established speech reception threshold, since the ear does not function at threshold in everyday communication, but at about 30 or 40 dB above the speech reception threshold first established with the spondee words. The words are grouped into lists of fifty, with each list containing most of the representative speech sounds used in everyday speech. The entire list should be presented to each subject. Figure 25 shows examples of these lists.

The tester notes the percentage of words the subject can repeat correctly at the above-threshold level, and this percentage is known as the discrimination score. For example, if 40 words out of 50 are repeated correctly, the discrimination score is 80 percent.

The principal use of speech hearing tests is to determine the handicapping effect of a hearing loss, perhaps for compensation purposes, for making diagnostic decisions, or for the fitting of a hearing aid. These speech tests have no definite place as yet in industrial hearing testing unless the industry is research minded or can forsee the value of such studies.

What the Audiometer Measures

A basic question to be considered in hearing testing is—"What is being measured with the pure-tone audiometer?" It is essential for the tester to appreciate that commercial audiometers are so calibrated and recording methods so standardized that what he measures is not a person's hearing acumen but actually his hearing *loss* in the frequencies tested. The audiometer is calibrated so that "0" dB loss is about the average normal hearing of the general population in the healthy age group from 20 to 29 years. If a person hears at "0" dB, then he has no hearing loss. If he cannot hear until the tone is 30 dB greater than "0," he has a loss of 30 dB. This is recorded on the audiogram as a 30 dB loss in hearing, *not* as the amount of hearing a person has remaining.

Despite the negative aspect of this approach—in that it measures hearing loss rather than actual hearing present—the pure-tone test is the best means yet devised for securing information which is vital to an effective conservation-of-hearing program. But unless the tester can produce reliable and valid audiograms, the audiometry is meaningless and the effectiveness of the entire conservation-of-hearing program is reduced. A standard manner of performing individual pure-tone audiometry in industry has been approved which, if observed, will help insure the production of valid results.

Who Should Do Audiometric Testing

The compensation aspects of occupational deafness have added considerable importance to the need for validity and reliability of audiograms. It is no longer satisfactory, or even safe, particularly for industry, to purchase an audiometer and allow an individual to conduct hearing tests solely on the basis of information supplied by the instrument salesman or the instructions accompanying the instrument. It is the convinced opinion of most authorities in the field that if hearing tests are to be done in any industrial situation they should be done accurately or not at all.

Obtaining an accurate hearing threshold in all personnel appears disarmingly simple. In order to perform satisfactory audiometry, however, a tester must be thoroughly trained, appreciate the importance of his responsibility, and have pride in his work. Inadequacies in any of these factors frequently result in unsatisfactory hearing studies, which may prove to be more of a liability than an asset.

Experience has shown that in many instances testers without adequate training, even though they may have performed many hundreds of audiograms and may consider themselves authorities on audiometry, are in fact making serious mistakes they do not recognize and are producing hearing tests that are neither reliable nor valid. This has been dramatically borne out by the report of the Z-24 X2 Committee of the American Standards Association (now American National Standards Institute, ANSI) which gathered many thousands of audiograms performed in industry, but could use only a very small percentage of them because of the manner in which they were performed.

Nurses, hospital technicians, safety engineers and many other individuals available in industry can be trained to perform excellent audiometry. Since in most industries hearing testing will occupy only a part of a technician's time, it is wise to select either the industrial nurse, if her other duties will permit, or some other interested person in the plant who can be thoroughly indoctrinated in all phases of hearing testing.

This indoctrination should include academic background in hearing and practical training in audiometry under the critical supervision of trained industrial audiologists and otologists. The suggested training program covers 15 hours of didactic and practical experience. However, there should be critical routine evaluations of the tester for several months after the initial training.

In recognition of the need for a program on the conservation of hearing that will be practical and economically feasible for the managements of both large and small industries, a practical course has been outlined for the training of audiometric technicians in industry. This course is recommended for use in training technicians to: (1) perform pure-tone air-conduction audiograms in industry; (2) administer a hearing protection program under the direction of a physician; and (3) assist physicians in planning and carrying out a hearing-conservation program in industry. The course is approved by the following societies: The American Speech and Hearing Association, The American Industrial Hygiene Association, The American Association of Industrial Nurses and The Industrial Medical Association.

Recommendations

It is recommended that these courses be planned through centers of learning with speech and hearing clinics directed by otologists and audiologists with experience in hearing conservation programs in commerce and industry.

Enrollment should be limited to 24 persons, with one clinician to supervise each 6 trainees during practice. A refresher course for at least one day is recommended 6 months to a year from the date of the original course.

Any nurse or technician who will be responsible for taking the audiograms and fitting the protective devices should participate in the training program.

Guide to Program

A detailed guide is being prepared to help instructors cover the most important features of each topic they discuss. The following is an outline for such a training program.

Guide for Training of Audiometric Technicians in Industry

First Day

Topic I (1 hr.)
- A. Hearing conservation in industry—why?
  1. Importance of hearing
  2. Social aspects
  3. Economic aspects
- B. Objective of training program
  1. Valid audiograms
  2. Effective ear protection
  3. Medical follow-up
- C. The technician's responsibility and limitations in hearing conservation

Topic II (1 hr.)

A. Basic discussion of how the ear functions (anatomy and physiology)

B. Causes of hearing problems and interpretation of audio-grams

Topic III (1 hr.)

A. Physics of sound and its measurement

B. Practical demonstration of noise measurement with noise level meter and analyzer

Topic IV (1 hr.)

The audiometer—what it is and how it works; its calibration and care

Lunch

Topic V (3½ hrs.)

A. Instruction to the subject (1 hr.)

1. Record keeping

2. Pitfalls

B. Supervised audiograms (2½ hrs.)

Each student to perform audiograms on numerous people

Second Day

Topic VI (3 hrs.)

A. A review of audiograms performed and additional practice

1. Types of audiograms—their significance and interpreta-tion (30 min.)

2. Practice (2 hrs.)

B. Film "A Hearing Conservation Program in Industry" (30 min.)

Topic VII (1 hr.)

Medicolegal aspects

Lunch

Topic VIII (3½ hrs.)

Hearing protection and noise control

Question and answer and general review

Written examination

Continued practice in taking audiograms for those who need more confidence

Certificate of attendance

The principal purpose of this type of program is to train the tester to utilize the best available audiometric technique and to fully appreciate all the potential pitfalls of hearing testing. It is not the responsibility of the technician to interpret results, but to do his work in such a manner that his hearing tests are valid. Such training is available in several institutions throughout the country, or by private concerns.

Generally speaking, it is unwise to assign the task to someone who will not enjoy the work, because before long unsatisfactory results will demonstrate his lack of interest.

A responsible person should be assigned to perform hearing tests. It may develop that a future compensation claim, or an important legal complication will be primarily based on an audiogram performed by the tester. If the test was valid, the disposition will be equitable; but if the test was poorly done, there may be complications for the industry or institution involved.

Small industries in which noise is a problem may find it more convenient to use the services of a local otologist or audiologist to do the hearing testing, and an otologist to interpret the results. Every industry doing hearing testing should have available the services of a competent otologist trained in industrial problems, who is able to evaluate hearing studies and to guide the conservation-of-hearing program.

Training of industrial personnel performing puretone threshold audiograms is necessary if the audiogram record is to have medicolegal validity.

Self-Recording Audiometry

This method of establishing pure tone thresholds permits the patient to trace his own audiogram as the tone or tones are automatically presented to him. Each ear is tested separately. The patient holds a hand switch and has on a set of earphones through which he hears the tone. As soon as he hears the tone he presses the switch, which causes the sound to decrease in loudness, and holds it down until the tone is no longer audible. When the tone is no longer audible, the patient releases the switch. This allows the tone to increase in intensity until it can be detected again, at which time he again presses the switch and holds it until the tone is gone. This procedure continues until the full range of frequencies have been tested.

The switch controls the attenuator of the audiometer that decreases or increases the intensity of the tone. A pen geared to the attenuator makes a continuous record on an audiogram blank of the patient's intensity adjustments. The audiogram blank is placed on a table which moves in relation to the frequency being presented. It is most advantageous to include 8,000 Hz in all audiometry because of its importance in diagnosis.

With proper instruction to the patient, self-recording audiometry can provide an accurate picture of threshold and also supply other valuable information to localize the site of lesions within the auditory system. A test routinely performed with Bekesy (continuous frequency) self-recording audiometry determines threshold, using both the pulsed and continuous tone presentations. If the pulsed tone is used first, a pen with a specific colored ink is placed in the pen holder and the thresholds are recorded. When the pulsed tone testing is completed, the pen is changed for one having a different color, the frequency is reset to the original point, and the switching is changed to provide a continuous tone. The patient then traces another audiogram, as he did for the pulsed tones. It is important that the patient not be able to see the equipment in operation, because the movements of the pen and operation of the hand switch may be mutually influencing and result in an invalid audiogram. By comparing the thresholds for the pulsed and continuous tones, the otologist is able to get a reasonably good indication of the site of the lesion, or at least additional information that would help in this determination.

There is some sentiment that hearing thresholds obtained with self-recording audiometers are legally acceptable even if the operator is not well-trained, because the operator cannot influence the data. This does not mean, however, that malingering does not occur and that a self-recorded audiogram is to be taken as valid and reliable. On the contrary, experience has shown that such audiograms can motivate more malingering than is possible when a tester is performing the audiogram manually.

A trained and experienced technician can generally recognize an unreliable self-recorded audiogram. Here again, certain clues may alert the operator: (1) Barring a language problem, an employee may refuse to follow the directions of the operator, or claim he doesn't understand the instructions as to his role in performing the hearing test. Repeated attempts to instruct the subject do not result in improved operation. (2) On repeat tests the employee may be unable to give reasonably similar responses, and this will result in a wide disparity between threshold tracings. (3) A malingerer may not respond at all to the tones, as though he were totally deaf, yet be able to carry on a normal conversation with the examiner. (4) Another indication of questionable responses is extremely wide tracings sweeps on the self-recorded audiogram, which makes it impossible to ascertain actual threshold. (5) Occasionally, an employee may show a moderate to severe, mostly flat loss which would ordinarily cause little doubt as to its reliability in the mind of the operator except for the fact that such a pattern is uncommon and should raise the suspicion that perhaps the subject was pressing and releasing his hand switch in a perfectly timed sequence. (6) In self-recording audiometry, it is possible to feign normal hearing by keeping the button depressed during the entire test sequence. If the operator has difficulty communicating with the subject (again barring a language problem) and yet his audiogram indicates extremely keen hearing, there is reason to doubt the accuracy of the audiogram.

More and more we are encountering a relatively high incidence of malingering (20-25%) in certain areas of industry, already restive, with compensation claims for industrial hearing loss. Malingering is seldom among salaried personnel.

The type of testing equipment used does not obviate the need for training the audiometric technician. There are other aspects to the hearing-conservation program with which the technician must have a working knowledge.

What Is an Audiogram?

An audiogram is a written record of an individual's threshold of hearing at certain specified frequencies. This record may be in graph form (Fig. 21 on page 73) or in block form, using numbers for the hearing loss at each frequency (Fig. 26). The audiogram obtained from most self recording audiograms is shown in Figure 27. The frequencies usually tested and recorded in industrial hearing testing are those at 500, 1,000, 2,000, 3,000, 4,000, 6,000, and 8,000 Hz. This overall range is used because it encompasses the frequencies important for understanding speech. The frequency of 250 Hz appears on many commercial audiogram forms, but for industrial testing the meager information derived from testing this frequency does not warrant its routine use. It is unfortunate that 8,000 Hz is frequently omitted in industrial hearing testing, the feeling being that thresholds at this frequency are not consistently reliable. Inclusion of 8,000 Hz is important in making a diagnostic decision from the general trend or slope of the threshold curve. Although some audiometers do not provide facilities to test the half octave frequencies of 3,000 and 6,000 cycles, these frequencies are important for early detection of industrial deafness and should be tested and recorded whenever possible.

The audiogram is a most important document and may acquire legal significance. Consequently, it should always be retained in its original form even if copies are made. Erasures should never be made on an audiogram. Errors

	250	500	1000	2000	3000	4000	6000	8000
LEFT EAR AIR CONDUCTION	5 / 5	0 / 0	0 / 0	0 / 0	30 / 25	45 / 45	20 / 20	0 / 0
RIGHT EAR AIR CONDUCTION	5 / 10	10 / 10	0 / 0	25 / 35	25 / 35	65 / 65	40 / 35	15 / 10

NAME _____ DATE _____ TESTER _____

Figure 26. Block and serial form of audiogram recording. Each independent threshold can be recorded at each frequency.

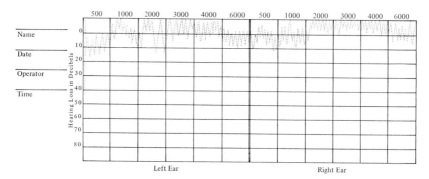

Figure 27. Discrete frequency self-recording audiometric threshold.

of the recorder, such as may be made by recording the threshold at 50 instead of at 60 dB should have a single line drawn through the incorrect figure and the correction should be initialed. If the threshold is once recorded and a recheck shows a variation at the same frequency, both thresholds obtained should be recorded, and the initial one should not be deleted. Obviously, after the initial examination, subsequent tests are recorded separately, regardless of differences from the original.

The audiogram always requires interpretation, and for this reason it should be shown to the subject with caution. Improper explanation or comment about an audiogram may sometimes cause unwarranted concern.

It is essential that each audiogram be properly dated, and the name of the tester and that of the subject be recorded. These records should be carefully kept by the medical department. In fact, hearing testing records should never be destroyed.

What Is Threshold?

The principle object of audiometry is to determine the weakest tone at certain frequencies which the subject can just detect by hearing. This weakest tone, or just audible sound, is called the threshold of hearing for that particular tone. Anyone who has had an audiometric hearing test, and this of course included all testers, will appreciate the difficulties of being certain that he does or does not hear all of the tones around the threshold. When the intensity of a tone gets low enough, the subject may hear the same intensity sometimes and not hear it at other times. The least intensity to which the subject responds 50 percent of the times it is presented is considered the threshold for that particular tone. For example, if the subject indicates 50 percent of the time that he hears at 20 dB, but not at 15 dB, the threshold is 20 dB. This distinction is not always so clear-cut, and often the subject will vary in his response to tones of the same intensity at around threshold. In such instances, record the weakest tone which is heard at least two out of three trials, not the sound to which he just fails to respond, as some testers are inclined to believe.

The precision with which an exact threshold of hearing can be obtained is influenced by many factors. Foremost is the fact that most pure-tone audiometers are calibrated in five-dB steps, so that a threshold may normally vary five decibles on either side of the level at which the subject responded. Threshold is often not a fine exact point, but rather a zone extending over a range of 10 dB, and even though the finest audiometric technique possible is used, a variation of plus or minus 5 dB around threshold can normally be expected.

Since determination of the hearing threshold is established by a subjective response from the subject, his cooperation and the method in which the tone is presented may influence the threshold values. Other influencing factors are the duration of the tone, the noise level in the testing room, the type of tone used (whether continuous or interrupted), and any pathological condition present in the subject's ear.

Despite all the variables that influence audiograms, it is possible and necessary for a threshold to be accurate and consistent to within approximately 5 dB, for reliable and valid audiometry. By reliable audiometry we mean that on repeated examination of a subject's hearing, using the same standard technique, the findings should be consistent with one another within this normally expected variation. If the results deviate more than five dB, further investigation is indicated for that particular subject. The causes for such inconsistency and variation are discussed in chapter 8.

By valid audiometry we mean that the hearing threshold obtained should be a measure of the subject's organic hearing acuity, and not merely a measure of the response mechanism. For example, a trained malingerer or a subject with hysterical deafness can repeatedly give the same audiometric findings irrespective of how many audiograms are done. The resulting audiogram is not really a valid one, however, because it is not an accurate measure of the subject's real hearing. Rather, it is a measure of the subject's responses. In industrial testing, audiograms must be reliable and valid.

The concept of threshold is a range derived on a statistical basis, rather than a fine exact point for which the subject strives by repeated testing around threshold level. Such persistent efforts are apt to have an exhausting effect on the subject, and do not conform with the best practice in industrial hearing testing.

The Initial Audiogram

The pre-employment hearing test is of primary importance, because it establishes the employee's hearing status prior to exposure to any noise produced in his new job. It also serves as a reference level with which to compare any changes in hearing that may occur in the future, and helps to establish the cause for such changes. It has been estimated that over 20 percent of applicants for jobs in noisy industry have some hearing loss.

The importance of securing an accurate initial threshold is demonstrated by our experience in several industrial plants. Hearing testing in these plants was previously done by a technician inadequately trained and unfamiliar with the pitfalls of industrial audiometry. On going over the records we found a significant number of employees with pre-employment normal audiograms, when in reality all of these employees had hearing losses of long duration completely unrelated to their present employment.

The inaccuracy of the initial audiogram was confirmed by the employees themselves, who admitted having long-standing hearing losses prior to employment and deliberately giving false responses to the previous tester. Some of the employees felt they would not be hired if their hearing was found to be defective, and by carefully watching the tester's technique they had devised methods by which they could falsely report normal hearing.

Instances are certain to arise in some industries when so many employees are hired in one day that it proves impossible to test all of them prior to their reporting for work. For this and other reasons, occasionally it may be advisable to perform pre-placement audiometry rather than pre-employment audiometry. This means that initial testing is performed only on employees when they are assigned to a job that has been classified as potentially hazardous to hearing.

The importance of the initial, pre-employment, or pre-placement audiogram as a legal document deserves special emphasis. Decisions of considerable importance may depend upon its validity. A single threshold determination is insufficient to establish an individual's reference hearing level. At least two, and possibly three, independent thresholds consistent with one another are necessary to establish a base line with which future comparisons can be made justifiably. These can be made independently at varying intervals. If there is any doubt about the consistency of any threshold, the subject should be asked to return for further examination. The audiogram with all pertinent information should be turned over to the plant physician or otologist for an evaluation prior if possible, to the subject's exposure to any intense industrial noise.

Instructions to Subject Prior to Audiometry

The instructions given each subject prior to audiometry must be concise, clear, and complete. The subject who has had previous audiometry will, of course, require little or no instructions. However, he should be reminded of the manner in which he is to respond to the tones.

The manner in which they are given will to a great degree determine the extent of the subject's cooperation and the efficiency with which the test can be performed. In the few minutes prior to adjusting the earphones, the tester must establish a pleasant rapport with the subject so he will be cooperative during the testing period. The instructions must be presented pleasantly and in a positive, definitive manner; they must also obviate any questions later arising in the mind of the subject, as questions are generally unnecessary and very time consuming.

The experience and personality of the tester are very influential in conducting the audiometric test. A successful opening approach is to ask:

"Have you ever had your hearing checked before?" Even if the answer is "yes," you will proceed with your instructions, as follows:

"Well, that is fine, but let me remind you of what you are to do. You will be listening for some tones. Each time you hear a tone, raise your finger (demonstrate). As soon as the tone stops, lower your finger (demonstrate). No matter how faint the sound, raise your finger when you hear it (demonstrate), and lower it when the tone stops (demonstrate).
Further:

"Can you hear better with one ear than the other?" If the subject specifies one ear as better, test the better ear first; otherwise, always start with the right ear, *advising the subject which ear is first being tested.*

As soon as this type of concise and clear instruction is completed, the tester should place the earphones over the subject's ears and start the test immediately. An opportunity to ask questions at this time should be avoided unless the subject seems very perplexed.

In some instances when large groups of subjects are to be tested, it may be possible to give verbal instructions to the entire group and demonstrate the method of response with a model subject. Under such circumstances each subject should require only a brief reminder prior to testing. Such instructions to a group are not often possible in industry, and generally individual instructions must be given to each new subject. Some testers use written instructions which they distribute to each individual just prior to his being tested. Although this may need to be done, it is not as satisfactory because in most cases it needs to be supplemented by additional verbal instructions. One of its disadvantages is that it prevents the tester from establishing as satisfactory a personal relationship with the subject as he can by oral presentation.

An important objective to the tester is to make the subject feel that the hearing test is being done for the subject's advantage. This need not be orally explained to each subject, but if the true purpose of audiometry is described to several of the subjects, it is generally promulgated throughout the industry, and the degree of cooperation and interest in the conservation of hearing program will be greatly enhanced.

How to Perform a Routine Audiogram

Before beginning the actual audiogram, it is necessary for the tester to give thorough consideration to the following preliminary steps to be certain that his audiogram will be valid.

Testing the Earphones

Prior to beginning a series of tests and at routine intervals the tester should place the earphones over his own ears, to be certain they are in proper working order. He should quickly determine if the thresholds are within reasonable calibration, as well as if the earphones are in their proper jacks. One phone is colored RED and the other BLUE to correspond with the control switch on the panel of the audiometer. The tester should try a tone in each ear to be certain that the phones correspond with the switch position.

In addition to checking the tones at generally normal threshold levels, the tester should try the loud tones as well and carefully note if the interrupter switch makes a clicking noise when it is depressed, since on occasion subjects will respond to such a click instead of to the pure tone. A clicking noise should not be present in a properly functioning instrument.

At all times the phones should be treated with care, and precautions taken that they not be dropped. It is important that the soft cushion around the phones be kept clean. This is particularly important when industrial personnel are being tested whose heads or ears are apt to be covered with debris (such as moisture, dust, etc.) from their occupation. Under such conditions the phones must be carefully cleaned after each subject is tested. Should a subject's ear be infected, it is also important to clean the cushion carefully after the testing. The intrusion of water or dirt into the diaphragm of the earphones must be meticulously avoided.

Checking the Audiometer

A routine check of the audiometer controls prior to placing the earphones upon the subject will considerably improve the efficiency of the tester in performing repeated audiograms. One of the more frequent errors which can thus be avoided is the possible production (with the attenuator inadvertently left at 100 dB) of unexpected very loud tone directly in the subject's ear, a situation which often results not only in ear discomfort for the subject but possibly in the creation of hostility by the subject for the tester.

A routine check of all the panel controls can be made in a very short time. The tester should be certain that:

1. The frequency selector is placed at the first tone to be tested.
2. The attenuator is turned down to 0 dB.
3. The audiometer is given time to warm up.
4. The earphone plugs are tightly inserted into their jacks.
5. The microphone switch, if one is present, is turned off.
6. The interrupter switch is adjusted so that a tone is produced only when the interrupter switch is pressed down.

In reference to item 6, it might again be noted that some audiometers are equipped with interrupter switches which work in an opposite pattern, so that pressing down the interrupter switch shuts off an otherwise constant tone produced by the audiometer. This type of audiometer is generally unsatisfactory for industrial testing. Most new audiometers have both systems available, and it is recommended that the audiometer be one which produced no constant tone and on which the tone is off except when the tester presses down the interrupter switch.

If the audiometer has a switch for converting to bone conduction, this switch should also be turned off. If a masking device is present, this too should be turned off.

Instructing the Subject

After the subject is seated in the booth the tester should make certain the subject has a clear and complete understanding of what his role is to be in performing the audiogram, with special emphasis on the manner by which the subject is to indicate he hears a tone.

If the subject has not previously been tested, it is advisable to let him hear a sample tone, such as the 1,000 cycle tone set at about 80 decibels, if necessary, in order to acquaint him with the general nature of the test tone. The tester should be cautious so that the sample tone is not so loud as to startle the subject or to produce a temporary auditory fatigue, which may occur in some ears following exposure to a loud tone.

The subject should be reminded to raise his finger when he hears the tone and to hold the finger up as long as the tone persists. When the tone stops, he should lower his finger immediately.

It is advisable for the tester to develop for himself a pattern of testing in which he consistently tests the same ear first during each test. The right ear is usually tested first because it is generally more natural for the subject to respond with the right hand. It is not uncommon to encounter subjects who indicate their responses with the right hand to tones in the right ear and with their left hand to tones in the left ear. It is often helpful in testing difficult cases for the tester to deliberately use such a method.

Placing the Earphones

The padded earphones act as ear protectors and block out some of the ambient noise in the booth and prevent distraction. The spring head band, holding the earphones, provides a uniform pressure on the ears. Care must be taken not to overstretch the spring in the head band, since this will alter the pressure with which the phones hug the ears.

It is most important that the earphones be snugly placed on the subject's ears so that no leakage exists between the phones and the side of the head and that the head band is adjusted to head size so that the phones are comfortable. The tester should ask that women subjects remove earrings and push back their hair from over the ears. Horned rimmed glasses, hearing aids, cotton, etc. should also be removed in all instances, since they prevent a snug fit of the receiver or can block out the test tones. The auricle of the ear should not be bent over by the phone, and the center of the phone should be directly aligned with the opening to the ear canal.

Care should be taken that the cord leading from the earphones is not draped over the front of the subject and thereby apt to be rubbed by movements of the subject, since this will introduce distracting noises.

When the tester places the earphones, he must be certain that the red phone is placed on the right ear and not on the left ear.

The earphones should be placed upon the subject until directions have been given to the subject and the tester is ready to proceed with the actual performance of the audiogram.

The Audiogram

The tester is to determine the subject's threshold at the specified frequencies in the following order: 1,000, 2,000, 3,000, 4,000, 6,000, 8,000, 1,000 (repeat) and 500 Hz. The 1,000 cycle tone is tested first because this is usually the easiest one for which to establish a definitive threshold. It is confirmed by repeating it, as the subject who has not previously had an audiogram may not have recognized it the first time at the lower levels. Both readings are recorded on the form. In industrial programs there will be more losses encountered at 2,000 Hz than at 1,000 Hz, and it is therefore advisable to begin the testing at 1,000 Hz.

With the subject seated in the booth in a position so subject and tester do not face each other, instructions given, and the audiometer and earphones carefully checked, the tester is ready to begin the actual testing.

With the earphone selector switch properly set, and the frequency dial at 1,000 Hz, turn on the tone and roll the hearing level dial slowly upward from 0 dB until the subject responds. Release the tone allowing the subject to lower his finger. Present the tone once again at this level to confirm the response. If he does respond, turn off the tone, and *decrease* the intensity by *10 dB.* Present the tone. Generally there should be no response to this 10 dB reduction in intensity. If no response, turn off the tone, *increase* intensity 5 dB and then present the tone. If there is a response to this 5 dB increase, turn off the tone and decrease by 5 dB. Present the tone. If no response, turn the tone off, *increase* by 5 dB, present the tone. If there is a response, this is threshold and record that number of last response. The objective is to get at least two "no," and two "yes" responses. For example: "yes," "no," "yes," "no," "yes," or "no," "yes," "no," "yes." Always have a "no" between each "yes" response. Always end on a "yes" response.

Most young subjects will have extremely good hearing and will respond to the tone while the hearing dial is still at 0 dB. It is good practice to obtain at least two or three responses in unison with presentation of the tones at these low levels.

If during the initial bracketing of threshold, there is confirmation of the first response, continue to roll the hearing dial up until there is a response and a confirmation. Then make the 10 dB reduction and proceed from that point.

A "yes" response requires the tone to be made softer until a "no" response is obtained. A "no" response requires the tone to be made louder until a "yes" response is obtained. This tracking up and down around threshold results in the pattern of responses described previously.

All tones which the tester presents to the subject should be brief bursts of sound and held for no longer than one second. At this point in the testing it is also wise for the tester to check to be certain that he is properly recording the threshold for the ear being tested and not for the opposite ear.

Avoid a rhythmical presentation of the tones either in space of interval or in intensity. There is, for instance a tendency on the part of some testers to make intensity changes and presentations of the tone at regular and therefore expected intervals. This regular presentation should be avoided, as it is an excellent means of producing an inaccurate threshold in routine industrial testing. Also the subject may continue to respond rhythmically with his finger long after the tone has ceased to be presented to the ear. This is particularly common in situations where many subjects are to be tested daily by a tester who is unfamiliar with the importance of his responsibility. It is essential to keep the time and intensity intervals between tones constantly varying.

When the threshold for the 1,000 Hz tone has been determined and recorded for one ear, the frequency selector is moved to 2,000 Hz and the threshold for the same ear at this frequency then determined in the manner outlined heretofore. This procedure is repeated for the frequencies of 3,000, 4,000, 6,000, and 8,000 cycles and the thresholds recorded. Following this, the threshold is again checked for the original 1,000 Hz tone. After this recheck of 1,000 Hz test 500 Hz.

When the tester has completed the recording of thresholds for one ear, the test tone is then switched to the opposite ear and the identical procedure repeated, starting with 1,000 Hz, and working upward as was done on the other ear, then do 500 Hz. It is also advisable to recheck the thresholds for those frequencies indicating a loss greater than 20 decibels. While this recheck is essential in pre-employment or pre-placement, it is also recommended for routine follow-up audiometry. The tester should always record on the audiogram all thresholds independently obtained.

When the thresholds for all frequencies have been properly determined and recorded for both ears, the routine audiogram is complete.

Explaining the Audiogram

Anyone showing a substantial change in hearing since his last audiogram should be given a repeat audiogram or called back on a different day. A good practice is to recheck the thresholds for all frequencies where the loss has become greater by 15 or more dB. If the repeat audiogram is consistent, referral to the plant physician is in order.

If a subject shows a consistent loss in only one ear of approximately 40 dB or more at all frequencies, this may be what is termed *"A Shadow Curve."* He may be totally deaf in this one ear and actually be responding when he hears the tones in the better ear. These cases require masking in the better ear to get an accurate audiogram. They should be referred to an otologist.

Interpret the audiogram findings to the subject cautiously in accord with the company's policy. Explain that the 500, 1,000, and 2,000 Hz are frequencies of the speech range and that any level of 25 dB (ISO) or less is considered within normal range. If the subject has a substantial hearing loss, explain that this could be for many reasons—heredity, infections, injury, age and so on—further evaluation by a physician will discuss these findings with him.

To a great extent the acceptance of the hearing conservation program will depend upon the skill of the examiner in her explanation of the audiogram to the subject. She should be positive in her approach, willing and competent to answer questions intelligently and clear up misconceptions which may exist.

Recording the Audiogram

A number of methods of recording the results of air conduction audiometry are in use at the present time. One method is to record the threshold at each frequency on a graph, such as supplied by manufacturers of audiometers, see Figure 21. Such a graph shows a curve of the individual's threshold. It is customary to record threshold for the right ear with a circle, and to use a red pencil to connect the circles with a continuous line. The results for the left ear are recorded with "X's" using a blue pencil and connecting them with a broken line. The different color for each ear is not essential but helps to distinguish more readily the thresholds of one ear from the other. If no threshold is obtainable at a certain frequency because the audiometer cannot be made loud enough for the subject to respond, this should be recorded by an arrow pointing downward signifying "out," using red for the right ear and blue for the left. At the bottom of each graph, a legend indicating that "O" refers to the right ear and "X" to the left should be included.

This type of graph is not satisfactory for industry. One of its chief disadvantages is the fact that should eight or ten audiograms be made during his years of employment, the subject's record becomes bulky and it is then difficult to compare one curve with another performed at a different date.

Another manner of recording audiograms, and one which obviates the use of an individual graph, is a serial audiogram sheet for each individual. A sample is shown in Figure 26. Here, instead of using one symbol for the right ear and another for the left, the number of decibels designating the threshold is recorded at each frequency. Each new audiogram is recorded below the previous one, so a series of tests taken over a period of months or even years can be compared at a glance. Also, a place for comments and a brief history should be available on this form of serial audiogram.

The use of serial audiograms further makes it easier to include several features, one of the most important being to record independently all thresholds obtained. For example, the hearing test is started at 1,000 Hz, a threshold is obtained, and after 8,000 Hz is tested another threshold is obtained at 1,000 Hz. Both these thresholds, even if alike, should be recorded one above the other in the space provided for the threshold at 1,000 Hz. In legal situations, this will confirm that the threshold was rechecked several times. It is important to record *every* threshold that is independently derived, even if there is considerable variation, for this may have considerable significance. It is important that every serial audiogram include the date and the signature of the tester, the serial number and calibration standard of the audiometer, as well as other information that may be placed under "comments." Industries actively concerned with a conservation of hearing program should carefully consider using this manner of recording.

Since there is always a possibility that the tester, in an attempt to complete the test quickly, may be influenced by a previously obtained threshold, it is advisable for the tester not to have before him the previous audiogram on the serial chart. For this reason it is helpful to have an assistant record, while the tester specifies the threshold obtained at each frequency. If a tester cannot obtain a satisfactory assistant for this purpose, he should place a card over all previously obtained readings so that previous results do not influence him in any way. A special mask which allows only the blank spaces on the audiogram to be seen can also be prepared. This type of self-restriction will insure to the tester's satisfaction that he is performing as objective a test as possible.

Review of Common Errors in Audiometry

Despite careful training in audiometry, hearing testers should routinely evaluate their technique with critical detachment. To aid the tester in this self-criticism, presented here is a check list of the most common errors and pitfalls the author has encountered among testers:

1. Taking too long to do an audiogram will fatigue the subject and result in inaccurate response. Adjustments from one frequency to another and from one intensity to another should be made quickly, and the entire audiogram should be performed as rapidly as possible without sacrificing the validity of the threshold.

2. Rushing through the test so rapidly that accurate thresholds are not obtained must be equally guarded against. The tester should appreciate that some subjects take longer than others to respond. Sufficient time must be given to each subject to respond to the stimulus. Faster and more definitive responses can be obtained if the directions are concise and explicit, prior to testing.

3. Allowing the subject to sit so that he can watch the control panel of the audiometer or motions of the tester may result in inaccurate responses. This also enhances the possibilities of malingering.

4. Placing the wrong receiver on the ear and recording the threshold for the wrong ear is another common error to be avoided. Repeated checks should be made to see that the phones are correctly placed and that they correspond with the switch on the control panel.

5. Presenting the signal and then looking up at the subject as if to ask whether he has heard the tone should be avoided. This is poor audiometric technique, and frequently the subject will respond even though he does not hear the tone.

6. Making intensity readings in less than the 5-dB steps, in which most audiometer attenuators are calibrated is incorrect and most likely will result in inaccurate thresholds. Readings should always be made on the intensity dial in multiples of 5 dB.

7. Presenting the sound signal for a long period of time, particularly if it is loud, may produce temporary fatigue and result in an inaccurate threshold. The tone should be produced in short bursts, and each tone should be presented for about the same length of time, such as $1/2$ to $3/4$ sec.

8. Taking too long to determine whether the threshold is at 0, –5, or –10 dB is unjustified in a conservation-of-hearing program. The significance of such a determination, as compared with other fac-

tors, does not warrant the time it consumes. A 5-dB threshold on either side is often an expected variation and does not indicate an uncooperative patient or a defective instrument. Occasionally, accurate threshold readings at the 8,000 Hz tone may be very difficult to obtain. Often, such difficulty is caused by the short wave length at this high frequency and the possible presence of standing waves. As a result, the threshold may fluctuate widely, particularly if the subject presses the earphone closer to his ears so that he can hear it better.

9. Failing to recheck the first signal presented at 1,000 Hz may often result in an inaccurate reading of this tone. The tester should always return to the initial 1,000 Hz tone for a recheck of the threshold.

10. During the testing of many subjects, if significant hearing losses are repeatedly found in the same frequencies on consecutive subjects, it is wise for the tester to recheck the earphones on himself to ascertain whether anything has gone wrong during the testing procedures.

11. If a subject shows a hearing loss, particularly in the low frequencies, and his threshold values fluctuate widely (such as 15, 20, or even 25 dB), the tester should have the ears of the subject examined to be sure that no impacted cerumen or other pathology is present. He should then suspect the presence of malingering, functional deafness, poor cooperation, or misunderstanding on the subject's part. The tester should note and record the widely fluctuating threshold levels reported by the subject, for they may have important significance to the otologist who interprets the audiogram.

12. It is necessary to avoid a rhythmic presentation of the signal, either in intensity or in time intervals.

13. If, during the testing of a subject or a number of subjects, the ambient noise level in a room increases so that it interferes with the threshold obtained, the tester should note this on the audiogram to show that the test was made under adverse condition.

14. Some subjects will complain, particularly after listening to very loud tones, that the tones continue to linger even after the signal itself has stopped. This so-called aftertone occurs occasionally in certain ears and must be taken into consideration. More time and more careful determination of threshold is indicated in such subjects.

15. Occasionally, a subject will be encountered who has tinnitus. Such a subject may state that his head noise interferes with accurate determination of his threshold at certain frequencies. If a threshold

cannot be determined in a routine manner to the tester's satisfaction, several other methods are available. One of these is to use several short, interrupted bursts of tone—say, two or three times instead of the single tone generally presented in the routine audiogram. Sometimes this will enable a subject to respond more accurately. A note should be made on such a subject's record on this change in technique and of the fact that the subject complains of tinnitus.

16. Occasionally, a subject will be encountered whose responses are so varied that an accurate threshold is not obtainable at that particular time. Rather than delay the entire testing schedule of the many other subjects who are waiting to be tested, it is wiser to recall this subject at a time when he can receive more individual attention. It is unsatisfactory for a tester to report a vague, general threshold on such a subject when accurate responses are not attainable. Such responses may be an indication of functional hearing loss, malingering, or some organic condition which requires further study.

17. In recording hearing losses at the frequencies of 250 Hz and 8,000 Hz, the tester should be careful not to record higher levels than the maximum output of the audiometer. The tester should be familiar with the limitations of his audiometer.

18. When depressing the interrupter switch, the tester must be particularly careful not to press this switch down so hard or let it spring back so quickly that it makes a clicking sound which might result in a subject's responding to the click rather than to the pure tone presented.

19. Neither the tester nor the subject should do any unnecessary talking during the test procedure, as this disturbs the subject's concentration. If instructions are properly given before the test, rarely should an occasion arise when a discussion is necessary during the test procedure.

20. Whenever possible, and particularly during the preplacement or preemployment audiograms, every threshold at each frequency should be rechecked two or three times independently. If a hearing loss is present, particularly at the frequencies of 1,000 or higher, each threshold should be rechecked after the entire audiogram is completed.

21. The tester should always keep foremost in mind that the results he is recording on the audiogram are of important medical significance, and that he will have to assume responsibility for their validity and reliability. No audiometric technician or tester should be satisfied with only fair results. Every audiogram should be

performed in the best possible manner, using the most reliable audiometric technique.

Tester's Work Records

In addition to recording the previous information on the individual audiogram charts, the tester should keep his own record of calibration checks. This can be kept on a large card available every time audiometry is performed. The information to be recorded should include the following:

1. The time of the day at which the audiometer was checked for calibration and on how many normal or other ears it was checked. Record the serial number of the audiometer for each of these biological calibration checks. Serial numbers of temporary replacement equipment should also be recorded.

2. Any marked changes in the ambient noise level during the daily testing procedure should be recorded. Hopefully, a very careful survey of all possible test sites will have resulted in selecting an area not subject to intrusion of plant or other noise sources into the test area.

3. If the audiometer seemed to go out of calibration but the tester continued to use it, a record of this should be made along with any correction factor which the tester has determined necessary to compensate for the improper calibration of the audiometer. For example, if one earphone becomes faulty during the testing and the test is completed with a single earphone by switching it from one ear to the other, this should be noted on the tester's work sheet.

4. When an audiometer is returned from the factory after being calibrated, the date should be recorded on the tester's record, with a note that he checked the accuracy of the calibration on several normal ears. A certificate of factory or shop calibration should also be obtained and kept with the daily biological calibration sheets.

5. If, on certain test days, the regular audiometer was away for repairs and another instrument was used, a note to this effect should be made on the tester's record, again recording the serial number of the replacement.

The tester should appreciate that each threshold or comment recorded may at any time be introduced as legal evidence in a medical-legal situation. Checking the calibration of the audiometer, and the method whereby this is done is of utmost importance on this work record sheet.

Figure 28 gives an example of a work record kept by a tester during an actual hearing testing program in one industrial plant.

Additional Information on Audiogram Record

On every audiogram record there should be a space in which to record comments and information which will enhance the reliability of the audiogram for legal purposes.

The comments should be concise, and the information should include at least the following:

TESTERS WORK RECORD

Biological Calibration
Instrument #

Date	
3/ 2/73	
3/ 5/73	✓
3/ 6/73	✓
3/ 7/73	✓
3/ 8/73	*
3/ 9/73	✓
3/15/73	✓
3/16/73	✓

Electronic Calibration

Date	2/10/73
By whom	Electronic Associates
Type of calibration	
Certificate of calibration	Received and checked
Reason for recalibration	
Annual or other	
Earphones replaced	
Audiometer failure	

*3/8/73 Right earphone broken. Audiometer sent for repair and calibration. Replacement of audiometer #1234 used and calibration tested.

Routine Listening Checks

No noise in phone	
No cross talk	
Earphone cords O. K.	
Jacks seated	
Jack panel O. K.	
Dials not loose	
Tones are clear	
Volume increases O. K.	
Tone presenter quiet	

Audiometric Test Room

Date   3/8/73 Noise analysis done
Reason   Low frequencies not accurate audiometer earphones broken.
Room noise levels meet ANSI requirements

OTHER COMMENTS

3/2/73 Excessive ambient noise in test room due to operation of new machine in next room for one day. Audiograms show a 10 dB additional loss at 500 Hz; correction made.

Figure 28. Work Record.

1. The amount of time which elapsed between the employee's leaving his noisy job and reporting for his hearing test. This information is necessary to evaluate the role of temporary threshold shift (auditory fatigue).

2. The presence of a head cold, allergy attack, ear infection, or head noise at the time the test is performed.

3. The date when the subject left a noisy job or assumed a different noisy job since the last audiogram.

4. The hearing tester should comment upon adverse conditions that may have occurred during the specific test; for example, some employees refuse to permit closing of the test booth door due to claustrophobia.

5. A comment should also be made if the subject claims to be using ear protectors. Experience has shown that information supplied by the subject in this regard is often unreliable, and a personal check during actual working conditions is advisable.

6. Other comments may include such items as exposure to gunfire during hunting, rifle practice, recent episode of fullness in the ears re-

(Use Ink Only)

FULL NAME _____ BIRTH DATE _____ S. S. # _____
LAST   FIRST   MIDDLE

SERVICE DATE _____ DEPT. _____ SHIFT _____

DATE	RIGHT EAR								LEFT EAR								SERIAL NUMBER STANDARD	JOB TITLE	Years On Present Job	NOISE LEVEL		Exposure Lapse	Protection Used	TESTER (Sign Here)	COMMENTS
	500	1000	2000	3000	4000	6000	8000		500	1000	2000	3000	4000	6000	8000					dBA	Hrs. Per Day				

HISTORY: Anyone in your Family have hearing loss? _____ Is your hearing—Good? _____ Fair? _____ Poor? _____
Ever had previous measurement? _____ Where? _____ Been in military service? _____
Exposed to any gunfire or loud noises? _____ Ever had infections (running ear)? _____
Ever had surgery on either ear? _____ Explain _____
What antibiotics or other drugs have you taken? _____ What contagious diseases have you had? _____
Ever worked at a very noisy job? _____ If yes, where, type job, length of time _____
Ever had dizziness? _____ What type, when does it occur? _____
Have you ever had noises in your ears? _____ What does it sound like? _____
Do you have any noisy hobbies? _____ Do you have a second job? _____

DATE	Comments following periodic or special audiograms (use reverse side for any comments, if necessary)

Figure 29. Serial audiogram devised by Hearing Conservation Noise Control, Inc. with information required to accompany initial hearing test.

sulting from an airplane trip (aero-otitis media) attacks of vertigo, recent illnesses, medications taken, and the like.

Figure 29 shows one manner of recording this information. Another method is to simply leave a blank space in which the tester may write his own comments. If individual audiograms are used, the information may be recorded on the reverse side or on an attached card.

Every time an audiogram is performed, this information should be recorded by the tester, and the comments should be dated to correspond with the audiogram on that specific day. This information is in addition to that already obtained during the medical examination.

Ear Examination and Histories

Ear examinations and detailed histories of ear trouble and previous noise exposure should be obtained on all personnel exposed to noisy jobs which have been classified as hazardous to hearing on the basis of physical noise measurements. These examinations should be done not only on new applicants for employment, but also on personnel already employed and on those to be transferred to noisy jobs.

The ear examinations can be made by the industrial physician, a local physician, or specially trained nurse who can also report on the otoscopic findings. Chart I provides the examining physician with a guide of the more important information to be obtained in a routine ear examination. Since this examination will probably precede any hearing testing on new applicants, the physician should take necessary steps to be sure the ensuing hearing tests will be reliable. Impacted cerumen should be removed, and if ear infection is present the hearing testing should be delayed or performed with full understanding of its limitations. Each industry should supply its own ear examination forms, not only for the convenience of the examining physician, but also in order to standardize the examinations. If the industry already has a general medical form, it may include the ear examination on it. It is preferable, however, to have a separate form so that all

the information needed for a hearing evaluation may be kept together.

Ear Examination

NAME   AGE

1. Describe any congenital or acquired ear malformations. (Atresias,
   Exostoses, Mastoidectomy Scars, or other Operative Procedures).

2. Cerumen Impacted (this should be removed by the physician).

3. Describe the presence of any external otitis or stenosis.

4. Describe abnormalities in Tympanic Membrane (Check Appropriately).

                                             Right   Left
           Normal
   (a) Thickened and Opaque
   (b) Retracted
   (c) Scarred
   (d) Calcareous deposit
   (e) Perforation present
   (f) Active infection
   (g) Other findings

5. Middle ear damage visible—Describe

Chart I

In performing the ear examination, the examiner recognizes
that the appearance of the eardrum can sometimes provide valuable information. He should appreciate, however, that it is possible to have practically normal hearing despite the presence of
marked pathology in the eardrum, including a large perforation.
Conversely, a marked conductive hearing loss due to ossicular
chain pathology may be present with little or no visible abnormality in the eardrum. For these and other reasons, decisions concerning an individual's hearing should be made only after careful consideration of the ear examination, medical examination,
medical and otological history and comprehensive hearing
studies.

Auditing Thresholds

It is generally impractical to examine the ears of each employee prior to every routine hearing test. In order to circumvent such
a problem, the hearing tester should always bring to the physi-

cian's attention all employees in whom any of the following findings are encountered during routine audiometry:

1. A change of 15 dB or more from the previous audiogram in any two or more frequencies, or 25 dB in any one frequency.
2. Inconsistent responses from the subject, such as thresholds that vary 15 dB or more when rechecking at each frequency.
3. A subjective complaint of ringing in the ears, deafness, dizziness, or other history of ear infection since the last examination.

Referral to Otologist

By promptly examining the ears of such employees the examining physician may account for some of these findings by discovering impacted wax or by diagnosing a head cold, allergic attack, ear infection or some other readily curable condition; or he may find that the hearing loss is more substantial and warrants further investigation. If the examining physician should encounter abnormal findings during the initial or subsequent ear examination, or if he should decide that a serious hearing loss exists, or a loss is progressing and needs more study, it is advisable to refer the employee to a competent otologist. When referring an employee, it would be helpful to supply the otologist with as much background information as possible, including results of previous ear examinations, previous serial audiograms, description of the noise to which the employee is exposed, otological and noise exposure history, and whether or not the subject being referred is a new applicant or one on whom no previous studies are available.

In return the otologist should, if possible, supply the industry with the following information:

1. What is the cause of the damage present?
2. Is the hearing loss present conductive or sensorineural?
3. Is the hearing loss of a progressive type?
4. Will exposure to the noise of the employee's proposed or present job have a greater tendency to impair his hearing than it would that of a normal hearing person?
5. What special precautions are necessary to protect the individual at his job, both from the standpoint of ear hygiene and ear protection?
6. How often should routine audiograms be repeated on the individual after he has started work?

7. Should the individual be permitted to work in the specified noisy environment?

The importance of the answers to these questions is obvious. The answers must be based not only on sound clinical experience, but generally on the following studies:

1. Complete otological examination, including complete medical and otological histories.
2. Examination with tuning forks, if indicated.
3. Repeated air and bone conduction studies, using proper masking, when necessary.
4. Speech reception testing for threshold and discrimination.
5. Recruitment and tone decay studies.
6. Others, if necessary.

Sometimes the otologist will not be able to answer all of the above questions immediately on the basis of his examination. He may then suggest hiring the employee, watching his hearing at specified intervals, and if changes occur referring him again to the otologist for further study. Often this is the best policy, because as yet scientific study has insufficient data available upon which to base answers to all of these questions. Clinical experience and close observation provide the best solution presently available.

Noise Exposure History

In addition to the ear examination, a careful history is needed on all employees exposed to intense noise. Again, each plant should compose its own history forms. A sample form containing information which has been found valuable in a hearing evaluation is shown in chart II. When properly prepared, these questionnaires can be answered in a very short time by the employee himself, unless a reading or language difficulty is present. Such a questionnaire does not impose on the already busy schedule of the doctor or nurse. Both the ear examination report and the history questionnaire should be prepared on standard size forms, such as paper or large cards $8\frac{1}{2}$ x 11 inches. If possible, audiogram forms should also be this size, for convenience of handling and reviewing information.

Despite the questionable reliability of any questionnaire answered by the tested individual, the otological history often provides invaluable information in establishing a diagnosis or cause of deafness. For example, previous exposure to gunfire often explains certain types of high tone hearing loss, and previous ear infection may explain a low tone hearing loss. Should medicolegal situations arise, it is often possible to confirm the reliability of the questionnaire by referring to previous audiograms and histories obtained either in the military services or other industries.

For greater convenience the medical department of the industry should keep the forms on the ear examination, histories, and audiograms. These should be kept separately from the general medical examination. This will make it possible to more readily evaluate an employee's hearing by having all related information together in one folder.

While the importance of doing all these studies on new employees is generally conceded, the value of their usefulness is often questioned for the many employees who have already been working for years in noisy places without having previous examination. The only satisfactory answer to this question is now being provided by the inequitable claims for occupational deafness. All employees, newly employed and long-time alike, who are exposed to hazardous noise should receive ear examination, histories, audiograms, and ear protection, and should be included in the overall conservation-of-hearing program.

Experience has shown that a large number of older employees tested will have little significant hearing loss despite years of exposure to moderately intense noise. For this large group, the initial examination will provide a satisfactory baseline for future comparison. For those older employees in whom hearing loss is discovered, the cause and indicated measures to stop further hearing damage can be established. Contrary to the opinion of industry and labor, any steps taken to protect hearing will be favorably received by the great majority of employees, and their full cooperation can be enlisted readily. As in all large programs, there will be a fringe group who may not wish to conform; but if the conservation-of-hearing program is properly conducted, this fringe group will be extremely small.

Functional Hearing Impairment

Functional hearing impairment exists when there is no organic basis for the patient's apparent deafness. This has become such an integral part of hearing conservation programs because of the compensation and legal aspects that a discussion of functional loss is included in this chapter. In functional deafness the patient's inability to hear results entirely, or chiefly, from psychological or emotional factors, and his hearing mechanism may be essentially normal. Although there may be some slight damage in the ear, the recorded hearing loss is disproportionate to the amount of actual damage.

Functional hearing loss may be the result of anxiety because of emotional conflict, and beyond the reasonable control of the individual. Hysterical deafness is an example of functional hearing impairment. Probably the classic example is that of the young soldier in battle who is too frightened to charge yet ashamed to retreat while his buddies bravely go forward. From the absence of a rational way out, his unconscious mind conjures up the concept of deafness or perhaps blindness. In many instances, the functional hearing loss may be superimposed on true organic deafness, in which case the term functional overlay is used. The problem then is to recognize the two components in the patient's hearing impairment. The history and the otologic examinations often provide important clues, such as the unrealistic attempts of a patient to account for his difficulty. For example, he may claim that his hearing was excellent until a physician cleaned out his ears with such force that he suddenly went stone deaf.

In a patient with unilateral functional deafness, there may be complete absence of bone conduction on the side of the bad ear, and the normal acuity on the side of the good ear. Such a patient may even disclaim hearing shouts directed at the bad ear in spite of the good hearing in the opposite ear. These inconsistencies help establish a diagnosis of functional hearing loss. There is another type of functional hearing loss called malingering in which the individual deliberately fabricates deafness, and this is becoming increasingly common especially in industry and in the military. In such situations the individual is motivated to seek some advantage, especially financial compensation.

Malingering

Unlike the neurotic individual who believes his symptoms are real, the malingerer who pretends deafness has no "pattern" in his alleged disability. His hearing tests are a crazy quilt of inconsistencies. When he is subjected to tests that he does not understand, he suspects he may be tripped up by the doctor and his testing machine. He wishes to preserve the fiction that he is deaf, but when asked whether he can hear a signal of a given strength, he does not know when to say, "yes," and when to say "no." He falters in his answers. Yesterday's audiogram may have shown a 70 dB hearing level, and today's a 35 dB. The record may indicate a 60 dB hearing loss for pure tone, but a loss of only 10 dB for speech reception. When the tests are repeated, his answers may vary by as much as 30 to 40 dB.

When a patient malingers to the extent of exaggerating a true organic hearing loss, the task of learning the truth becomes more difficult. Such a problem may assume considerable importance in medicolegal cases, particularly if they involve compensation claims for occupational deafness.

Malingerers in industrial hearing testing may fall into two major categories:

1. The individual who already has a hearing loss and attempts to conceal it in order to be hired may subsequently attempt to attribute his hearing loss to the exposure of industrial noise at his new job.

2. The individual who has normal hearing, or a lesser loss, and pretends to be more hard of hearing than he actually is, so that his compensation will be greater than the amount to which he may be entitled.

It is conceivable that some industries may become so harassed by the fear of legal entanglements from industrial deafness claims that they will be hesitant to employ any person having significant hearing impairment. This would be most unfortunate if practiced without due consideration to each individual case. Such practice might also induce some employees to feign normal hearing, hiding their hearing losses in order to secure employment.

Instances of this have already been encountered in industry and are not uncommon in the military services. In all fairness to individuals who resort to this method, it must be said that many may not initially do it with the intent of claiming compensation for any hearing loss existing prior to their employment. Unfortunately, in some instances circumstances may later induce a few of these individuals to claim compensation for an already existing hearing loss, particularly if a successful claim for compensation has been made by a fellow employee. Another factor is failure of the industry to perform pre-employment hearing testing or to perform it accurately. Erroneous results may be more damaging than not testing at all. There are some companies for example, that still use whispered and spoken voices as the sole hearing tests. The inaccuracies of this kind of test, particularly in the hands of untrained testers, are well established. Inaccurate testing with an audiometer can also result in inaccurate audiograms, a fact which may become a great liability both to the employee and to the industry.

The special importance of the initial or pre-employment audiogram can well be appreciated. At least two independent hearing thresholds should be obtained on every initial test. This applies not only to subjects with hearing loss, but even those with normal hearing. In this manner it will often be possible to detect subjects who do not give reliable responses.

As the paying of compensation for industrial deafness becomes more common, there will most likely be an increasing number of incidents in which employees exaggerate their hearing losses intentionally for personal gain. This type of malingering will not be the responsibility of the industrial hearing tester, since it may become a medicolegal problem. Rather, it will be the responsibility of the otologist, who will establish the true hearing threshold by means of other tests and examination.

Management of Malingering

The principal responsibility of the hearing tester in industry is to learn to suspect or detect personnel who do not seem to produce reliable hearing thresholds. This is particularly important in the pre-employment testing. Certain clues may alert the tester. The attitude and cooperation of the subject are often of aid in detecting a malingerer. Experience will more clearly define these attitudes. The most important clue is inconsistent threshold on repeat testing. For example, if a subject responds to 30 dB at one time and does not respond until 50 dB another, and perhaps 60 dB the next time, it should lead the tester to suspect the patient of being uncooperative. Another common clue is being able to carry on a normal conversation with the tester's mouth hidden from the subject's view to prevent lip reading. In some instances when malingering is suspected, if the tester deliberately lets the subject watch his hands while presuming to produce tones without actually doing so, a reasonably positive proof of malingering can be established if the subject responds to the visual rather than the auditory stimulus. Repeated complete audiograms performed with excellent technique are the best means of detecting and preventing malingering.

The question as to what a tester in industry should do when he suspects or detects malingering is of prime importance. The tester should be constantly aware that it is not his responsibility to accuse the subject of being a malingerer. As a matter of fact, such an accusation is not only a serious mistake but may lead to serious complications, since many of the clues suggesting malingering (such as inconsistency) may also be present in conditions other than malingering. The only responsibility of the tester is to suspect that the audiogram does not represent the accurate threshold of hearing of the individual tested; but he should give the subject no indication whatsoever of his suspicion. He should, instead, treat the subject as he does others, and bring the results of the tests and his comments to the attention of the physician in charge of the hearing-testing program. It is the responsibility of the physician, if he is suitably trained, or of the otologist retained as a consultant to investigate the subject more completely and to establish a hearing threshold and diagnosis. Very frequently a subject who is inclined to malinger when tested by a technician will give accurate responses when tested by a trained audiologist. This will significantly reduce the number of malingerers and avoid many complications.

The tester must always remember that his responsibility is to test and to evaluate intelligently, but not to interpret audiograms. He should leave this for a physician who can integrate the history, physical examination, and otological data, including many special tests.

RECOMMENDED READINGS

Davis, Hallowell and Silverman, S. Richard: *Hearing and Deafness,* 3rd Edition. New York, Holt, Rinehart, and Winston, 1970.

Emerick, Lon L.: *A Workbook in Clinical Audiometry.* Springfield, Thomas, 1971.

Engelberg, Marvin W.: *Audiological Evaluation for Exaggerated Hearing Level.* Springfield, Thomas, 1970.

Glorig, Aram, Editor: *Audiometry: Principles and Practices.* Baltimore, Williams and Wilkins, 1965.

Hirsh, Ira J.: *The Measurement of Hearing.* New York, McGraw-Hill, 1952.

Jerger, James J., Ed.: *Modern Developments in Audiology.* New York, Academic Press, 1963.

Katz, Jack, Editor: *Handbook of Clinical Audiology.* Baltimore, Williams and Wilkins, 1971.

Miller, Maurice H. and Polisar, Ira A.: *Audiological Evaluation of the Pediatric Patient.* Springfield, Thomas, 1971.

Newby, Hayes A.: *Audiology: Principles and Practice,* 2nd Edition. New York, Appleton-Century-Crofts, 1964.

O'Neill, John J. and Oyer, Herbert J.: *Applied Audiometry.* New York, Dodd, Mead, 1966.

Rasmussen, Grant L. and Windle, William F.: *Neural Mechanisms of the Auditory and Vestibular Systems.* Springfield, Thomas, 1965.

Ventry, Ira R., Chaiklin, Joseph B. and Dixon, Richard F.: *Hearing Measurement, A Book of Readings.* New York, Appleton-Century-Crofts, 1971.

Chapter 8

INTERPRETATION OF AUDIOGRAMS

THE REASON FOR DISCUSSING interpretation of audiograms is to acquaint the industrial medical department with some of the procedures the otologist uses in establishing a diagnosis. For detailed information of audiometric interpretation the reader is referred to the author's (JS) book, *Hearing Loss* (Lippincott).

The otologist encounters many difficulties in his search for the cause of an individual case of deafness. He cannot determine the medical cause for a hearing loss merely by examining the audiogram. He must also study the patient's history, medical and otological findings, and the results of many special tests before he can attempt to make a diagnosis. Even with all this information available, it is not possible to make an accurate diagnosis in every instance.

Examination of the audiogram pattern provides considerable help to the otologist seeking the site and cause of the hearing damage. Other clues also become evident during the actual hearing testing. For instance, if thresholds vary widely at each frequency (such as 10 dB or more) it may be due to an ear infection or even malingering. If the end point thresholds are sharp it suggests the presence of sensorineural deafness. A one-sided flat hearing loss of about 50 or 60 dB with normal hearing in the other ear indicates the need for retest with masking in the good ear. Any one-sided nerve deafness of over 20 dB in all the frequencies suggests the need for ruling out a tumor of the auditory nerve. In self-recording audiometry wide fluctuations indicate the patient does not know how to respond to thresholds or the possibility of malingering. Frequently such tests have to be repeated.

The audiometric pattern provides only a reasonable clue as to the type of deafness present (conductive or nerve). Figure 30 shows the audiometric pattern characteristic of conductive hearing loss (the damage is in the outer or middle ear). The greater loss of hearing occurs in the low frequencies and is due to causes such as ear infections and otosclerosis. Figure 31 shows the audiometric pattern characteristically found in nerve deafness such as caused by old age, drugs, viruses, etc. The greater loss occurs in the high frequencies. These characteristic patterns can provide helpful guidance in seeking the cause of a hearing loss. How-

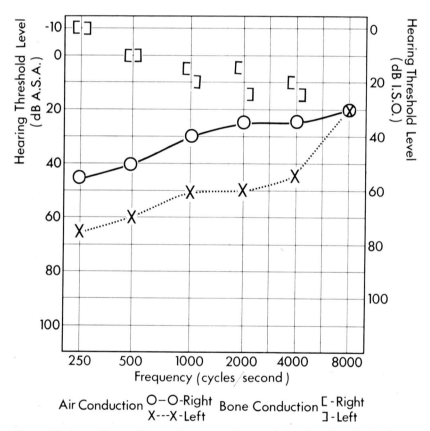

Air Conduction O–O-Right Bone Conduction C-Right
X---X-Left   ꓕ-Left

Figure 30. Ascending audiometric pattern characteristic of conductive deafness.

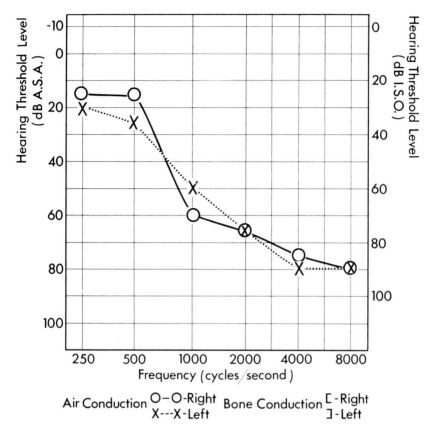

Figure 31. Descending audiometric pattern characteristic of sensorineural deafness.

ever, basing an individual diagnosis on the shape of the audiogram alone is hazardous. For example, the low frequency pattern characteristic of conductive loss is also found in Meniere's disease where the damage occurs to the inner ear and it is considered nerve, or "sensorineural," rather than conductive hearing loss. Simply establishing a diagnosis on this particular pattern would lead to an erroneous classification of the type of hearing loss. Similarly, a high frequency loss is not always indicative of nerve deafness since a similar pattern can be produced when a normal ear canal is filled with an oily solution or with wax. Fluid in the middle ear can also cause the high frequency loss without involv-

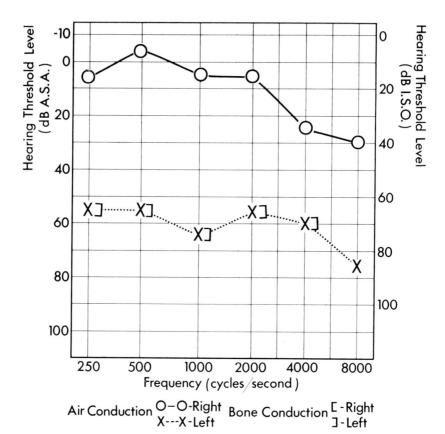

Figure 32. Audiometric pattern showing a flat loss that can be produced by many different causes.

ing the sensorineural mechanism. Here, again, the diagnosis would be wrong if it were based exclusively on the shape of the audiogram.

As a further example of the hazards involved in making a diagnosis solely from an audiogram, let us consider the air conduction audiogram shown in Figure 32. This is the audiogram of a 37-year-old individual, whose type of hearing curve is commonly encountered among employees in certain noisy industrial plants. When the otologist looks at this audiogram, he must consider any one of the following diagnoses as being possible:

1. Congenital hearing loss
2. Otosclerosis
3. Progressive hereditary nerve deafness
4. Presbycusis
5. Meniere's Disease
6. Impacted wax in the ears
7. Infection
8. Acoustic nerve tumor
9. Occupational deafness caused by noise
10. Malingering
11. Functional deafness
12. Toxic reaction from drugs
13. Other causes, such as systemic diseases (syphilis, Paget's disease etc.)

Only by further careful and comprehensive study is it possible for the otologist to establish definitely which of the above causes has produced the deafness in this particular patient. Let us follow the otologist as he considers the characteristic features and tests that help him make an accurate diagnosis.

Examination by the Otologist

When examining a patient referred by an industry, most otologists usually follow a standardized procedure which includes the following essential elements:

1. History
2. Otological examination
3. Tuning fork tests
4. Audiometric tests
5. Special tests

History

A penetrating medical history is obtained which seeks to uncover all possible clues that might account for the hearing loss. The otologist usually asks the patient the following important questions:

1. Is there a family history of hearing loss that might resemble the present type of loss? Such information may help to confirm the presence of conditions, such as otosclerosis or an inherited tendency to progressive nerve deafness.
2. Does the patient admit having trouble in hearing? If so, in which

situations is this loss most noticeable: speaking on the telephone, listening in a quiet or a noisy place?

3. Was the hearing loss of sudden or gradual onset? Strangely enough some patients may have a profound hearing loss in one ear for years without being aware of it, until one day they try to use the telephone on the bad ear. They then feel the onset was on that particular day, not realizing that the loss was actually present for a long time. Also, some persons may even have moderate degrees of hearing loss in both ears for many years without being aware of a hearing handicap. Perhaps a head cold or other infection may cause a further hearing loss, and the patient attributes his total loss to that incident. Most of us ordinarily use speech loud enough to overcome a minor hearing loss, so the subject may be unaware of his handicap. Some persons may subconsciously refuse to admit having any hearing difficulty, even though they are aware they miss parts of conversation. For this reason, the question of onset must be critically evaluated by the otologist. Certain conditions cause sudden deafness while others cause gradual onsets.

4. Is the deafness accompanied by ear noises? Does the patient have attacks of dizziness; such as feeling his head spin, or the room turn around? This has important bearing on disorders of the inner ear and nerve.

5. What is the character of the ear noises and of the dizziness?

6. Has the patient ever had ear infections? If so, what kind?

7. What fevers and other systemic diseases has the patient had?

8. Does the patient have headaches, difficulty in seeing, double vision, or does he lose his balance? These symptoms sometimes suggest the presence of a serious infection or tumor inside the skull.

From the answers to these questions and many others, the otologist begins to narrow down his diagnosis and to decide which further special studies outside the field of otology such as eye examination, blood examinations, brain wave studies, spinal fluid studies, etc., are essential and which may be eliminated safely.

DIAGNOSTIC REASONING

1. If the cause were congenital hearing loss, the patient might admit or betray a sibilant speech defect, with the letter "S," a common finding in those born with high tone hearing loss in both ears. The reason for this speech defect is the difficulty in hearing certain consonants and the inability, therefore, to learn to imitate their production correctly. There may also be a history of similar congenital deafness in the family.

The medical and ear examinations in such instances are generally normal unless the patient has had superimposed complications. A bone conduction test would show reduced bone conduction.

2. In otosclerosis there may be a family history of hearing loss, the onset of which would have been from early adulthood. Characteristically, the bone conduction would be excellent, and the patient would speak in a very soft, subdued voice since he hears his own voice more acutely by bone conduction and is not aware of how softly he speaks. He might also have disturbing noises in his ears (tinnitus). Careful questioning would show that he hears better in noisy than in quiet places. Speech discrimination tests would give excellent results. Otological findings would also generally be normal. Recruitment of loudness would be absent.

3. If this were progressive hereditary nerve deafness in all likelihood there would be similar losses in other members of his family. The earliest and greatest changes would occur in the highest frequencies in contradistinction to the dips found in industrial deafness. Response to the frequencies 10,000, 12,-000 and 14,000 Hz would be practically gone. Bone conduction also would be reduced. This is often a difficult diagnosis to establish, except by elimination of other possibilities.

4. Such a severe loss as shown in Figure 32 would rarely be expected in an average case of presbycusis, since low tones are not generally affected to this degree. However, it might be a mixed deafness consisting of presbycusis and some middle ear damage. History, examination, and the age of the patient would aid in this differentiation.

5. Meniere's disease (labyrinthosis) would be characterized by recurrent attacks of vertigo and tinnitus. Bone conduction would be reduced and speech discrimination quite poor. Recruitment of loudness would be present. The ear examination would generally be normal, but testing the labyrinth response (balance mechanism in the ear) might offer diagnostic information. The end points of the audiogram curve during audiometry would be unusually definite and clear cut.

6. Impacted wax could readily be detected by an otological ex-

amination. In order to be certain that the ear wax is the sole cause of hearing loss, the audiogram should be repeated after the wax is removed. Sometimes the wax may be hiding a middle ear infection, or there may be an entirely unrelated deafness present.

7. Infections of the ears would be determined by the history and examination. The bone conduction is usually normal if ear infection is the sole cause of the deafness.

8. A tumor on the nerve of hearing rarely causes hearing loss in both ears at the same time. In this instance, however, the otologist would consider the possibility that the hearing loss in one ear might be caused by an infection, while the loss in the opposite ear could be due to a tumor in the nerve. Neurological studies, tone decay, recruitment studies, and labyrinthine studies are essential if a tumor is suspected.

9. Occupational deafness would be established by the history, normal otological findings, reduced bone conduction, and perhaps recruitment of loudness. In this type of deafness, the hearing loss would be in both ears.

10. Malingering and psychogenic deafness would be detected by inconsistent findings, particularly between the repeated audiograms and speech reception tests. Many other tests are available to establish malingering and other forms of psychogenic deafness. The Psycho-galvanic skin resistance test and cortical responses are noteworthy among these tests.

11. The hearing loss could be the result of previous treatment with dihydrosteptomycin, neomycin, or other drugs. This would be determined from the patient's history.

12. The general medical examination would help rule out such causes as syphilis, Paget's disease, hypotension, and others.

Otological Examination

A complete examination is then performed. The otologist examines the throat, and with a small mirror looks behind the soft palate into the nasopharynx, which is the area behind the nose and above the palate. Here he observes the opening to the Eustachian tubes, which lead to the ears, to see if they appear normal from this angle. He examines the ears including the mobility of the eardrums. The nasal passages are inspected and with an instrument called a nasopharyngoscope passed far back into one of the nasal passages; the otologist again examines the nasopharynx, this time from a different angle. The presence of any adenoid tissue or tubal obstruction is particularly noticeable through the nasopharyngoscope. A careful ear examination is not complete without an accurate evaluation of the nasopharynx.

Tuning Fork Tests

By means of a tuning fork the otologist obtains a preliminary opinion of the type of hearing loss present; that is, whether the loss is conductive, neural, or a mixture of both. Three basic tests usually help establish this opinion.

1. The Rinne Test compares the patient's ability to hear the tuning fork by air-borne sound with his ability to hear it by bone conduction. The vibrating fork is first placed about an inch from the ear, and the patient is requested to note its loudness. Then the base of the fork is quickly pressed against the mastoid bone. The patient is then asked in which position the fork sounds louder.
2. The Weber Test determines which ear, if either, hears the tuning fork better by bone conduction. The base of the vibrating fork is held on the center of the forehead or upper front teeth and the patient is asked in which ear the fork sounds louder.
3. The Schwabach Test compares the patient's ability to hear the fork by bone conduction through the mastoid bones, with a normal hearing patient's ability to hear the fork in the same position. Usually, the normal-hearing listener is the otologist himself.

By a critical interpretation of the results obtained from these three tests, it is possible in most situations to obtain an indication as to whether the hearing loss is due to a conductive impairment, a neural deafness, or perhaps a mixture of both.

A word of caution is in order concerning tuning fork testing. This is a most difficult procedure to perform, and to interpret accurately. The frequency of the tuning fork used and the manner in which it is held and struck, either next to the ear or on the mastoid bone, greatly influence the results obtained. Quite frequently the same tests, performed in a slightly different manner by various individuals may result in completely contradictory impressions. A great deal of clinical experience is needed to do accurate testing with tuning forks. Furthermore, such tests are not done for quantitative measurements, but only to determine the qualitative nature of a hearing loss. Tuning fork tests supplement, but do not replace accurate audiometry.

The otologist will more than likely report to the industrial physician how the patient's hearing by bone conduction compares with his hearing by air conduction. Usually if the patient hears better by bone conduction than by air conduction, his hearing loss is conductive in character. If bone conduction tests show a marked reduction, the loss is probably sensorineural.

Audiometric Tests

Quantitative air and bone conduction audiometry are next performed. First, the otologist performs an air conduction audiogram using the same basic audiometric technique described previously and repeatedly checks each threshold to establish its accuracy.

The otologist next performs bone-conduction audiometry, a most difficult procedure to perform and to interpret accurately. It should be done only by a trained audiologist or otologist and must be done with proper masking noise in the ear opposite from the one being tested. The type of masking noise used and its intensity must be accurately controlled. Masking is necessary because the skull so readily transmits sound from one side to the other with almost no loss in sound energy (attenuation). As a matter of fact, if a normal listener places a tuning fork over one of his mastoid bones and puts his finger in his opposite ear, the tuning fork will sound much louder in the occluded ear than it will in the one nearer the tuning fork. This demonstrates how readily the sound on one side of the head is conducted to the other, through the skull. To be sure that a tester is testing only the one ear by bone conduction and is not getting carry-over to the opposite side, the otologist must mask out the opposite ear with a sufficient amount of noise. The type of noise most commonly used is known as *white noise* because it has an equal distribution of all audible frequencies. It is often difficult to determine the intensity of white noise required. If the noise is too low, it will not mask sufficiently. However, if the masking noise is too loud, it too may carry over across the skull and affect the ear whose bone conduction is being determined.

On occasion a patient is encountered who has almost total hearing loss in one ear and no loss in the other. When the routine audiogram is obtained, however, it will show normal hearing in one ear, and only about a 50 or 60 dB loss in the other. In such a situation, it is essential that adequate masking be used in the ear with normal hearing to assess the actual hearing in the bad ear. Adequate masking is essential not only for air conduction, but for bone conduction as well. Only the otologist is trained to interpret the results accurately.

Special Tests

Speech Reception Test

Depending on findings already obtained, certain special hearing tests may also be indicated. If a substantial hearing loss is present, it is always advisable for the otologist to do a speech *reception* test, using spondee words on each ear individually. The results of this test are reported as a speech reception threshold and generally compare favorably with the decibel loss obtained by pure tone testing in the frequencies 500, 1,000 and 2,000 Hz. For example, a speech reception of 30 dB, as determined with spondee words, generally indicates that the patient has about a 30 dB loss in these frequencies. Such a loss is the level at which an individual often begins to have noticeable difficulty in hearing everyday conversation and at which he may require a hearing aid.

Another important consideration in evaluating an audiogram is to recognize that the audiometric threshold does not establish the handicapping effect of the hearing impairment. The threshold gives only an indication of how the individual hears (extremely soft) tones. Since we do not use such weak tones in everyday communication, it is more important to determine how the person hears at "above threshold" rather than solely at threshold level; and generally such information is not obtainable from the simple air conduction routine audiograms performed in industrial hearing testing. For example, an individual with an audiogram as shown in Figure 8-3 may hear and understand everyday speech reasonably well, even in a noisy room. Yet another individual with precisely the same type of audiogram may have a great deal of difficulty understanding speech, and find it almost impossible to carry on everyday conversation. The former's hearing loss may be due to ear infection and the latter's to Meniere's disease or surgical severance of part of the auditory nerve. Furthermore, the conductive loss can be well compensated with a hearing aid, but the loss due to Meniere's disease or nerve severance cannot. Therefore, it is inadvisable to present an accurate evaluation of the handicapping extent of a person's hearing impairment merely from an audiogram. Supplementary tests using speech are essential.

Discrimination Test

One of the most important of these studies is called *discrimination* testing, using a list of phonetically balanced words (PB). Used in conjunction with the speech reception and other tests, the results of the discrimination test help establish the individual's ability to hear and understand speech, and to communicate in his daily social and business life. The discrimination score is reported in percentages of words correctly heard at a certain level of loudness above the individual's speech reception threshold.

For example, a patient may understand only 50 percent of PB words given him at 20 dB above the speech reception threshold. At 40 dB above the threshold he may get 70 percent of the words. In certain hearing disorders such as conductive losses, the louder the level at which the PB words are presented the more words the subject will hear correctly. However, in certain other hearing disorders (congenital losses for instance), patients may not discriminate any better at 40 dB above the threshold than they do at a lower level. In still some other conditions, such as Meniere's disease, patients may be less able to discriminate as the loudness of speech is increased. This discrimination curve, or ability to understand at various levels of loudness, helps to establish not only the site of the damage in the ear, but it is also most useful in evaluating the handicapping effects of the hearing loss for each individual. This is important for compensation purposes.

Recruitment Test

Another test the otologist is frequently obliged to use concerns itself with a complicated phenomenon called recruitment of loudness. Increasing clinical experience is leading to a fuller understanding of this phenomenon which requires consideration, particularly in some occupational cases, because of its increasing importance as a diagnostic criterion. Recruitment of loudness occurs in some partially deaf ears. It is essentially an increase in the patient's sensation of loudness out of proportion to the increase in the physical intensity of the signal. For example, when the audiometer produces a tone which is only 20 dB above threshold, to an individual with a recruiting ear, the tone may sound to him as loud as a tone 50 dB above threshold in a normal ear. The patient whose ear recruits generally presents some of the following symptoms:

1. Distortion—the patient will often complain that voices, music, and certain sounds are tinny, hollow, fuzzy.
2. Diplacusis—this is a technical term describing a condition in which the same musical note sounds different in pitch in each ear, usually sounding higher in the ear with recruitment.
3. The patient usually cannot tolerate moderately loud noises which seem otherwise well tolerated by a normal ear. He will be disturbed, for example, by trolley squeaking, brake squeals, and similar sounds.
4. The patient with a recruiting ear usually has very sharp and more definite audiometric end points than a person with a conductive loss.
5. In Meniere's disease (labyrinthosis), in which recruitment is most evident, the hearing may fluctuate markedly. It may be poor for days or months.

It is generally believed that a recruiting ear localizes damage in the organ of Corti. Recruitment is generally not present in a lesion restricted to auditory nerve fiber. Where damage exists in both the organ of Corti and nerve pathway, probably recruitment will be present if the proportion of hair cell damage is greater than the proportion of nerve fiber involvement. If this ratio is reversed, recruitment may not be present.

Since the presence of recruitment may be helpful in distinguishing occupational deafness from other forms of deafness, the otologist should be familiar with methods of determining recruitment. Presently the *alternate binaural loudness balance test* is the most practical method for this purpose. This test requires at least a 30 dB difference in the frequency threshold being tested between the two ears.

Abnormal Tone Decay

Just as recruitment is usually indicative of damage in the inner ear, abnormal tone decay (abnormal auditory fatigue) is usually a sign of pressure or damage to the auditory nerve fibers. Of particular importance in this phenomenon is the fact that it can be an early sign of an acoustic neuroma or some other tumor occupying space in the posterior part of the skull. The test for abnormal tone decay is very simple to perform and should be done routinely in every case of unilateral sensorineural deafness, especially when no recruitment is found.

The test is based on the fact that an individual with normal hearing can continue to hear a steady threshold tone for at least one minute, whereas the patient who has a tumor pressing on his auditory nerve is unable to maintain a threshold tone for this length of time. The test is performed with an audiometer. A frequency that shows reduced threshold is selected, and the patient is instructed to raise his finger as soon as the tone comes on and to keep it raised as long as he can hear it. The tone is then presented at 5 dB (or above threshold) and a stop watch is started with the presentation of the tone. Each time the patient lowers his finger the intensity is increased 5 dB, and the time noted for that period of hearing. The tone interrupter switch is never released from the "on" position during any of the intensity changes. The test is one minute in duration, and a person with no abnormal tone decay will usually continue to hold up his finger during the entire 60 seconds. Occasionally he may require a 5 or 10 dB increase during the first part of the test, but he then maintains the tone for the remainder of the time. A patient who has abnormal tone decay may lower his finger after only about 10 seconds, and when the tone is raised 5 dB he may lower his finger again after another 10 seconds, and continue to indicate that the tone fades out repeatedly, even though after 60 seconds there may be an increase of 25 dB or more above the original threshold. Some patients may even fail to hear the tone at the maximum intensity of the audiometer after one minute, whereas originally they may have heard the threshold tone at 25 dB. This finding of abnormal tone decay is highly suggestive of pressure on the auditory nerve fibers.

Malingering

When *malingering* is suspected, a battery of special tests will need to be considered. In such instances the ingenuity, experience, and training of the otologist is of utmost importance. Among the special tests now used in this situation are: (a) Stenger, (b) Doerfler Stewart, (c) Psychogalvanic skin resistance test. For a detailed description of these and other tests for malingering, the reader is referred to any of the excellent books on otology and audiology.

RECOMMENDED READINGS

Davis, Hallowell and Silverman, S. Richard: *Hearing and Deafness,* 3rd Edition. New York, Holt, Rinehart, and Winston, 1970.

Littler, T. S.: *The Physics of the Ear.* New York, Pergamon Press, 1965.

Sataloff, Joseph: *Hearing Loss.* Philadelphia, J. B. Lippincott Co., 1966.

Sensorineural Hearing Loss, *Ciba Foundation Symposium.* Baltimore, Williams and Wilkins, 1970.

Ventry, Ira R., Chaiklin, Joseph B. and Dixon, Richard F.: *Hearing Measurement, A Book of Readings.* New York, Appleton-Century-Crofts, 1971.

Chapter 9

NOISE CRITERIA AND LEGAL ASPECTS OF OCCUPATIONAL HEARING LOSS

Noise Criteria and Their Shortcomings

I T IS GENERALLY AGREED that very intense noise can produce deafness, but there is considerable difference of opinion as to the "boundary line" that separates harmless from harmful noises. This boundary line has been called the *critical noise level* or the *maximum safe intensity level,* assuming that intensity was solely responsible for the hazardous quality of noise. For many years investigators tried to determine this maximum safe intensity level by evaluating the deafening effect of an industrial noise solely on the basis of overall measures of intensity. It became obvious that this approach was inadequate, especially since the ear is far more sensitive to certain frequencies than to others. Two different noises may each have about the same overall sound-pressure level, but they do not necessarily have the same effect upon hearing. If one of the noises has a spectrum similar to that shown in Curve A (Fig. 33), with most of its sound energy in the lower frequencies, it will probably have little or no effect upon hearing. The other noise of the same overall intensity having most of its sound energy in the higher audible frequency range, Curve B, could produce substantial hearing damage. In addition to the intensity, the spectrum and duration of a noise must be carefully analyzed before its deafening effect can be determined.

The numerous conflicting experimental conclusions concerning

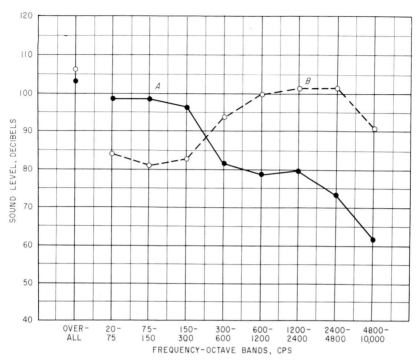

Figure 33. Spectra of two different noises.

"critical noise levels," were no doubt the results of failure to take into account these factors as well as additional criteria that must be considered before accurate conclusions can be drawn. For example, sound-level meters and noise analyzers used for sound measurement must be of the proper type and be calibrated accurately at the time of use. The limitations of each piece of equipment must be understood fully by the person using it, especially when microphones are used under conditions of differing temperatures and pressures. In hearing testing and calibration of audiometers, the ambient noise level of the test room must be measured accurately and evaluated properly prior to performing audiometry.

Often, investigators having an excellent appreciation of the electronic and physical aspects of sound measurement take for granted the apparent simplicity of performing and interpreting audiograms. Similarly, the competent otologist or audiologist, assuming that he has merely to read a meter, may draw conclusions that are to be based on inaccurate sound measurements.

Undoubtedly the greatest cause for the lack of valid experimental conclusions relating industrial noise and hearing acuity is the failure of the investigator to appreciate the limitations of the audiogram. In a cross sectional investigation it is generally inadvisable to draw conclusions concerning the employee's hearing acuity on the basis of a single threshold, especially when a large number of subjects are tested one after another. At least two independent consistent thresholds are essential to establish a threshold of hearing for research purposes in industry.

The attitude and interest of the technician are also important factors in determining thresholds. Taking routine manual or self-recorded audiograms one after another for numerous subjects can be conducive to poor audiometry.

Many reports represent much labor and thousands of hearing tests; but all too frequently the tests were not made under standard conditions and were not reliable determinations of the subject's thresholds.

In a long-range study of the deafening effects of noise, it is also important to consider the time of day when the hearing test is given. For example, if a subject is employed as a chipper, his hearing threshold in the morning prior to work will differ considerably from his hearing threshold after six hours of exposure to noise. Temporary hearing loss must be excluded if comparison of audiograms is to be valid. In studying the permanent effects of long-term noise exposures, it is misleading to compare hearing thresholds taken in the morning with those taken in the evening after noise exposure.

In addition to these criteria, in studying the deafening effect of noise upon hearing one must consider factors such as the time relations of a sound stimulus, its period of continuity, its fluctuation, its rate of buildup, and its release of sound energy.

Damage-risk Criterion

The need to consider so many factors led investigators to introduce the concept of damage-risk criterion. The most important factors influencing the capability of a noise to produce hearing loss are its intensity, its frequency spectrum, its time pattern, and the duration of an individual's exposure. Within certain limits, the risk of hearing damage increases with increasing intensity, longer duration of exposure, and with continuous as opposed to interrupted noise. It is also known that noises of predominently higher frequencies (above 1,000 Hz) are more damaging than those of lower frequencies (below 1,000 Hz).

Federal Noise Regulation

Recognizing the urgent need for practical noise criteria, representatives from five major societies concerned with noise and hearing formed an Intersociety Committee to establish noise guidelines. The committee included delegates from the American Industrial Hygiene Association (AIHA), Industrial Medical Association (IMA), American Academy of Ophthalmology and Otolaryngology (AAOO), the American Conference of Government Industrial Hygienists (ACGIH), and the American Academy of Occupational Medicine (AAOM). This Intersociety Committee, along with a subcommittee of the American Standards Association (now called American National Standards Institute— ANSI), on the basis of available data, produced a series of socalled "risk-curves." These curves show what percentage of population could be expected to develop hearing impairment (more than 15 dB, ASA, or 26 dB, ANSI average in the frequencies 500,

A-weighted Sound Level (Continuous Noise)	Percentage of Population Having Impaired Hearing (a) by Age Groups				Source of Information (b)
dB	20-29	30-39	40-49	50-59	
Non-Noise	3	5	10	20	13
General Population	2	5	14	24	14
80	1	3	6	19	17
85	3	7	13	27	17
90	6	14	21	37	17
92	3	9	15	28	14
95	10	22	32	47	17
96 (c)	3	10	19	-	13
97	7	22	32	48	15
100	16	36	46	60	17
102	10	18	30	45	13
104	5	21	35	57	16
105	24	50	62	75	17

(a)   Average hearing threshold level in excess of 15 dB at 500, 1,000 and 2,000 Hz.

(b)   Refers to a list of references.

(c)   Estimated level.

Figure 34. Percentage of population having hearing impairment by age groups.

1,000 and 2,000 Hz) with habitual exposure to industrial noise eight hours daily for a "life-time of work" (Fig. 34).

In May of 1969 the United States Department of Labor published in the Federal Register regulations based on these curves to prevent occupational deafness. These regulations applied to all industries having government contracts of $10,000 or more. The Noise Regulation included in the Federal Register of May 1969 is as follows:

50-204.10—Occupational Noise Exposure

a. Protection against the effects of noise exposure shall be provided when the sound levels exceed those shown in Table 1 of this section when measured on the A scale of a standard sound level meter at slow response. When noise levels are determined by octave band analysis the equivalent A-weighted sound level may be determined as follows:

Equivalent sound level contours. Octave band sound pressure levels may be converted to the equivalent A-weighted sound level by plotting them on the graph and noting the A-weighted sound level corresponding the point of highest penetration into the sound level contours. This equivalent A-weighted sound level, which may differ from the actual A-weighted sound level of the noise, is used to determine exposure limits from Table 1.

b. When employees are subjected to sounds exceeding those listed in Table 1 of this section, feasible administrative or engineering controls shall be utilized. If such controls fail to reduce sound levels within the levels of the table, personal protective equipment shall be provided and used to reduce sound levels within the levels of the table.

c. If the variation in noise level involves maxima at intervals of 1 second or less, it is to be considered intermittent. In such cases, where the duration of the maxima are less than a second, they shall be treated as of 1-second duration.

d. In all cases where the sound levels exceed the values shown herein, a continuing effective hearing conservation program shall be administered.

The hearing damage percentages shown in Figure 34 are based chiefly on audiometric data from only one field investigation on a population of American workers.

The other studies used by the Intersociety Committee were chiefly laboratory rather than field studies. Scrutiny of representative audiometric data taken from the original field study re-

TABLE II

PERMISSIBLE NOISE EXPOSURES*

Duration Per Day, Hours	Sound Level dBA
8	90
6	92
4	95
3	97
2	100
1½	102
1	105
½	110
¼ or less	115

* When the daily noise exposure is composed of two or more periods of exposure of different levels, their combined effect should be considered rather than the individual effect of each. If the sum of the following fractions: C1/T1 C2/T2..+..Cn/Tn exceeds unity, then the mixed exposure should be considered to exceed the limit value. Cn indicates the total time of exposure at a specified noise level, and Tn indicates the total time of exposure permitted at that level. Exposure to impulsive or impact noise should not exceed 140 dBA peak sound pressure level.

veals several shortcomings limiting its usefulness for National Standards. For example, there are thresholds recorded above the limits of the audiometer, the study did not exclude conductive and other causes of hearing loss and many low frequency losses suggest higher than permissable ambient noise levels in the test room.

In spite of these shortcomings these data can be used as presently recommended by the Intersociety Committee and the Occupational Safety and Health Act (OSHA) as guides for starting hearing conservation programs. However, more valid studies are needed to confirm the relationship of hearing loss to noise exposure especially in the 84 dBA to 92 dBA range.

An essential requirement of OSHA is that any industry in which employees are exposed daily to continuous noise levels exceeding 90 dBA for an eight-hour working day over many years must either reduce the noise or protect the hearing of exposed personnel by instituting a hearing conservation program.

In all likelihood 90 dBA is to become a very much used and abused number. Those unfamiliar with noise measurement, for instance, will occasionally omit the A and simply state 90 dB; an

Hearing Conservation

incorrect application. There may be even more serious misuses in medicolegal situations.

The 90 dBA level specified in the OSHA is the level at which conservation of hearing should be started. It is not a damage-risk criterion to be used in compensation or legal cases. Facts are not yet available to establish definitive noise criteria that are valid for all individual cases. The 90 dBA applies to exposure to continuous noise. Information on impact noise and intermittent noises is even less available. Certain guidelines have been proposed for intermittent and part-time exposure to noise. These are described as follows by the Intersociety report.

In using the damage-risk curves that have been suggested, a number of qualifications should be applied:

1. The contours should not be taken too literally, since deviations of the order of 1 or 2 dB in either direction can be disregarded. Contours should generally be interpreted as zones with some uncertainty attending the measurement of the exposure stimulus, and the biological variability modifying the probability of damage.
2. The levels are considered to be safe in terms of exposures during working days for durations up to a lifetime.
3. The criterion levels apply to exposure noise that has a reasonably continuous time character with no substantial sharp energy peaks.
4. For wide-band noise, the curve designated "octave bands" should

TABLE III

ACCEPTABLE EXPOSURES TO NOISE IN DBA AS A FUNCTION OF THE NUMBER OF OCCURRENCES PER DAY

Daily Duration		Number of Times the Noise Occurs Per Day						
Hours	Minutes	1	3	7	15	35	75	160 up
8		90	90	90	90	90	90	90
6		91	93	96	98	97	95	94
4		92	95	99	102	104	102	100
2		95	99	102	106	109	114	
1		98	103	107	110	115		
	30	101	106	110	115			
	15	105	110	115				
	8	109	115					
	4	113						

To use the Table, select the column headed by the number of times the noise occurs per day, read down to the average sound level of the noise, and locate directly to the left in the first column the total duration of noise permitted for any 24 hour period. If necessary it is permissible to interpolate noise levels in dBA.

be used. For pure tones or for noise in which the major portion of the energy is concentrated in a band narrower than the critical band, the curve designated "critical bands" should be used.

5. This damage-risk criterion is a statistical concept and must be interpreted as such without discrimination, and without application to individual situations. Furthermore, it is a very complex concept involving variables that are incompletely understood, such as individual susceptibility to noise, its cumulative effect, and the relation of auditory fatigue to permanent deafness.

Compensation and Legal Aspects of Occupational Hearing Loss

One of the primary reasons for the increased interest in industrial noise problems is payment of compensation for occupationally caused loss of hearing. It has been known for many years that excessive noise can cause hearing loss. Certain types of deafness have even become associated with a specific noisy job such as "boilermaker's deafness," "airplane deafness," and "gunfire deafness." For many years it has been possible for workers to collect compensation for hearing loss in some states. However, the filing of large numbers of claims did not occur until after judicial interpretations in New York and Wisconsin established the principle of payment of compensation for partial loss of hearing without loss of earnings. These were the first instances in the compensation field in which payments were made for a partial loss of function as an occupational disease without direct economic loss.

The original basic concept of workmen's compensation was to provide payment for loss of earnings and for medical costs of injury arising out of employment. Under this concept, the employer gave up his common-law defenses of assumption of risk, contributory negligence, and negligence of a fellow employee. In return, the employee gave up his right to sue for whatever he could collect. Specific limits were placed on the amounts of liability. In addition to payments of compensation for lost earnings and payment of medical costs, specific awards were established for the loss of specific members—fingers, arms, legs, etc.—by accident.

Subsequent to the enactment of legislation for the above purposes, provision was made for payment of compensation for occupational diseases. Under the occupational disease provisions, there were no scheduled awards for loss of function only. Claimants had to establish a disability and sustain a loss of earnings in order to be compensated for an occupational disease.

The approach to the problem of compensation for partial hearing loss is based on the assumption that partial deafness, which develops over a period of time as a result of exposure to noise, is an occupational disease. Deafness caused by a single incident, such as an explosion, is generally considered as an accident.

This concept is not without exception in its application, however. In the State of Georgia in 1962, the court ruled that an employee's hearing loss resulted from the cumulative effect of a succession of injuries caused by each daily noise insult on the ear. On the basis of this type of reasoning, the court felt that the hearing loss was compensable under the accidental injury provisions of the law. This is a concept of "gradual injury" applied to hearing loss. It is a unique application of the concept of hearing loss in the United States. The case referred to in Georgia and the conclusions reached open serious questions, particularly since most informed people disagree with the otologic findings in this particular case.

In 1948 the New York Court of Appeals ruled in a hearing loss case that the claimant was entitled to compensation under a schedule award, even though he had not lost time and had suffered no loss of earnings. This decision established the concept of a schedule loss in an occupational disease without loss of time or loss of earnings. This departure from the wage-loss concept resulted in the filing of a large number of claims for loss of hearing in New York.

The influx of cases created a major problem for industry and insurance carriers through the principle of *accrued liability*—liability for injury which occurred prior to the Appellate Court decision. During this period many people were exposed to noise, but since it was not considered as compensable, self-insured industry had accumulated no reserves and insurance companies had collected no premiums from which to make payments. It posed a major economic problem.

An administrative directive by the Workmen's Compensation Board in New York provided that since hearing-loss measurements made while a person is still employed in a noisy environment represent a combination of both temporary and permanent hearing loss, no compensation should be paid unless the claimant had medical proof of permanent defective hearing. This provision was based on the theory that some recovery of hearing occurs following removal from the offending noise exposure.

In Wisconsin, which has also figured prominently in the development of the industrial noise story, the Workmen's Compensation Act provided for scheduled payments for loss of hearing— 133⅓ weeks ($12,000) for bilateral loss. In spite of the fact that the Act had been in force since 1931, the first significant number of claims was filed in 1951. During 1951 and 1952 a large number of claims developed. One of these was appealed to the Wisconsin Supreme Court to clarify several questions. The Industrial Accident Board made an award; the Circuit Court of Dane County reversed the Board's findings on the basis that hearing loss is an occupational disease and therefore not subject to a schedule award. In addition, the court found that no "last day of work" had been established.

Following this reversal, the Wisconsin legislature passed "stop-gap legislation" which provided for payment of compensation for hearing loss based on wage loss, with a maximum of $3,500. This law became effective July 1, 1953.

Just before this law went into effect several hundred claims totaling several million dollars were filed.

A few months later the Supreme Court of Wisconsin reversed the decision of the Circuit Court in the test case. This reversal caused considerable confusion.

As a result of many months of study and with the recommendation of the Wisconsin Industrial Commission Advisory Committee on Workmen's Compensation, a bill establishing a schedule payment for occupational hearing loss was passed by the Wisconsin legislature. It became effective July 1, 1955.

With respect to occupational deafness, this section of the Workmen's Compensation Act establishes a schedule for deafness in one ear, 160 weeks for total deafness in both ears, with proportionate compensation for permanent partial disability. It also provides that an employee must wait six months after the "time of injury" before filing a claim. The "time of injury" is defined as any one of the following: (1) transfer because of occupational deafness to non-noisy employment by an employer whose employment has caused occupational deafness; (2) retirement; (3) termination of the employer-employee relationship; or (4) layoff that is complete and continuous for one year.

Paragraph 7 of the new section is of special interest in its bearing upon preplacement hearing tests, and the opportunity these tests afford the employer to control his loss experience. An employee may not appeal for loss of hearing against an employer for whom he has not worked a total of at least 90 days (par. 6). However, (7) an employer shall become liable for the entire occupational deafness to which his employment has contributed; *but if previous deafness is established by a hearing test* or by other competent evidence, whether or not the employee was exposed to noise within the past six months preceding such test, the employer shall not be liable for previous loss so established, nor shall he be liable for any loss for which compensation has previously been paid or awarded. There is further provision that:

> No employee shall, in the aggregate, receive greater compensation from any or all employers for occupational deafness, than that provided in this section for total occupational deafness.

In many states where partial hearing loss due to noise exposure is not covered under workmen's compensation, and there are no specific provisions made for hearing loss compensation whether caused by accident or disease, it is often possible for compensation to be paid under "common law action." The economics and legal complications of such common-law action can be quite extensive and even alarming. In the state of New Jersey such an action has been taken on the basis that employers are negligent in failing to warn or protect employees in regard to their noise exposure. The results of this case in New Jersey have caused considerable apprehension and concern to management.

In summary, compensation for hearing loss resulting from occupational noise exposure can be collected under a variety of methods including:

(1) As an occupational disease specifically covered under Workmen's Compensation Law.
(2) As a "gradual injury" specified under accidental injury provisions.
(3) As an occupational injury covered by general workmen's compensation law.
(4) Under common-law action.

There is little doubt that on the basis of scientific evidence and practical experience the best method for compensating an occupational hearing loss is as a disease covered by specific legislation under the Workmen's Compensation Act.

Table II shows a 1970 compilation of the status of compensation for hearing loss in the states throughout the country. The differences in many of the states are quite marked, and a review of the various laws shows that those states having passed the most recent legislation tended to correct inequities and difficulties found in the application of laws of those states having passed earlier legislation.

Perhaps the most advanced legislation is that passed in the State of North Carolina. It includes certain advantages to both management and labor. It could well serve in many respects as a working "model law" for these states which still have not yet enacted special legislation for occupational hearing loss. The law passed in North Carolina is as follows:

GENERAL ASSEMBLY OF NORTH CAROLINA
1971 SESSION
RATIFIED BILL
CHAPTER 1108
SENATE BILL 674

AN ACT TO AMEND G.S. 97-53 RELATING TO COMPENSATION FOR OCCUPATIONAL DEAFNESS.

The General Assembly of North Carolina enacts:

Section 1. G.S. 97-53 is hereby amended by adding a new subsection at the end of such section as follows:

" (28) Loss of hearing caused by harmful noise in the employment. The following rules shall be applicable in determining eligibility for compensation and the period during which compensation shall be payable:

(a) The term 'harmful noise' means sound in employment capable of producing occupational loss of hearing as hereinafter defined. Sound of an intensity of less than 90 decibels, A scale, shall be deemed incapable of producing occupational loss of hearing as defined in this section.

(b) 'Occupational loss of hearing' shall mean a permanent sensorineural loss of hearing in both ears caused by prolonged exposure to harmful noise in employment. Except in instances of pre-existing loss of hearing due to disease, trauma, or congenital deafness in one ear, no compensation shall be payable under this act unless prolonged exposure to harmful noise in employment has caused loss of hearing in both ears as hereinafter provided.

(c) No compensation benefits shall be payable for temporary total or temporary partial disability under this act and there shall be no award for tinnitus or a psychogenic hearing loss.

(d) An employer shall become liable for the entire occupational hearing loss to which his employment has contributed, but if previous deafness is established by a hearing test or other competent evidence whether or not the employee was exposed to noise within six months preceding such test, the employer shall not be liable for previous loss so established, nor shall he be liable for any loss which compensation has previously been paid or awarded and the employer shall be liable only for the difference between the percent of occupational hearing loss determined as of the date of disability as herein defined and the percentage of loss established by the pre-employment and audiometric examination excluding, in any event, hearing losses arising from non-occupational causes.

(e) In the evaluation of occupational hearing loss, only the hearing levels at the frequencies of 500, 1,000 and 2,000 cycles per second shall be considered. Hearing losses for frequencies below 500 and above 2,000 cycles per second are not to be considered as constituting compensable hearing disability.

(f) The employer liable for the compensation in this section shall be the employer in whose employment the employee was last exposed to harmful noise in North Carolina during a period of 90 working days or parts thereof, and an exposure during a period of less than 90 working days or parts thereof shall be held not to be an injurious exposure; provided, however, that in the event an insurance carrier has been on the risk for a period of time during which an employee has been injuriously exposed to harmful noise, and if after insurance carrier goes off the risk said employee has been further exposed to harmful noise, although not exposed for 90 working days or parts thereof so as to constitute an injurious exposure, such carrier shall, nevertheless, be liable.

(g) The percentage of hearing loss shall be calculated as the average, in decibels, of the thresholds of hearing for the frequencies of 500, 1,000 and 2,000 cycles per second. Pure tone air conduction audiometric instruments, properly calibrated according to accepted national standards such as American Standards Association, Inc. (ASA), International Standards Organization (ISO), or American National Standards Institute, Inc. (ANSI), shall be used for measuring hearing loss. If more than one audiogram is taken, the audiogram having the lowest threshold will be used to calculate occupational hearing loss. If the losses of hearing average 15 decibels (26 dB if ANSI or ISO) or less in the three frequencies, such losses of hearing shall not constitute any compensable hearing disability. If the losses of hearing average 82 decibels (93 dB if ANSI or ISO) or more in the three frequencies, then the same shall constitute and be total or 100 percent compensable hearing loss. In measuring hearing impairment, the lowest measured losses in each of the three frequencies shall be added together and divided by three to determine the average decibel loss. To allow for the average amount of hearing loss from aging and non-occupational causes found in the population at a given age, there shall be deducted, before determining the percentage of hearing impairment, from the total average decibel loss $\frac{1}{2}$ decibel for each year of the employee's age over 38 at the time of last exposure to harmful noise. For each decibel of loss exceeding 15 decibels (26 dB if ANSI or ISO) an allowance of $1\frac{1}{2}$ percent shall be made up to the maximum of 100 percent which is reached at 82 decibels (93 dB if ANSI or ISO). In determining the binaural percentage of loss, the percentage of impairment in the better ear shall be multiplied by five. The resulting figure shall be added to the percentage of impairment in the poorer ear, and the sum of the two divided by six. The final percentage shall represent the binaural hearing impairment.

(h) There shall be payable for total occupational loss of hearing in both ears 150 weeks of compensation, and for partial occupational loss of hearing in both ears such proportion of these periods of payment as such partial loss bears to total loss.

(i) No claim for compensation for occupational hearing loss shall be filed until after six months have elapsed since exposure to harmful noise with the last employer. The last day of such exposure shall be the date of disability. The regular use of employer-provided protective devices capable of preventing loss of hearing from the particular harmful noise where the employee works shall constitute removal from exposure to such particular harmful noise.

(j) No consideration shall be given to the question of whether or not the ability of an employee to understand speech is improved by the use of a hearing aid. The employer shall not be obligated to furnish the employee with hearing aids, including accessories and replacement, in cases of occupational hearing loss.

(k) No compensation benefits shall be payable for loss of hearing caused by harmful noise after the effective date of this act if employee fails to regularly utilize employer-provided protection device or devices, capable of preventing loss of hearing from the particular harmful noise where the employee works."

It has been established that exposure to damaging noise produces damage in the inner ear causing a type of hearing loss classified as sensorineural nerve deafness. Consequently, it is advisable that every compensation act specify that the type of hearing impairment present in an employee be diagnosed as noise induced sensorineural loss, in order that the compensation act be applicable. This will help eliminate unwarranted claims due to conductive hearing loss and sensorineural losses of non-occupational origins.

Another feature of considerable importance is the problem of unilateral and bilateral deafness. Many states include in their workmen's compensation law a clause that hearing loss can be compensated if it constitutes deafness in one or both ears. These laws originally were written to cover accidental injury and not habitual noise exposure. However, the concept has been carried over to apply to occupational hearing loss in these acts. Since it is well established that in a free noise field where both ears are exposed to the same kind of noise, the hearing loss in both ears is equal or almost equal; it is advisable to stipulate that compensation for occupational hearing loss should be paid only in cases where both ears are impaired. In case of unilateral deafness due to noise of accidental origin, compensation is covered by accidental injury laws already available in practically all states.

An interesting feature of the North Carolina law is that it specifies that 90 dBA as the noise level below which a noise should not be considered hazardous enough to cause impaired hearing in both ears. (Assuming that the exposure must be for a full day's work over a period of many months and years.) This refers to continuous and not intermittent noise exposure. The North Carolina law also specifies that occupational hearing loss refers to "permanent" sensorineural loss, and consequently designates some waiting period to be able to definitely rule out any temporary hearing loss that may be present. The waiting period is generally accepted as 6 months from the last exposure. This time period has been based on important economic considerations in behalf of the employee and employer, rather than on scientific evidence. It helps to spread out the payment of claims and helps to establish the permanence of a hearing loss.

Establishing "last" day of injury is an important provision because of statute of limitation. Since it is difficult to set a specific date when a hearing loss was last caused, it is generally conceded that this loss takes place on the last day of employment and is revalued six months after the employee's removal from injurious noise.

The problem of apportioning parts of a hearing loss to the employee while in the plant where the hearing loss occurred is an important provision. Employers feel that should not be held accountable for hearing loss or part of a hearing loss that occurred while the employee was working for another company. Usually, compensation laws provide for the pattern of apportionment.

An essential part of a compensation act is the manner of calculating how much compensation an employee should receive for a specific amount of hearing loss. It is first necessary to distinguish the concepts of impairment and disability. Impairment is a medical concept that concerns "loss of living power" or reduction in the individual's enjoyment of daily living. More specifically, hearing impairment has been designated as an average loss of the three frequencies 500, 1,000, 2,000 cycles or more than 15 decibels (ASA). Disability involves many non-medical factors and includes a concept of loss of ability to earn a daily livelihood. Hearing impairment contributes to a disability but there are many other factors involved. Compensation law deals with paying compensation for disability.

Each state has its own method of paying for disability. The Subcommittee on Noise of the American Academy of Ophthalmology and Otolaryngology, developed a formula that has been generally accepted throughout the country as a basis for the compensating of occupational hearing loss.

The ultimate test in any formula for determining hearing disability is the ability to understand speech. But since speech audiometry has not been developed sufficiently for practical use, pure tone audiometry is utilized. The most important frequencies for hearing speech have been accepted as 500, 1,000, 2,000 Hz. A so-called "low-fence" of 15 dB ASA (26 dB ANSI) has been determined. Below these averages a hearing loss is considered insufficient to warrant compensation. Above these averages compensation is generally paid.

The following method for measuring hearing impairment for compensation has been adopted from a report prepared by the Subcommittee on Noise of the Committee on the Conservation of Hearing of the American Academy of Ophthalmology and Otolaryngology. It provides a method for measuring and calculating binaural hearing impairment. The hearing level for each frequency is the number of decibels that the listener's threshold of hearing lies above the standard audiometric zero for that frequency. It is the reading on the so-called "hearing level" dial of an audiometer.

The hearing level for speech is a simple average of the hearing levels at the three frequencies of 500, 1,000 and 2,000 Hz.

In order to evaluate the hearing impairment, it must be recognized that the range of impairment is not nearly as wide as the audiometric range of human hearing. Audiometric zero—which is presumably the average normal threshold level—is not the point at which impairment begins. If the average hearing level at 500, 1,000 and 2,000 Hz is 15 decibels or less (ASA) usually no impairment exists in the ability to hear everyday speech under everyday conditions. At the other extreme however, if the average hearing level at 500, 1,000 and 2,000 Hz is over 81.7 decibels, the impairment for hearing everyday speech should be considered total.

Example:

Cycles Per Second	Threshold Level Right Ear	Threshold Level Left Ear
500	35	20
1,000	40 } 120 dB	30 } 90 dB
2,000	45	40
3,000	45	45
4,000	50	50
6,000	60	60

$$\frac{120 \text{ dB}}{3} = 40 \text{ dB estimated hearing level for speech (right ear)}.$$

$$\frac{90 \text{ dB}}{3} = 30 \text{ dB estimated hearing level for speech (left ear)}.$$

To convert estimated hearing level for speech to percent impairment of hearing:

    40 dB

−15 dB hearing level for speech which is the upper limit of the no-impairment range

  25 dB right ear hearing level

  25 dB × 1.5% per decibel = 37.5% impairment of hearing in the right ear.

  30 dB estimated hearing level for speech (left ear).

−15 dB hearing level for speech which is upper limit of the no-impairment range

  15 dB hearing level of left ear.

  15 dB × 1.5% per decibel = 22.5% impairment of hearing in left ear.

To convert monaural impairments to binaural percentage impairment, the formula is:

  ((percent impairment in better ear × 5) + (percent impairment in worse ear)) divided by 6

Therefore:

  ((22.5% × 5) + 37.5%)) divided by 6 = 25% binaural impairment
  (112.5% + 37.5% divided by 6 = 25%)

Since it is well known that hearing sensitivity deteriorates with aging, it has been felt by many states that a deduction should be made for the natural deterioration of hearing due to sensorineural deafness before paying compensation for hearing impairment in older employees. The number of decibels usually deducted from the average hearing level is about half of a dB for each year beyond the age of 40, or in some states beyond the age of 50. Since there is still some contention as to the advisability and the amount of the deduction, each state has to decide the best course to follow.

Another important consideration in writing a compensation law for occupational hearing loss is establishing the accuracy of the audiograms presented. It is not uncommon in any court case to have two physicians present audiograms on the same individual with such varied thresholds as to perplex the judge and jury. Compensation acts should state that the best threshold should be used on which to calculate compensation. However, every effort must be made to be certain of the competence of the audiometric technician, and the competence of the physician interpreting the results.

REFERENCES

Background for Loss of Hearing Claims, American Mutual Insurance Alliance, 20 N. Wacker Drive, Chicago, Illinois (1964).

Committee on Medical Rating of Physical Impairment: Guides to Evaluation of Permanent Impairment; Eye, Nose, Throat and Related Structures, J Amer Med Assoc 177:489, Aug. 1961.

Guide for Conservation of Hearing in Noise. Supplement to the Transactions of the American Academy of Ophthalmology and Otolaryngology, AAOO Subcommittee on Noise Research Center, 3819 Marple Avenue, Dallas, Texas, Revised 1964.

Guidelines for Noise Exposure Control, Intersociety Committee on Guidelines for Noise Exposure Control.

Guidelines to the Department of Labor's Occupational Noise Standards for Federal Supply Contracts, Bulletin 334, U. S. Department of Labor, Workplace Standards Administration, Bureau of Labor Standards.

Guides for the Evaluation of Hearing Impairment, Trans. Amer. Acad. Ophthal. and Otolaryng., pp. 167-168, March-April 1959.

Industrial Noise Manual, American Industrial Hygiene Association, Detroit, Michigan, 2nd Edition, 1965.

Kryter, K. D.: The Effects of Noise on Man. Monograph Supplement #1, J Speech and Hearing Disorders, Wayne University, Detroit, Michigan, Sept. 1950.

Safety and Health Standards for Federal Supply Contracts, Under the Walsh-

Healey Public Contracts Act, and Federal Service Contracts under the McNamara-O'Hara Service Contract Act, Title 41, Part 50-204 of the Code of Federal Regulations, U. S. Department of Labor.

The Relations of Hearing Loss to Noise Exposure, Report of Explanatory Committee 2-24-x-2, American National Standards Institute, 1430 Broadway, New York, New York.

The Williams Steiger Occupational Safety and Health Act of 1970. U. S. Department of labor, Occupational Safety and Health Administration.

Chapter 10

PHYSICS OF SOUND

THE SENSATION OF SOUND is produced when pressure variations having a certain range of characteristics reach the ear. These pressure variations may be produced by any object that vibrates in a conducting medium with the proper cycle rate, or frequency, and amplitude. Sound may consist of a single frequency and amplitude; however, common noise spectra have many different frequency components with many different amplitudes.

Terminology

AMPLITUDE. The amplitude of sound may be described by the quantity of sound produced at a given location away from the source, or in terms of the overall ability of the source to emit sound. The amount of sound at a location away from the source is generally described by the sound pressure or sound intensity, while the ability of the source to produce sound is described by the sound power of the source.

FREE FIELD. A free field exists in a homogeneous, isotropic medium free from boundaries. In a free field, sound radiated from a source can be measured accurately without influence from the test space. True free-field conditions are rarely found except in expensive anechoic (echo-free) test chambers; however, approximate free-field conditions may be found in any homogeneous space where reflecting surfaces are at great distances from the measuring location as compared to the wavelengths of the sound being measured.

FREQUENCY (f). The frequency of sound describes the rate at which complete cycles of high and low pressure regions are produced by the sound source. The unit of frequency is the cycle

174

per second (cps) which is also called the hertz (Hz). The frequency range of the human ear is highly dependent upon the individual and the sound level, but a normal-hearing ear will have a range of approximately 20 to 20,000 cps at moderate sound levels. The frequency of a propagated sound wave heard by a listener will be the same as the frequency of the vibrating source if the distance between the source and the listener remains constant; however, the frequency detected by a listener will increase or decrease as the distance from the source is decreasing or increasing (Doppler effect).

LOUDNESS. The loudness of a sound is an observer's impression of its amplitude which includes the characteristics of the ear.

NOISE AND SOUND. The terms noise and sound are often used interchangeably, but generally, sound is descriptive of useful communication or pleasant sounds such as music while noise is used to describe discourse or unwanted sound.

PERIOD (T). The period is the time required for one cycle of pressure change to take place; hence, it is the reciprocal of the frequency. The period is measured in seconds.

PITCH. Pitch is used as a measure of auditory sensation that depends primarily upon frequency but also upon the pressure and wave form of the sound stimulus.

PURE TONE. A pure tone refers to a sound wave with a single simple sinusoidal change of level with time.

RANDOM NOISE. Random noise is made up of many frequency components whose instantaneous amplitudes occur randomly as a function of time.

RESONANCE. Resonance of a system exists when any change in the frequency of forced oscillation causes a decrease in the response of the system.

REVERBERATION. Reverberation occurs when sound persists after direct reception of the sound has stopped. The reverberation characteristics of a space is specified by the "reverberation time" which is the time required after the source has stopped radiating sound for the rms sound pressure to decrease 60 dB from its steady state level.

ROOT-MEAN-SQUARE (rms) SOUND PRESSURE. The root-mean-square (rms) value of a changing quantity, such as sound pressure, is the square root of the mean of the squares of the instantaneous values of the quantity.

SOUND INTENSITY (I). The sound intensity at a specific location is the average rate at which sound energy is transmitted through a unit area normal to the direction of sound propagation. The units used for sound intensity are joules per square meter per second. Sound intensity is also expressed in terms of a level (sound intensity level L_I) in decibels referenced to 10^{-12} watts per square meter.

SOUND POWER (P). The sound power of a source is the total sound energy radiated by the source per unit time. Sound power is normally expressed in terms of watts. Sound power is also expressed in terms of a level (sound power level L_P) in decibels referenced to 10^{-12} watts.

SOUND PRESSURE (p). Sound pressure normally refers to the rms value of the pressure changes above and below atmospheric pressure when used to measure steady state noise. Short term or impulse-type noises are described by peak pressure values. The units used to describe sound pressures are newtons per square meter (N/m^2), dynes per square centimeter (d/cm^2), or microbar. Sound pressure is also described in terms of a level (sound pressure level L_p), in decibels reference to 2×10^{-5} newtons per square meter.

VELOCITY (c). The speed at which the regions of sound-producing pressure changes move away from the sound source is called the velocity of propagation. Sound velocity varies directly with the square root of the density and inversely with the compressibility of the transmitting medium as well as with other factors; however, for practical purposes, the velocity of sound is constant in a given medium over the normal range of conditions. For example, the velocity of sound is approximately 1,130 ft/sec in air, 4,700 ft/sec in water, 13,000 ft/sec in wood, and 16,500 ft/sec in steel.

WAVELENGTH (λ). The distance required for one complete pressure cycle to be completed is called one wavelength. The wavelength (λ), a very useful tool in noise control work, may be calculated from known values of frequency (f) and velocity (c):

$$\lambda = c/f. \tag{1}$$

WHITE NOISE. White noise has an essentially random spectrum with equal energy per unit frequency bandwidth over a specified frequency band.

Noise Measurement and Calculations

THE DECIBEL (dB). The range of sound pressures commonly encountered is very wide. For example, sound pressures well above the pain threshold (about 20 newtons per square meter, N/m^2) are found in many work areas, while pressures down to the threshold of hearing (about 0.00002 N/m^2) are also of wide interest. This range of more than 10^6 N/m^2 cannot be scaled linearly with a practical instrument because such a scale might be many miles in length in order to obtain the desired accuracy at various pressure levels. In order to cover this very wide range of sound pressures with a reasonable number of scale divisions and to provide a means to obtain the required measurement accuracy at extreme pressure levels, the logarithmic decibel (dB) scale was selected. By definition, the dB is a dimensionless unit related to the logarithm of the ratio of a measured quantity to a reference quantity. The dB is commonly used to describe levels of acoustic intensity, acoustic power, hearing thresholds, electric voltage, electric current, electric power, etc., as well as sound-pressure levels; thus, it has no meaning unless a specific reference quantity is specified.

SOUND PRESSURE AND SOUND-PRESSURE LEVEL. Most sound-measuring instruments are calibrated to provide a reading of root-mean-square (rms) sound pressures on a logarithmic scale in decibels. The reading taken from an instrument is called a sound-pressure level (L_p). The term "level" is used because the pressure measured is at a level above a given pressure reference. For sound measurements in air, 0.00002 N/m^2* commonly serves

---

* An equivalent reference 0.0002 dynes per square centimeter is often used in older literature. The microbar is also used in older literature interchangably with the dyne per square centimeter.

as the reference sound pressure. This reference is an arbitrary pressure chosen many years ago because it was thought to approximate the normal threshold of human hearing at 1,000 Hz. The mathematical form of the L_p is written as:

$$L_p = 20 \log \frac{p}{p_o} \text{ dB,} \qquad (2)$$

where p is the measured rms sound pressure, p_o is the reference sound pressure, and the logarithm (log) is to the base 10. Thus, L_p should be written in terms of decibels referenced to a specified pressure level. For example, in air, the notation for L_p is commonly abbreviated as "dB re 0.00002 N/m²."

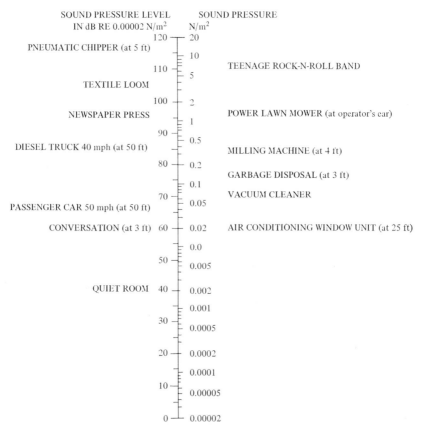

Figure 35. Relationship Between A-Weighted Sound-Pressure Level in Decibels (db) and Sound pressure in N/m².

Figure 35 shows the relationship between sound pressure in N/m² and sound pressure level in dB re 0.00002 N/m², and illustrates the advantage of using the dB scale rather than the wide range of direct pressure measurements. It is of interest to note that any pressure range over which the pressure is doubled is equivalent to six decibels whether at high or low levels. For example, a range of 0.00002 to 0.00004 N/m², which might be found in hearing measurements, and a range of 10 to 20 N/m², which might be found in hearing conservation programs, are both ranges of six decibels.

The L_p referenced to 0.00002 N/m² may be written in the form:

$$L_p = 20 \log (p/0.00002)$$
$$= 20 [\log p - \log 0.00002]$$
$$= 20 [\log p - (\log 2 - \log 10^5)]$$
$$= 20 [\log p - (0.3 - 5)]$$
$$= 20 (\log p + 4.7)$$
$$= 20 \log p + 94 \text{ re } 0.00002 \text{ N/m}^2. \tag{3}$$

SOUND INTENSITY AND SOUND-INTENSITY LEVEL. Sound intensity (I) at any specified location may be defined as the average acoustic energy per unit time passing through a unit area that is normal to the direction of propagation. For a spherical or free-progressive sound wave, the intensity may be expressed by

$$I = \frac{p^2}{\rho c}, \tag{4}$$

where p is the rms sound pressure, ρ is the density of the medium, and c is the speed of sound in the medium. It is obvious from this definition that sound intensity describes, in part, characteristics of the sound in the medium, but does not directly describe the sound source itself.

Sound intensity units, like sound pressure units, cover a wide range, and it is often desirable to use dB levels to compress the measuring scale. To be consistent with Equations (2) and (4), intensity level (L_I) is defined as

$$L_I = 10 \log \frac{I}{I_0} \text{ dB}, \tag{5}$$

where I is the measured intensity at some given distance from the source and I_0 is a reference intensity. The reference intensity commonly used is 10^{-12} watts/m². In air, this reference closely corresponds to the reference pressure 0.00002 N/m² used for sound-pressure levels.

SOUND POWER AND SOUND-POWER LEVEL. Sound power (P) is used to describe the sound source in terms of the amount of acoustic energy that is produced per unit time. Sound power may be related to the average sound intensity produced in free-field conditions at a distance r from a point source by

$$P = I_{avg} \ 4\pi r^2, \qquad (6)$$

where I_{avg} is the average intensity at a distance r from a sound source whose acoustic power is P. The quantity $4\pi r^2$ is the area of a sphere surrounding the source over which the intensity is averaged. It is obvious from Equation (6) that the intensity will decrease with the square of the distance from the source; hence, the well-known inverse-square law.

Power units are often described in terms of decibel levels because of the wide range of powers covered in practical applications. Power level L_P is defined by

$$L_P = 10 \ \log \frac{P}{P_o}, \qquad (7)$$

where P is the power of the source, and P_o is the reference power. The arbitrarily chosen reference power commonly used is 10^{-12} watt. Figure 2 shows the relationship between sound power in watts and sound-power level in dB re 10^{-12} watt.

RELATIONSHIP OF SOUND POWER, SOUND INTENSITY, AND SOUND PRESSURE. Many noise-control problems require a practical knowledge of the relationship between pressure, intensity, and power. An example would be the prediction of sound-pressure levels that would be produced around a proposed machine location from the sound-power level provided for the machine.

Example:

Predict the sound-pressure level that would be produced at a distance of 100 feet from a pneumatic chipping hammer. The manufacturer of the chipping hammer states that the hammer has an acoustic power output of 1.0 watt.

From Equations (4) and (6) in free field for an omnidirectional source:

$$P = I_{avg} \ 4\pi r^2 = \frac{p^2_{avg} \ 4\pi r^2}{\rho c} \ , \qquad (8)$$

where

$$P_{avg} = \sqrt{\frac{P\rho c}{4\pi r^2}} \ . \qquad (9)$$

If P is given in watts, r in feet, and p in N/m², then, with standard conditions, Equation (9) may be rewritten as

$$P_{avg} = \sqrt{\frac{3.5P \times 10^2}{r^2}} \ , $$

and, for this example,

$$P_{avg} = \sqrt{\frac{3.5 \times 1.0 \times 10^2}{(100)^2}} = 0.187 \ N/m^2.$$

The sound-pressure level may be determined from Equation (2) to be:

$$L_p = 20 \ \log \frac{0.187}{0.00002} = 79.4 \ dB \ re \ 0.00002 \ N/m^2.$$

Noise levels in locations that are reverberant can be expected to be somewhat higher than predicted because of the sound reflected back to the point of measurement.

COMBINING SOUND LEVELS. Often, it is necessary to combine sound levels (dB). An example is the combination of frequency-band levels to obtain the overall or total sound-pressure level. Another example is the estimation of total sound-pressure level resulting from adding a machine of known noise spectrum to an existing noise environment of known characteristics. Simple addition of individual sound-pressure levels, which are logarithmic quantities, constitutes multiplication of pressure ratios; therefore, the sound pressure corresponding to each sound-pressure level must be determined and added with respect to existing phase relationships.

For the most part, industrial noise is broadband with nearly random phase relationships. Sound-pressure levels of random

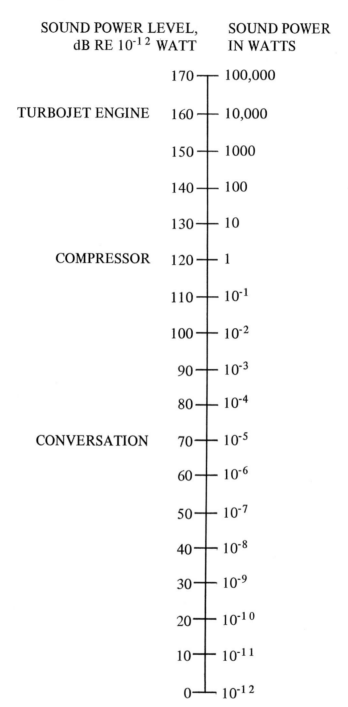

Figure 36. Relationship between sound power level in decibels (db) and sound power in watts.

noises can be added by converting the levels to pressure, then to intensity units which may be added arithmetically, and reconverting the resultant intensity to pressure and finally to sound-pressure levels in dB. Equations (2) and (4) can be used in free-field conditions for this purpose.

A more convenient way to add the sound-pressure levels of two separate random noise sources is to use Table IV. To add one random noise level $L_p(1)$, measured at a point to another, $L_p(2)$, measured by itself at the same point, the numerical difference between the levels, $L_p(2)—L_p(1)$, is used in Table IV to find the corresponding value of $L_p(3)$ which, in turn, is added arithmetically to the larger of $L_p(1)$ or $L_p(2)$ to obtain the resultant of $L_p(1) + L_p(2)$. If more than two are to be added, the resultant of the first two must be added to the third, the resultant of the three sources to the fourth, etc., until all levels have been added, or until the addition of smaller values do not add significantly to the total.

Example:

The overall sound-pressure level produced by a random-noise source can be calculated by adding the sound-pressure levels measured in octave bands shown in the following table:

Octave band center frequency (Hz)	31.5	63	125	250	500	1,000	2,000	4,000	8,000
Sound-pressure level (dB)	85	88	94	94	95	100	97	90	88

A good procedure for adding a series of dB values is to begin with the highest levels so that calculations may be stopped when lower values are reached which do not add significantly to the total. In this example, the levels of 100 and 97 have a difference of 3 that corresponds with $L_p(3) = 1.8$ in Table IV. Thus, 100 dB + 97 dB = 100 + 1.8 = 101.8 dB. Combining 101.8 and 95, the next higher level, gives 101.8 + 0.8 = 102.6 dB which is the total of the first three bands. This procedure is continued with one band at a time until the overall sound-pressure level is found to be about 104 dB.

The overall sound-pressure level calculated in the above example corresponds to the value that would be found by reading a sound level meter at this location with the frequency weighting set so that each frequency in the spectrum is weighted equally.

Common names given to this frequency weighting are flat, linear, 20 kc, and overall.

The corresponding A-weighted sound-pressure level (dBA) found in many noise regulations may also be calculated from octave band values such as those in the above example if the adjustments given in Table V are first applied. For example, the octave band levels with A-weighting corresponding to the above example would be:

Octave band center
  frequency (Hz) 31.5   63   125   250   500   1,000   2,000   4,000   8,000
Sound-pressure level
  (A-weighted) (dB) 45.8 61.9 77.8 85.4 91.7   100   98.2   91.0   86.9

These octave band levels with A-frequency weighting can be added by the procedure described above to obtain the resultant A-weighted level which is about 103 dBA.

A large majority of industrial noises have random frequency characteristics and may be combined as described in the above paragraphs. However, there are a few cases of noises with pitched or major pure-tone components where these calculations will not hold, and phase relationships must be considered. In areas where pitched noises are present, standing waves will often be recognized by rapidly varying sound-pressure levels over short distances. It is not practical to try to predict levels in areas where standing waves are present.

When the sound-pressure levels of two pitched sources are added, it might be assumed that the resultant sound-pressure level $L_p(R)$ will be less as often as it is greater than the level of a single source, however, in almost all cases, the resultant $L_p(R)$ is greater than either single source. The reason for this may be seen if two pure-tone sources are added at several specified phase differences (see Figure 37). At zero phase difference, the resultant of two like pure-tone sources is 6 dB greater than either single level. At a phase difference of 90°, the resultant is 3 dB greater than either level. Between 90° and 0°, the resultant is somewhere between 3 and 6 dB greater than either level. At a phase difference of 120°, the resultant is equal to the individual levels; and between 120° and 90°, the resultant is between 0 and 3 dB greater than either level. At 180°, there is complete cancellation of

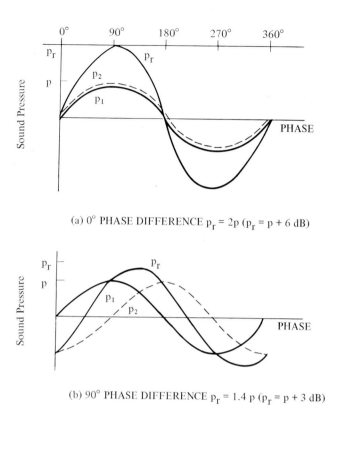

(a) 0° PHASE DIFFERENCE $p_r = 2p$ ($p_r = p + 6$ dB)

(b) 90° PHASE DIFFERENCE $p_r = 1.4$ p ($p_r = p + 3$ dB)

(c) 120° PHASE DIFFERENCE $p_r = p$ ($p_r = p + 0$ dB)

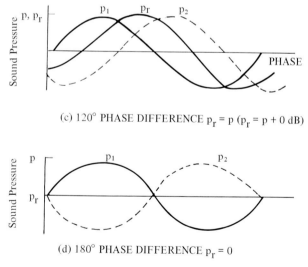

(d) 180° PHASE DIFFERENCE $p_r = 0$

Figure 37. Combinations of two pure tone noises (p_1 and p_2) phase differences.

sound. Obviously, the resultant $L_p(R)$ is greater than the individual levels for all phase differences from 0° to 120°, but less than individual levels for phase differences from 120° and 180° —a factor of 2:1. Also, most pitched tones are not single tones but combinations thereof; thus, almost all points in the noise fields will have pressure levels exceeding the individual levels.

FREQUENCY BANDWIDTHS. The most common frequency bandwidth used for industrial noise measurements is the octave band. A frequency band is said to be an octave in width when its upper band-edge frequency f_2 is twice the lower band-edge frequency f_1:

$$f_2 = 2f_1. \tag{10}$$

Octave bands are commonly used for measurements directly related to the effects of noise on the ear and for some noise-control work because they provide the maximum amount of information in a reasonable number of measurements.

When more specific characteristics of a noise source are required, such as might be the case for pinpointing a particular noise source in a background of other sources, it is necessary to use narrower frequency bandwidths than octave bands. Half-octave, third-octave and narrower bands are used for these purposes. A half-octave bandwidth is defined as a band whose upper band-edge frequency f_2 is the square root of 2 times the lower band-edge frequency f_1:

$$f_2 = \sqrt{2} f_1. \tag{11}$$

A third-octave bandwidth is defined as a band whose upper band-edge frequency f_2 is the cube root of 2 times the lower band-edge frequency f_1:

$$f_2 = \sqrt[3]{2} f_1. \tag{12}$$

The center frequency f_m of any of these bands is the square root of the product of the high and low band-edge frequencies (geometric mean):

$$f_m = \sqrt{f_2 f_1}. \tag{13}$$

It should be noted that the upper and lower band-edge frequencies describing a frequency band do not imply abrupt cutoffs at these frequencies. These band-edge frequencies are conventionally used as the 3-dB-down points of gradually sloping curves that meet the American Standard Specification for Octave, Half-Octave, and Third-Octave Band Filter Sets S1.11-1966.[3]

COMPARING LEVELS HAVING DIFFERENT BANDWIDTHS. Noise-measurement data (rms) taken with analyzers of a given bandwidth may be converted to another given bandwidth *if* the frequency range covered has a continuous spectrum with no prominent changes in level. The conversion may be made in terms of sound-pressure levels by

$$L_p(A) = L_p(B) - 10 \log \frac{\Delta f(B)}{\Delta f(A)}, \tag{14}$$

where

$L_p(A) = $ the sound-pressure level, in dB, of the band having a width $\Delta f(A)$ Hz.

$L_p(B) = $ the sound-pressure level, in dB, of the band having a width $\Delta f(B)$ Hz.

Sound-pressure levels for different bandwidths of flat continuous spectrum noises may also be converted to spectrum levels. The spectrum level describes a continuous-spectrum wide-band noise in terms of its energy equivalent in a band one cps wide, assuming that no prominent peaks are present. The spectrum level L_p (S) may be determined by

$$L_p(S) = L_p(f) - 10 \log \Delta f, \tag{15}$$

where

$L_p(\Delta f) = $ the sound-pressure level of the band having a width of f Hz,

$\Delta f = $ the bandwidth in Hz, and

$f = $ the center frequency of the band Δf Hz wide.

It should be emphasized that accurate conversion of sound-pressure levels from one bandwidth to another by the method described above can be accomplished only when the frequency bands have flat continuous spectra.

Noise Propagation Characteristics—Practical Solutions

The sound-power level supplied by the manufacturer of noise-making equipment can be used to predict sound-pressure levels that will be produced by the equipment in surrounding work areas if the acoustical characteristics of the work area are known. These calculations are complex if all factors are considered, but simple approximate solutions to general cases are often helpful to estimate levels.

NOISE SOURCE IN FREE FIELD. A free field has been defined as one in which the sound pressure decreases inversely with the distance from the source. These ideal acoustical conditions are rarely found in work environments because of the reflecting surfaces of equipment, walls, ceilings, floors, etc.; however, free-field conditions may sometimes be approached outdoors or in very large rooms. For standard free-field conditions, the sound-pressure level L_p at a given distance r from a small omnidirectional noise source can be written in terms of the sound-power level L_p of the source as

$$L_p = L_p - 20 \log r - 0.5, \qquad (16)$$

where r is in feet, L_p is in dB referenced to 0.00002 N/m², and L_P is in dB referenced to 10^{-12} watts.

Many noise sources have pronounced directional characteristics; that is, they will radiate more noise in one direction than another. Therefore, it will be necessary for the equipment manufacturer to provide the directional characteristics of the source, as well as the power levels, to predict the sound-pressure levels. The directional characteristics of the source are generally given in terms of the directivity factor Q. Q is defined as the ratio of the sound power of a small, omnidirectional, imaginary source to the sound power of the actual source where both sound powers produce the same sound-pressure level at the measurement position. The directivity factor may be added to Equation (16) in the form

$$L_p = L_P - 20 \log r - 0.5 + 10 \log Q, \qquad (17)$$

where $10 \log Q$ is called the directivity index.

Example:

Predict the sound-pressure level that will be produced in a free field at a distance of 100 feet directly in front of a particular machine. A directivity factor of 5 is provided by the machine manufacturer for this location. The noise source has a continuous spectrum and a sound power of 0.1 watt.

From Equation (17):

$$L_p = 10 \log \left(\frac{0.1}{10^{-12}} \right) - 20 \log 100 - 0.5 + 10 \log 5$$
$$= 10 (\log 0.1 - \log 10^{-12}) - 20(2) - 0.5 + 10(0.7)$$
$$= 10(-1 + 12) - 40 - 0.5 + 7$$
$$= 76.5 \text{ dB re } 0.00002 \text{ N/m}^2.$$

NOISE SOURCE IN REVERBERANT FIELD. In reverberant fields where a high percentage of reflected sound energy is present, the sound-pressure levels may be essentially independent of direction and distance to the noise source. Levels in these reverberant areas depend upon room dimensions, object size and placement in the room, and upon the acoustical absorption characteristics of sur-

TABLE IV

A-FREQUENCY WEIGHTING ADJUSTMENTS[2]

$f(Hz)$	Correction
25	−44.7
32	−39.4
40	−34.6
50	−30.2
63	−26.2
80	−22.5
100	−19.1
125	−16.1
160	−13.4
200	−10.9
250	− 8.6
315	− 6.6
400	− 4.8
500	− 3.2
630	− 1.9
800	− 0.8
1,000	0.0
1,250	+ 0.6
1,600	+ 1.0
2,000	+ 1.2
2,500	+ 1.3
3,150	+ 1.2
4,000	+ 1.0
5,000	+ 0.5
6,300	− 0.1
8,000	− 1.1
10,000	− 2.5
12,500	− 4.3
16,000	− 6.6
20,000	− 9.3

faces in the room. Additional complications may be present in the form of regions of enforcement and cancellation of sound pressure, standing waves, caused by strong pure-tone components being reflected. Thus, it is extremely difficult to predict sound-pressure levels at a particular point in a reverberant area.

SOUND ABSORPTION. A room's acoustical characteristics are strongly dependent upon the absorption coefficients of its surface areas. A surface that absorbs all energy incident on its surface is said to have an absorption coefficient of one, while a surface that reflects all incident energy has an absorption coefficient of zero.

A rule of thumb that may be used to determine the amount of noise reduction possible from the application of acoustically absorbent material on room surfaces is as follows:

$$\text{dB reduction} = 10 \log \frac{\text{absorption units after}}{\text{absorption units before}},$$

where the absorption units are the sum of the products of surface areas and their respective noise absorption coefficients.[4, 5, 6]

TRANSMISSION LOSS (TL) OF BARRIERS. Sound transmission loss (TL) through a barrier may be defined as ten times the logarithm (to the base 10) of the ratio of the acoustic energy transmitted through the barrier to the incident acoustic energy. The TL of a barrier is a physical property of the material used for a given wall construction. The TL for continuous, random noise commonly found in industry increases about 5 dB for each doubling of wall weight per unit of surface area, and for each doubling of frequency.

Multiple wall construction with enclosed air spaces provides considerably more attenuation than the single-wall mass law would predict.[7, 8, 9] However, considerable care must be taken to avoid rigid connections between multiple walls when they are constructed or any advantages in attentuation will be nullified.[10, 11]

Noise leaks which result from cracks or holes, or from windows or doors, in a noise barrier can severely limit noise reduction characteristics of the barrier. In particular, care must be exercised throughout construction to prevent leaks that may be

TABLE V

TABLE FOR COMBINING DECIBEL LEVELS OF NOISES
WITH RANDOM FREQUENCY CHARACTERISTICS

Sum (L_R) of dB Levels L_1 and L_2		
Numerical Difference Bewteen Levels L_1 and L_2	L_3: Amount to Be Added to the Higher of L_1 or L_2	
0.0 to 0.1	3.0	Step 1: Determine the difference
0.2 to 0.3	2.9	between the two levels to be
0.4 to 0.5	2.8	added (L_1 and L_2).
0.6 to 0.7	2.7	
0.8 to 0.9	2.6	Step 2: Find the number (L_3)
1.0 to 1.2	2.5	corresponding to this differ-
1.3 to 1.4	2.4	ence in the Table.
1.5 to 1.6	2.3	
1.7 to 1.9	2.2	Step 3: Add the number (L_3) to
2.0 to 2.1	2.1	the highest of L_1 and L_2 to
2.2 to 2.4	2.0	obtain the resultant level
2.5 to 2.7	1.9	($L_R = L_1 + L_2$).
2.8 to 3.0	1.8	
3.1 to 3.3	1.7	
3.4 to 3.6	1.6	
3.7 to 4.0	1.5	
4.1 to 4.3	1.4	
4.4 to 4.7	1.3	
4.8 to 5.1	1.2	
5.2 to 5.6	1.1	
5.7 to 6.1	1.0	
6.2 to 6.6	0.9	
6.7 to 7.2	0.8	
7.3 to 7.9	0.7	
8.0 to 8.6	0.6	
8.7 to 9.6	0.5	
9.7 to 10.7	0.4	
10.8 to 12.2	0.3	
12.3 to 14.5	0.2	
14.6 to 19.3	0.1	
19.4 to ∞	0.0	

caused by electrical outlets, plumbing connections, telephone lines, etc., in otherwise effective barriers.

REFERENCES

1. Holliday, D. and R. Resnick: *Physics* (p. 512), New York, John Wiley, 1967.
2. American Standard Specification for Sound Level Meters, S1.4-1971, American National Standards Institute, 1430 Broadway, New York, N. Y. 10016.

3. American Standard Specification for Octave, Half-Octave, and Third-Octave Filter Sets, S1.11-1966, American National Standards Institute, 1430 Broadway, New York, N. Y. 10016.
4. Beranek, L. L.: *Acoustics.* New York, McGraw-Hill, 1954.
5. "Performance Data Architectural Acoustical Materials," issued annually by Acoustical and Insulating Materials Association (AIMA), 205 W. Touhy Ave., Park Ridge, Illinois 60068 (Bulletin XXX issued 1970).
6. "Sound Absorption Coefficients of the More Common Acoustic Materials," National Bureau of Standards, U. S. Department of Commerce, Letter Circular L C 870.
7. "Guide to Airborne, Impact and Structureborne Noise Control in Multi-Family Dwellings," U. S. Department of Housing and Urban Development, September, 1967 (U. S. Government Printing Office, FT/TS-24).
8. "Field and Laboratory Measurements of Airborne and Impact Sound Transmission," ISO/R 140—1960(E), International Organization for Standardization, 1 Rue de Varembe, Geneva, Switzerland.
9. "Recommended Practice for Laboratory Measurement of Airborne Sound Transmission Loss of Building Floors and Walls," American Society for Testing Materials (ASTM), 1916 Race Street, Philadelphia, Pennsylvania 19103, Designation E-90-70 (1970).
10. Bonvallet, G. L.: Retaining High Sound Transmission Loss in Industrial Plants. Noise Control *3* (2), 61-64 (1957).
11. Beranek, L. L.: *Noise Reduction.* New York, McGraw-Hill, 1960.

Chapter 11

NOISE MEASUREMENT

AIRBORNE SOUND PRESSURE levels from a wide range of frequency spectra can be measured with a sound level meter if the levels do not change rapidly. The characteristics of rapidly changing sound levels must be measured with an oscilloscope or peak reading instruments designed for this purpose. If information on sound pressure distribution over the frequency spectrum is required, analyzers or filters must be used in conjunction with a sound level meter.

The Sound Level Meter

Basically, the sound level meter consists of a microphone, an amplifier-attenuator circuit, and an indicating meter. The microphone transforms airborne acoustic pressure variations into electrical signals with the same frequency and amplitude characteristics, and feeds the electrical signals to a carefully calibrated amplifier-attenuator circuit. The electrical signals are then directed through a logarithmic weighting network to an indicating meter where the sound pressure is displayed in the form of levels above 0.00002 newtons per square meter.

Most sound-measuring instruments present the sound-pressure levels in terms of its root-mean-square (rms) value which is defined as the square root of the mean squared displacements during one period. The rms value is useful for hearing conservation purposes because it is related to acoustic power and it correlates with human response. Also, the rms value of a random noise is directly proportional to the bandwidth; hence, the rms value of any bandwidth is the logarithmic sum of the rms values of its component narrow bands. For example, octave-band levels may be added logarithmically to find the overall level for the frequency range covered. The rms value of pure tones or sine waves is equal to 0.707 times the maximum value (see Figure 38).

Rms values cannot be used to describe prominent peak pressures of noise which extend several dB above a relatively constant background noise. Maximum, or peak, values are used for this purpose. On the other hand, peak readings are of relatively little

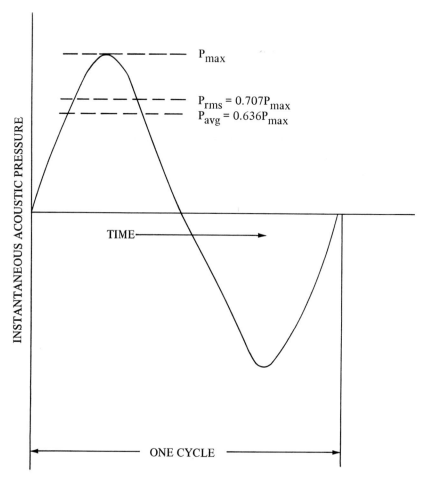

P_{max}

$P_{rms} = 0.707P_{max}$
$P_{avg} = 0.636P_{max}$

TIME

INSTANTANEOUS ACOUSTIC PRESSURE

ONE CYCLE

Figure 38. A comparison of maximum (P_{max}) or peak, root-mean-square (P_{rms}), and rectified-average (P_{avg}) values of acoustic pressure.

value for measuring sustained noises unless the waveform is known to be sinusoidal because the peak reading's relationship to acoustic power changes with the complexity of the wave. As the waveform becomes more complex, the peak value can be as much as 25 dB above the measured rms value.

In addition to the rms and peak values, a rectified average value of the acoustic pressure is sometimes used for noise measurements. A rectified average value is an average taken over a period of time without regard to whether the instantaneous signal values are positive or negative. The rectified average value of a sine wave is equal to 0.636 times the peak value. For complex waveforms, the rectified average value may fall as much as 2 dB below the rms value. In some cases, rectified average characteristics have been used in sound level meters by adjusting the output to read 1 dB above the rms level for sine wave signals, so that the average reading will always be within 1 dB of the true rms value. Figure 1 shows a comparison of root-mean-square, maximum, and rectified average values of a sinusoidal wave.[1, 2, 3]

METER INDICATION AND RESPONSE SPEED. The indicating meter of a sound level meter may have ballistic characteristics that are not constant over its entire dynamic range, or scale, which will result in different readings depending upon the attenuator setting and the portion of the meter scale used. When a difference in readings is noted, the reading using the higher part of the meter scale (the lowest attenuator setting) should be used, since the ballistics are generally more carefully controlled in this portion of the scale.

Most general-purpose sound level meters have fast and slow meter response characteristics that may be used for measuring sustained noise.[4] The fast response enables the meter to reach within 4 dB of its calibrated reading for a 0.2 second pulse of 1,000 cps; thus, it can be used to measure with reasonable accuracy noises whose levels do not change substantially in periods less than 0.2 second. The slow response is intended to provide an averaging effect that will make widely fluctuating sound levels easier to read; however, this setting will not provide accurate readings if the sound levels change significantly in less than 0.5 second.

FREQUENCY-WEIGHTING NETWORKS. General-purpose sound level meters are normally equipped with three frequency-weighting networks, A, B, and C, that can be used to approximate the frequency distribution of noise over the audible spectrum.[4] These three frequency weightings shown in Figure 39 were chosen because (1) they approximate the ear's response characteristics at different sound levels and (2) they can be easily produced with a few common electronic components. Also shown on Figure 39 is a linear or flat response that weights all frequencies equally.

The A-frequency weighting approximates the ear's response characteristics for low level sound, below about 55 dB re 0.00002 n/m². The B-frequency weighting is intended to approximate the ear's response for levels between 55 and 85 dB, and the C weighting corresponds to the ear's response for levels above 85 dB.

In use, the frequency distribution of noise energy can be approximated by comparing the levels measured with each of the frequency weightings. For example, if the noise levels measured using the A and C networks are approximately equal, it can be

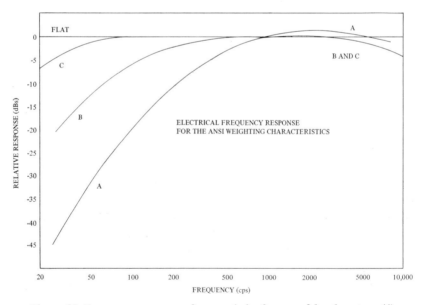

Figure 39. Frequency-response characteristics for sound level meters (4).

reasoned that most of the noise energy is above 1,000 Hz because this is the only portion of the spectrum where the weightings are similar. On the other hand, if there is a large difference between these readings, most of the energy will be found below 1,000 Hz.

Many specific uses have been made of the individual weightings besides the frequency distribution of noise. In particular, the A network has been given prominence in recent years as a means for estimating annoyance caused by noise and for estimating the risk of noise-induced hearing damage.

Microphones

The three basic types of microphones commonly used for noise measurements are: piezoelectric, dynamic, and condenser. Each of these types has advantages and disadvantages that depend upon the specific measurement situation; all three types can be made to meet the American Standard Specification for General Purpose Sound Meters, S1.4.1961.[4] The dynamic and piezoelectric microphone designs are normally less expensive than the condenser type and are provided as standard equipment with most low- and medium-priced sound measuring instruments.

FREQUENCY RESPONSE CHARACTERISTICS. Piezoelectric microphones used with sound measuring equipment have reasonably flat response characteristics for low and middle audible frequencies; however, the high-frequency responses are not as flat, nor do they extend as far, as dynamic or condenser types. Good quality piezoelectric microphones are normally acceptable for a frequency range of from about 15 to 8,000 Hz. A few dynamic microphones have a somewhat more uniform frequency response than the piezoelectric type above 1,000 Hz and their upper range may extend above 12,000 Hz. Various condenser microphone sizes may be used with sound measuring instruments to cover a very wide frequency range from a few Hz to well over 100,000 Hz. Tolerance limits for sound level meters (including the microphone) are included in the ANSI Specification for General-Purpose Sound Level Meters.[4]

SOUND LEVEL RANGE. Most of the one-inch microphones supplied as standard equipment with sound level meters have a dynamic range of about 20 to 145 dB re 0.00002 n/m^2 but the sound level meter circuitry may limit low measurements to levels greater than 40 dB. Special purpose microphones designed for use at high noise levels usually will have approximately the same dynamic range but their lower overall sensitivity shifts the upper limit to higher levels than possible with the standard microphones. For example, the ½-, ¼-, and ⅛-inch condenser microphones may have dynamic ranges of about 30 to 160 dB, 50 to 175 dB, and 60 to 185 dB.

TEMPERATURE AND HUMIDITY EFFECTS. The Rochelle-salt microphones that were supplied with older sound measuring equipment are easily damaged by heat or humidity extremes. These piezoelectric microphones can be permanently damaged by heat such as that produced in a closed car on a hot day; therefore, extreme care should be taken in their use and storage. The piezoelectric microphones made with barium titanate or lead zirconate titanate that are furnished with most sound measuring equipment today are not damaged by exposure to normal ranges of temperature and humidity. However, temporary erroneous readings may result from condensation if they are moved from very cold to warm humid areas.

The dynamic microphone's response characteristics are somewhat dependent upon the ambient temperature, but over most of the audible frequency range, the variation is less than about 1 dB for 50°F change in temperature. The dynamic microphone is affected relatively little by humidity extremes, except for temporary erroneous readings that may result from condensation. Specific temperature correction information for each microphone should be available from the manufacturer.

The condenser microphone is not permanently damaged by exposure to humidity extremes, but high humidity may cause temporary erroneous readings. The variation of sensitivity of condenser microphones with temperature is approximately −0.04 dB per degree F. Here again, correction information for a specific microphone should be obtained from the manufacturer.

MICROPHONE DIRECTIONAL CHARACTERISTICS. Most noises encountered in industry are produced from many different noise sources and from their reflected energies. Therefore, at any given position in these areas, noise will be coming from many different directions and often may be considered to be randomly incident upon any plane where a microphone diaphragm might be placed. For this reason, microphones are sometimes calibrated for randomly incident sound; however, depending upon the design and purpose of the microphone, they may be calibrated for grazing incidence, perpendicular incidence, or for use in couplers (pressure calibration). Thus, care must be taken to use microphones in the manner specified by the manufacturer in order to obtain the highest accuracy.

Microphones commonly used with sound-measuring equipment are nearly omnidirectional for frequencies below 1,000 Hz; however, directional characteristics become important for frequencies above 1,000 Hz (see Figure 40). Therefore, when measurements are to be made of high frequency noise produced by a directional noise source, i.e. where a high percentage of the noise energy is coming from one direction, the orientation of the microphone becomes very important even though this microphone may be described as omnidirectional. For a microphone calibrated with randomly incident sound, the microphone should be pointed at an angle to the major noise source that is specified

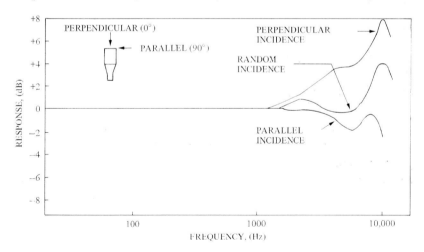

Figure 40. Directional Characteristics of a Piezoelectric Microphone.

by the manufacturer. An angle of about 70° from the axis of the microphone is often used to produce similar characteristics to randomly incident waves, but the angle for each microphone should be supplied by the manufacturer. A free-field microphone is calibrated to measure sounds perpendicularly incident to the microphone diaphragm; thus, it should be pointed directly at the source to be measured. A pressure-type microphone is designed for use in a coupler such as those used for calibrating audiometers; however, this microphone can be used to measure noise over most of the audible spectrum if the noise propagation is at grazing incidence to the diaphragm and the microphone calibration curve is used.

Directional characteristics of microphones may be used to advantage at times. For example, an improved signal-to-noise ratio may be obtained for sound pressure-level measurements of a given source by using 0° incidence when high background levels are being produced by sources at other locations. Erroneous readings caused by reflected high-frequency sound emitted by other sources but coming from the same direction may be checked with directional microphones by rotating the microphone about an axis coinciding with the direction of incident sound. Reflected energy will be evidenced by a variation in level as the microphone is being rotated. The microphone orientation corresponding to the lowest reading should be chosen since the reflection error would be a minimum at this position.

Special-purpose microphones with sharp directional characteristics may be used to advantage in some locations. These microphones are particularly useful for locating specific high-frequency noise sources in the presence of other noise sources.

MICROPHONE CABLES. Standard microphone cable with shielded and twisted wires should be used with a dynamic microphone to minimize electrical noise pickup. Usually, no correction is needed when this cable is used between a dynamic microphone and its matching transformer unless the cable is longer than 100 feet.

Cable corrections may, or may not, be required for condenser microphones depending upon the preamplifier design and the overall calibration. Some condenser microphones are calibrated when mounted directly on the sound-measuring equipment; others are calibrated with cables attached. Instructions with the microphones should provide this information.

A correction is normally required when a titanate-type piezo-electric microphone is used with a cable unless the microphone has a built-in circuit to lower its output impedance. For the case where there is no built-in impedance-reducing circuit, a correction of about +7 dB must be added to the titanate microphone output when used with a 25-foot cable. The exact correction factor should be supplied with the microphone.

A correction factor that is a function of temperature must be applied when a Rochelle-salt microphone is used with a cable. These correction factors are found in instruction manuals supplied by the instrument manufacturers.

Frequency Analyzers

In many instances, the rough estimate of frequency-response characteristics provided by the sound level meter weighting networks does not give enough information. In these cases, the output of the sound level meter can be fed into a suitable analyzer which will provide more specific frequency distribution characteristics of the sound pressure.[5] The linear network of the sound level meter should be used when the output is to be fed to an analyzer. If the sound level meter does not have a linear network, the C network may be used for analyses over the major portion of the audible spectrum (see Figure 2).

OCTAVE-BAND ANALYZERS. The octave-band analyzer is the most common type of filter used for noise measurements related to hearing conservation. Octave-bands are the widest of the common bandwidths used for analyses; thus, they provide information of spectral distribution of pressure with a minimum number of measurements.

An octave band is defined as any bandwidth having an upper band-edge frequency f_2 equal to twice the lower band-edge frequency f_1. The center frequency (geometric mean) of an octave band, or other bandwidths, is found from the square root of the product of the upper and lower band-edge frequencies. The spe-

cific band-edge frequencies for octave bands are arbitrarily chosen. The older instruments usually have a series of octave bands
extending from 37.5 to 9,600 Hz (37.5 to 75, 75 to 150, 150 to
300, . . . 4,800 to 9,600). Newer octave-band analyzers may be designed for octave bands centered at 31.5, 63, 125, 250, 500, . . .
8,000 Hz according to American Standard Preferred Frequencies
for Acoustical Measurements (S1.6-1960).[6] Octave band-edge frequencies corresponding to the preferred center frequencies can
be calculated using two equations with two unknowns. The first
equation comes from the definition of an octave band, the upper
band-edge frequency is equal to twice the lower band-edge frequency $(f_2 = 2f_1)$. The second equation describes the center frequency f_c in terms of the band-edge frequencies $(f_c = \sqrt{f_1 f_2})$.
For example, the band-edge frequencies corresponding to a center frequency of 1,000 cps can be calculated as follows:

$$f_c = \sqrt{f_1 f_2} \tag{1}$$

and

$$f_2 = 2f_1. \tag{2}$$

From Equation (1), $f_c = 1,000 = \sqrt{f_1 f_2}$ and substituting Equation
(2) into Equation (1), $1,000 = \sqrt{f_1 \times 2f_1} = f_1 \sqrt{2}$. Therefore,
$f_1 = 1,000/1.414 = 707$ cps and, from Equation (2), $f_2 = 2 \times 707 =$
1,414 cps.

Most combinations of sound level meter and octave-band analyzer have separate attenuators on each instrument. In these
cases, it is always important to take a measurement of the overall
noise on the sound level meter first and leave its attenuator at
this position for all analyzer measurements. This procedure prevents overloading of the sound level meter and resulting erroneous readings. If the overall level changes during a series of measurements, the entire procedure must be repeated.

HALF-OCTAVE AND THIRD-OCTAVE ANALYZERS. When even more
specific information of the pressure spectral distribution is desired than that provided by octave bands, narrower-band analyzers must be used. The number of measurements necessary to cover the overall frequency range will be directly related to the
bandwidth of the analyzer; thus, a compromise must be reached
between the resolution required and the time necessary for the
measurements.

Half-octave and third-octave filters are the next steps in resolution above octave-band analyzers. A half-octave is a bandwidth with an upper-edge frequency equal to the $\sqrt{2}$ times its lower-edge frequency. A third-octave has an upper-edge frequency that is $\sqrt[3]{2}$ times its lower-edge frequency.

ADJUSTABLE-BANDWIDTH BROADBAND ANALYZERS. Some analyzers are designed with independently adjustable upper and lower band-edge frequencies. This design permits a selection of bandwidths in octaves, multiples of octaves, or fractions of an octave. The smallest fraction of an octave usually available on these adjustable-bandwidth analyzers is about one-tenth, and the largest extends up to the overall reading.

In addition to the obvious advantage of being able to select the proper bandwidth for a particular job, these analyzers permit the selection of any octave band, rather than a preselected series of octaves. For example, they can be adjusted to the older series of octaves (75—150, 150—300, etc.) or to bands with preferred center frequencies described in recent American Standards (125, 250, 500, etc.).[6] The disadvantage of these instruments is their relatively large size.

NARROW-BAND ANALYZERS. Analyzers with bandwidths narrower than tenth-octaves are normally referred to as narrow-band analyzers. Narrow-band analyzers are usually continuously adjustable, and they are classified either as constant-percentage bandwidth or as constant-bandwidth types.

The constant-percentage narrow-band analyzer is similar to the broad-band fractional octave analyzer in that its bandwidth varies with frequency. As its name indicates, the bandwidth of the constant-percentage analyzer is a constant percentage of the center frequency to which it is tuned. Typically, a bandwidth of about $\frac{1}{30}$-octave might be selected with these analyzers.

The bandwidth of a constant-bandwidth analyzer remains constant for all center frequencies over the spectrum. Provision may be made on some instruments to vary the bandwidth, but typically, the bandwidth of a constant-bandwidth analyzer remains constant at a few hertz.

The constant-bandwidth analyzer normally provides a narrower bandwidth and better discrimination outside the passband than the constant-percentage analyzer; therefore, it is often the best choice when discrete frequency components are to be measured. Also, it usually covers the entire spectrum with a single dial sweep, thus facilitating coupling to recorders for automatic analysis. Most constant-percentage analyzers require band switching to sweep the audible spectrum. On the other hand, caution must be used when constant-bandwidth analyzers are used to analyze noises which have frequency modulation, or warbling, of components for serious errors may result.[7] Frequency-modulated noises are commonly produced by reciprocating-type noise sources in some machinery. Frequency-modulated noise is not a major problem if constant-percentage analyzers are used.

Impulse—or Impact-Noise Measurement

The inertia of the indicating meters of general purpose sound level meters prevents accurate, direct measurements of single-impulse noises which have significant level changes in less than 0.2 second. Typical noises with short time constants are those produced by drop hammers, explosives, and others with short, sharp, clanging characteristics. A low inertia device such as an oscilloscope must be used to measure these impulse-type noises if detailed information is required.

Measurement of impulse noise characteristics may be taken directly from a calibrated oscilloscope with a long persistence screen, or photographic accessories may be used to obtain permanent records. The oscilloscope is usually connected to the output of a sound level meter having a wide frequency response and calibrated with a known sound level of sinusoidal characteristics. The screen of the oscilloscope is calibrated directly in decibels (rms) by comparing the oscilloscope deflection produced by a sinusoidal signal with the sound level meter reading. Several calibration points may be fixed on the oscilloscope screen by providing various signal levels into the sound level meter, or the scale may be determined from a single calibration level by using linear equivalents to decibels. For example, for a sine wave signal, half of a given deflection on the oscilloscope will be equivalent to a 6 dB drop in level, and 0.316 times the deflection will be the equivalent to a 10 dB drop in level. These equivalent values may be calculated from the equation

$$\text{Drop in Level (dB)} = 20 \log_{10} \frac{d_1}{d_2},$$

where d_1 and d_2 are the small and large linear screen deflectors being compared. It should be noted that this calibration using a sine wave is for convenience, and that there is a constant factor of 3 dB that must be added to the rms calibration to obtain the true instantaneous peak values for sine waves. The relationship of rms to peak values is more complex for nonsinusoidal waves.[1, 2, 3]

Care should be taken while using an oscilloscope driven by a sound level meter to prevent errors resulting from overloading. If the oscilloscope deflections show a sharp clipping action at a given amplitude, the attenuator settings on one or both instruments may require adjustment upwards. Also, a check should be made to determine if the indicating meter of the sound level meter affects the waveform produced on the oscilloscope. This may be done by switching the meter out of the circuit, to a battery check position, and observing the waveform. If the oscilloscope waveform is changed in any way by the indicating meter, it should be removed from the circuit each time a deflection is measured on the oscilloscope.

The oscilloscope is inconvenient to use in many field applications because it is relatively large and complex. Also, most oscilloscopes require a.c. power and, in the field, the supply may vary and cause changes in calibration. For these applications, it is often convenient to use peak-reading impact-noise analyzers which may be connected to the output of a sound level meter. These battery-driven instruments do not provide as much information as the oscilloscope trace, but they are often adequate. The electrical energy produced by an impulse noise is stored for a short time by these instruments in capacitor-type circuits so that information may be gained on the maximum peak level, on the average level over a period of time, and on the duration of the impact noise. As with the oscilloscope, care must be taken not to overload the sound level meter driving these impact-noise meters.

Magnetic Field and Vibration Effects

The response of sound level meters and analyzers may be affected by the strong alternating magnetic fields found around some electrical equipment. Dynamic microphones, coils, and transformers are particularly susceptible to hum pickup from these fields. Some of the newer dynamic microphones have hum-bucking circuits that minimize this pickup, but caution should be used in all cases. To test for hum pickup, disconnect the suspected component and check for a drop in level on the indicating meter. It is good practice to follow the equipment manufacturer's procedure for this check.

The magnetic fields produced by dynamic microphones may attract metal filings that will change the frequency response characteristics; therefore, dynamic microphones are not a good choice for measurements in metal shop areas.

Vibration of the microphone, or measuring instrument, may cause erroneous readings and, in some cases, strong vibrations may permanently damage the equipment. It is always good practice to mechanically isolate sound-measuring equipment from any vibrating surface. Holding the equipment in your hands or placing it on a foam rubber pad is satisfactory in most cases. Possible effects of vibration can be checked by observing the meter reading while the noise is shut off if this can be done without changing the vibration. If the meter reading drops by more than 10 dB, the effects of vibration are not significant. If the noise cannot be shut off without changing the vibration, the same result can be obtained by replacing the microphone cartridge with a dummy microphone. The equipment manufacturer can supply information necessary to build a dummy microphone.

Tape Recording of Noise

It is sometimes convenient to record a noise so that an analysis may be made at a later date. This is particularly helpful when lengthy narrowband analyzes are to be made, or when very short, transient-type noises are to be analyzed. However, extreme care must be taken in the calibration and use of recorders to avoid errors. Also, direct sound pressure measurement and analysis should be made during the recording procedure so that the operator will be aware when additional measurements or data are necessary.

Many of the professional, or broadcast-quality, tape recorders are satisfactory for noise-recording applications; however, care must be taken that the microphone has the proper characteristics. Many times, the specifications given for a tape recorder do not include the microphone characteristics and the microphone may be of very poor quality. When the tape recorder is not specifically built for measuring noise, it is usually good practice to connect the recorder to the output of a properly calibrated sound level meter. As is the case when attaching any accessory equipment to sound level meters, it is important that the impedances are properly matched. The bridging input of a tape recorder is satisfactory for the output circuits of most sound level meters.

When a tape recorder is used to record noises that have no high prominent peaks, the recording level usually should be set so that the recorder meter (VU meter) reads between −6 and 0 dB. This setting assumes that a sinusoidal signal reading of +10 dB on the VU meter will correspond to about 2 or 3 percent distortion according to standard recording practice.

If the recorded noise has prominent peaks, it is good practice to make at least two additional recordings with the input attenuator set so that the recording levels are between −6 and 0, −16 and −10, and −26 and −20. If there is less than 10 dB between any two of these adjacent 10 dB steps, overloading has occurred at the higher recorded level and the lower of the two should be used.

It is important to calibrate the combination of tape recorder and sound level meter at known level and tone control settings throughout the frequency range before the recordings are made. Prior to each series of measurements, a pressure level calibration should be made by noting the overall sound pressure level reading corresponding to the recording along with a notation of the tape recorder dial settings. Also, it is good practice to note the type and serial numbers of the microphone and sound level meter, the location and orientation of the microphone, the description of the noise source and surroundings, and other pertinent information for each recording. It is often convenient to record this information orally on the tape to be sure that the information will not be lost or confused with other tapes.

Graphic Level Recording

A graphic level recorder may be coupled to the output of a sound level meter, or analyzer, to provide a continuous written record of the output level. Recent graphic level recorders provide records in the conventional rms logarithmic form used by sound level meters; thus, the data may be read directly in decibels. Some older recorders use rectified average response characteristics, so corrections must be made to convert these recordings to true rms values. As with sound level meters, these recorders are intended primarily for the recording of sustained noises without short or prominent impact-type peak levels. The equipment manufacturer or instruction manuals should be consulted to determine the limitations of each graphic level recorder.

Instrument Calibration

If valid data are to be obtained, it is essential that all sound-measuring and analyzing equipment be in calibration. When this equipment is purchased from the manufacturer, it should have been calibrated to the pertinent American Standards Specifications.[4, 5] However, it is the responsibility of the equipment user to keep the instrument in calibration by periodic checks.

Most general-purpose sound-measuring instruments have built-in calibration circuits that may be used for checking electrical gain. Most sound level meters have built-in, or accessory, acoustical calibrators that may be used to check the overall acoustical and electrical performance at one or more frequencies. These electrical and acoustical calibrations should be made according to the manufacturer's instructions at the beginning and at the end of each day's measurements. A battery check should also be made at these times. These calibration procedures cannot be considered to be of high absolute accuracy, nor will they detect changes in performance at frequencies other than that used for calibration; however, they will serve to warn of the most common instrument failures, thus preventing a long series of invalid measurements.

Periodically, sound-measuring instruments should be sent back to the manufacturer, or to a competent acoustical laboratory, for a complete overall calibration at several frequencies throughout the instrument range. These calibrations require technical competence and the use of expensive chambers and equipment which cannot be justified by the normal user of sound-measuring equipment. The frequency of these more complete calibrations depends upon the purpose of the measurements and how roughly the instruments have been used. In most cases, it is good practice to have a complete calibration performed every six months, or at least once each year. In any case, a complete calibration should be made if any unusual change (more than 2 dB) is seen in the daily calibration.

REFERENCES

1. Snow, W. E.: Significance of reading of acoustical instrumentation, *Noise Control,* 5:40, September 1959.
2. Beranek, L. L.: *Acoustic Measurements.* New York, Wiley, 1949.
3. Harris, C. M.: *Handbook of Noise Control.* New York, McGraw-Hill, 1957.
4. American Standard Specification for General-Purpose Sound Level Meters, S1.4-1961: American National Standards Institute, Inc., 1430 Broadway, New York, N. Y. 10018.
5. American Standard Specifications for Octave, Half-Octave, and Third-Octave Filter Sets: S1.11-1966, American National Standards Institute, Inc., 1430 Broadway, New York, N. Y. 10018.
6. American Standard for Preferred Frequencies for Acoustical Measurements, S1.6-1960: American National Standards Institute, Inc., 1430 Broadway, New York, N. Y. 10018.
7. Scott, H. H.: The degenerative sound analyzer, *J Acoust Soc Am,* 11:225 (1939).

Chapter 12

NOISE SURVEYS

THE IMPORTANCE of accurate and stable instrumentation for noise measurement is obvious. Not so obvious, but just as important, is the need for careful planning of the survey to make sure that all objectives will be satisfied from the measurement data collected.

The need for a comprehensive definition of the purpose and scope of a noise survey cannot be over-emphasized. The choice of instruments, measurement techniques and locations, and data recording procedures will be determined from this survey design.

Purpose and Scope

The purpose and scope of noise surveys may vary considerably; however, there are four general types that may be considered:

1. A survey to determine hearing damage risk.
2. A survey to determine speech interference levels.
3. A survey to determine disturbance levels.
4. A survey for noise control purposes.

The first three survey types require somewhat similar measurement procedures for these measures of man's reaction to noise. The fourth survey type usually requires a more detailed analysis of the noise, and measurement procedures are somewhat different than the first three types.

HEARING DAMAGE RISK SURVEYS. Current rules, regulations and guidelines concerned with noise-induced hearing loss specify that the A-frequency weighting and slow meter response on sound-level meters be used to measure noise exposure levels.[1] Most of these specifications are also concerned with time and level patterns of exposures. Therefore, the purpose and scope of a survey is often defined broadly by the pertinent safety regulation specification.[2-5]

Sound-level meter measurements are generally required only at the positions that will be occupied by persons exposed to noise in hearing damage risk surveys. The time necessary for the survey is determined by the time necessary to establish meaningful time and level patterns of noise exposure. If a man is exposed to a noise having nearly the same level continuously, or if there is a predictable on-off time pattern, a very short noise measurement sample should be adequate. If the on-off time, or levels, are not predictable, many days may be required to determine a meaningful exposure pattern.

Data-recording methods will vary depending upon the time-level exposure patterns. For simple time-level patterns, direct manual readings and recordings are adequate. These measurements need not be repeated until some change in noise sources, job locations, or other changes in time-level patterns are indicated. Unexpected shifts in monitored hearing thresholds would, of course, be another indication for the need of additional noise measurements. Complicated time-level noise-exposure patterns may require an unreasonable amount of manual recording time, so that automatic recording of sound levels will be desired.

SPEECH INTERFERENCE LEVEL SURVEYS. Speech interference level surveys may be made with narrow-band, octave-band, A-frequency weighting, or other frequency weightings.[6] For many instances, the relatively simple A-frequency weighting is adequate (see Chapter 13). The purpose and scope of the survey and the physical characteristics of the noise will determine the degree of detail and, hence, the means of measuring the noise.

The positions of measurement will be fixed at the locations where speech must be understood. As with the measurements made for damage-risk assessment, the number of measurements will be determined by the noise-exposure pattern. Data recording will also be similar to the methods used in recording damage-risk data.

DISTURBANCE LEVEL SURVEYS. Considerable flexibility is re-

quired in rules for estimating disturbances caused by noise because of the many psychological, physiological, and physical variables involved in most situations (see Chapter 13). Disturbances
may vary from minor annoyances caused by very low noise levels
to physical alterations in vision or tactile abilities caused by high
levels of noise.[7, 8]

In specific cases, a particular measuring means may be indicated for the best correlation of noise levels with man's response to
noise; however, in many instances, one of several different measuring means will provide satisfactory data. If a particular noise
source has a characteristic spectrum with a high percentage of energy in narrow frequency bands, a third-octave or narrow-band
analysis may provide much better correlation with responses to
this noise than would measurements with wider frequency bands.
Narrow frequency bands may also be required to measure or pinpoint the contribution of a particular source to a high background noise if the relationship of the listener and the source
are bad. For example, if a man lives near a factory that has recently fired a member of his family, the noise made by this factory may be much more disturbing to him than higher levels produced by other sources such as traffic. Thus, measurements must
be made to differentiate between the contributions of the various sources. However, in a very large number of cases where
common broad-band noises are involved, measurements using
A-frequency weighting, octave-bands, or other frequency weightings are just as effective as narrow-band analyses for measuring
disturbance levels.

The positions and number of measurements will be determined by the purpose of the survey and the variability of the
noise characteristics. A general survey will normally include measurements at the boundaries of all properties near the noise
source and at other locations where complaints might be expected. A survey to investigate a specific complaint might be restricted to a single location. An adequate number of measurements
should be made in each area to determine the level and time patterns produced by the particular source under investigation and
the relationship of this source noise to background noises. This

information is generally required for daytime, evening, and night for all conditions of source operation.

Data-recording requirements are much the same as for damage-risk and speech intelligibility. For simple noise exposure patterns, manual recording is satisfactory, but automatic recording is necessary to assess complex exposure patterns.

NOISE CONTROL SURVEYS. Noise control surveys normally require octave or narrow-band analyses to pinpoint and describe individual source contributions. Narrow-band analyses are required to differentiate between two or more major contributors to the overall noise levels when these contributors are closely spaced, or when noise control work is to be done on a particular source located in high background noise.

The locations for measurements in a noise control survey will differ depending upon the purpose. Two general purposes of noise surveys are: (1) to pinpoint and describe a particular noise source so that effective noise control measures can be selected, and (2) to determine the acoustical power output of a noise source so that noise levels can be predicted in other locations. Details of these measurement procedures are given later in this chapter.

The on-off time pattern of a given noise source is usually well-known or easily controlled during noise control procedures so that relatively short samples of noise are generally meaningful. When on-off time patterns are predictable, manual recording of data is normally satisfactory; however, automatic recording means may be helpful when narrow band analyses are used or when multiple point measurements are made in anechoic or reverberation chambers.[9]

Measurement Techniques

SELECTION OF INSTRUMENT AND MEASUREMENT LOCATIONS. The kind of instruments needed for a particular survey should be determined from the purpose and scope as described earlier. Measurement positions are also described generally by the purpose and scope, although each individual situation should be considered carefully to be sure that objectives of the survey will be met. Additional measurement locations, or measuring means, may be indicated by unexpected results during the survey. For example, if a reading is unexpectedly high when the microphone is pointed in one direction, it may be desirable to make additional measurements around that point. A survey must be flexible so that full advantage can be taken from leads provided by measurement data as the survey progresses.

LABORATORY PREPARATION PROCEDURES. Each piece of noise measuring equipment should be checked thoroughly before noise measurements are made. Much time may be wasted if the equipment is not in good working condition. To be sure that the equipment will be checked, calibrated, and operated properly, it is strongly recommended that the operator read the manufacturer's instruction books carefully.

Adjustments, modifications, battery replacements or recharging, etc., are much easier to do in the laboratory than in the field. Thus, it is very important that the following checks be made in the office or laboratory just prior to making a field trip.

> 1. Connect all equipment as it will be used in the survey, turn the power on, and allow sufficient time for stabilization (see equipment instruction manuals).
> 2. Check battery condition and replace or recharge if necessary.
> 3. Calibrate the equipment electrically and acoustically (see instruction manuals). Check each instrument separately and check the combination of instruments to be used.
> 4. Measure some familiar wide-band noise for a gross check on analyzer band performances.
> 5. Replace the microphone with a suitable dummy load (see instruction manual) and measure electrical background noise.

The first three steps listed above provides a satisfactory check of the sound-level meter portion of the equipment. Step 4 is needed only when octave- or narrow-band analyzers are to be used. Step 5 should be done periodically and, in particular, whenever low sound-pressure levels are to be measured.

Special preparation procedures may be required in some instances. For example, if measurements are to be made outdoors where wind may cause erroneous readings, a wind screen should be provided for the microphone, and proper corrections must be applied to any data taken while using the wind screen. Data corrections must also be applied if microphone cables, microphone accessories, or combinations of equipment are to be used. In most cases, these corrections may be found in instruction books provided for the equipment; however, the safest procedure is to recheck and recalibrate all equipment in the exact manner it is to be used immediately prior to leaving for a noise survey.

TRAVEL AND ON-SITE PREPARATION PROCEDURES. All noise measurement instrumentation should be hand-carried throughout transportation from the laboratory to the survey site. Many pieces of this equipment may be damaged or its operational characteristics may be changed by excessive vibration, mechanical shock, humidity, and temperature cycling that might be encountered during normal shipping procedures. When traveling by public conveyance, the equipment should be carried in the passenger space. When traveling by automobile, the equipment should be placed on the seat or on resilient pads to reduce vibration and shock.

Extremes of temperature and humidity should be avoided at all times, but, in particular, just prior to measurement. Microphones supplied with most modern noise measurement equipment will not be permanently damaged by exposure to normal temperature and humidity extremes; however, condensation that may result from bringing a cold instrument into a warm room may change the microphone response characteristics temporarily. For example, this condition may result when an instrument is taken from a car, where it had been stored overnight in cool temperatures, into a warm and humid area where the survey is to be made.

ON-SITE CHECKS. All measurement equipment should be rechecked and recalibrated on location before beginning measurements and at two-hour intervals during the survey. Care must be taken during field calibrations to be sure that the acoustical calibration signal is at least 10 dB higher than the background noise measured with the calibrator (not operating) mounted on the microphone. It should be remembered that both electrical and

NOISE SURVEY DATA SHEET

DATE_____

LOCATION ➤							Sound Measuring Equipment: Type _____ Model #_____ Serial #_____ Type #_____ Model #_____ Serial #____
OCTAVE BAND (Center Freq.)	DECIBELS	DECIBELS	DECIBELS	DECIBELS	DECIBELS	DECIBELS	OCTAVE BAND (Center Freq.)
Overall-Linear							Overall-Linear
A - Frequency Weighting							A - Frequency Weighting
31 Hz							31 Hz
62 Hz							62 Hz
125 Hz							125 Hz
250 Hz							250 Hz
500 Hz							500 Hz
1000 Hz							1000 Hz
2000 Hz							2000 Hz
4000 Hz							4000 Hz
8000 Hz							8000 Hz
	Time: _____ Remarks:	Time: _____ Remarks:	Time: _____ Remarks:	Time: _____ Remarks:	Time: _____ Remarks:	Time: _____ Remarks:	FIELD CALIBRATION Cal. Type _____ Correct Cal. Level ___ Freq (Hz) / Meas Cal / Lev dB — 125 / 250 / 500 / 1000 / 2000 / TIME
Taken By: _____							

acoustical calibrations are needed and that acoustical calibrations should be made with the microphone mounted on a cable, extension, or directly as it is to be used during the survey.

Field calibrations should always be made with calibrators recommended for the particular microphone in question. Other calibrators may be the right physical size; however, a physical fit does not assure accuracy. Also, in some cases, a microphone cartridge may be permanently damaged from the use of calibrators intended for other microphones.

To serve as a reminder to perform the calibrations, and for medical-legal purposes, the field calibration data should be recorded along with noise measurement data. Unless the field calibration is recorded serially as an integral part of a noise survey, many operators will neglect this calibration and much measurement time may be wasted.

REFERENCES

1. American National Standard Specification for Sound Level Meters, ANSI S1.4-1971, American National Standards Institute, New York, N. Y. (1971).

2. American Conference of Governmental Industrial Hygienists. Threshold Limit Values of Physical Agents Adopted by ACGIH for 1970.

3. Safety and Health Standards for Federal Supply Contracts. U. S. Department of Labor. *Federal Register 34*:7948-49 (May 20, 1969).

4. Guidelines for noise exposure control, *Am Ind Hyg Assn J 28*:418-424 (Sept.-Oct. 1967).

   ibid., *Arch Environ Health, 15*: 674-678 (November 1967).

   ibid., *J Occup Med, 9*:571-575 (November 1967).

   ibid., *Am Assn Ind Nurses J 16*:17-21 (May 1968).

5. Occupational Safety and Health Standards (Williams-Steiger Occupational Safety and Health Act of 1970). U. S. Department of Labor. *Federal Register, 36*:10518 (May 29, 1971).

6. Webster, J. C.: SIL—Past, present and future. *Sound and Vibration,* 22-26, August 1969.

7. Anticaglia, J. R. and A. Cohen: Extra-Auditory Effects of Noise as a Health Hazard, *Am Ind Hyg Assn J, 31*:277-281, May-June, 1970.

8. Glorig, A.: Noise and Your Ear. Grune and Stratton, New York, 1958.

9. ISO R.140 Field and Laboratory Measurements of Airborne and Impact Sound Transmission. International Organization for Standardization. Rue de Varembé, Geneva, Switzerland.

Chapter 13

NOISE SPECIFICATIONS
FOR INDOOR SPACES

A NY INDOOR NOISE limit specification obviously must limit levels so that there is no danger of noise-induced hearing impairment.[1, 2, 3] In addition, these specifications should cover noise disturbances that may take many forms including interference with communication, annoyance, distraction, and interference with work or relaxation.

Speech Interference Guidelines

The frequency range from 200 to 6,000 Hz, which contains most of the information in speech, may be divided into a large number of frequency bands each having equal importance to speech intelligibility. If a dynamic range of about 30 dB is maintained above threshold in each of these bands, intelligibility scores approaching 100 percent should be possible for normal-hearing persons.[4] A restriction of this speech range in any band will limit intelligibility scores. For example, a dynamic range of 15 dB will limit a specific speech contribution to about 50 percent of its potential value. The overall contribution of all bands in this range may be expressed in terms of the average of the contributions in each band. This single number percentage of the total possible contributions to speech is called the articulation index.[4, 5]

The masking of speech by noise has the effect of increasing a person's threshold of hearing with varying degrees at different frequencies depending upon the spectra of the masking noise.

218

Thus, speech must be made louder in some noise backgrounds if a high level of intelligibility is to be maintained. If it is impossible to maintain the required dynamic range of speech pressure levels because of distortion or potential danger from overloading the ear, or because of inadequate speech power, the overall speech intelligibility will be reduced.

PRACTICAL SPEECH INTERFERENCE CALCULATIONS. Measurements and calculations of the dynamic range of speech for a large number of frequency bands is not practical in many instances for other than research activities. Thus, many attempts have been made to develop simple procedures for predicting speech intelligibility in various noise backgrounds.

One of the most widely accepted simplified procedures for determining the effect of noise on speech intelligibility makes use of the arithmetic average of three octave band sound pressure levels measured from the background noise. The average sound pressure level in the original three octave bands (600 to 1,200, 1,200 to 2,400, and 2,400 to 4,800 Hz) was proposed by Beranek as speech interference levels (SIL)[6-9] which could be used to determine when speech communication is easy, difficult, or impossible under specified conditions.

Recently, Webster has proposed that the SIL octave bands be shifted slightly to conform with ANSI preferred frequencies which are commonly used in modern instrumentation design.

TABLE VI

SPEECH INTERFERENCE LEVEL CRITERIA

Background Noise Levels That Cannot Be Exceeded if Face-To-Face Speech Is to Be Intelligible at the Distances and Speech Levels Specified*

Speaker to Listener Distance in Feet	Speech Interference Level Ratings in dB re 0.00002 n/m²							
	Normal Speech		Raised Voice		Very Loud Speech		Shouting	
	PSIL	dBA	PSIL	dBA	PSIL	dBA	PSIL	dBA
1	70	75	76	81	82	87	88	93
3	60	65	66	71	72	77	78	83
6	54	59	60	65	66	71	72	77
12	48	53	54	59	60	65	66	71

* These values are intended for normal-hearing persons located in common broadband background noises that do not have a high percentage of energy in narrow frequency bands.

The arithmetic average of the sound pressure levels in the new octave bands centered at 500, 1,000, and 2,000 Hz is called preferred octave speech interference levels (PSIL).[10]

Other measures of noise, such as the A-frequency weighting, have also been shown to provide reasonably good estimates of speech interference levels for many common background noise spectra.[10-12] The A-frequency weighting measure (dBA) is particularly appealing because it is an easily obtained single number and because of its widespread use in various rules, regulations, and standards pertaining to hearing conservation, noise control, and community noise control.

Tables VI and VII show some guidelines in terms of PSIL and dBA for maximum noise levels that can be tolerated if everyday speech is to be intelligible to normal-hearing persons when face-to-face and when using the telephone.

Caution must be used when applying the sound pressure level limits shown in Tables VI and VII. These data are intended only for common broadband background noises that do not have a high percentage of energy in narrow frequency bands. Also, the data are based on male voices and for normal-hearing listeners.

OTHER COMMUNICATION INTERFERENCE FACTORS. Unfortunately, that portion of the speech frequencies containing most of the consonant power (above 2,000 Hz), which provide much of the information in speech, is relatively easily masked with background noise because of the low speech power levels in these fre-

TABLE VII

SPEECH INTERFERENCE LEVEL CRITERIA

Background Noise Levels That Cannot Be Exceeded
for Acceptable Telephone Conversation

| Quality of Telephone Speech Intelligibility | Speech Interference Level Ratings in dB re 0.00002 n/m² | | | |
| | Calls Within a Single Exchange | | Multiple Exchange Calls | |
	PSIL	dBA*	PSIL	dBA*
Satisfactory	68	73	63	68
Difficult	68-83	73-88	63-78	68-83
Unsatisfactory	<83	<88	<78	<83

* These values are intended for normal-hearing persons located in common background noises that do not have a high percentage of energy in narrow frequency bands.

quencies. Thus, background noise may be particularly bother-some to those persons with high frequency, sensori-neural hearing losses in this same frequency range.

Background noise can also mask warning signals; thereby, cre-ating a potential injury hazard. It is impossible to set reasonable guidelines on the masking of warning signals unless their spectra and the acoustical characteristics of the space are defined. Some guidance may be provided by critical band relationships.[17]

Indoor Noise Limits for Purposes Other Than Speech Communication

The many psychological, physiological, and physical variables involved in defining annoyance, distraction, and interference with work or relaxation that are found for different individuals in different noise exposure situations make it impossible to estab-lish a single set of applicable rules or guidelines based on sound pressure levels alone. For example, a dripping faucet, a hushed conversation, a child crying, or a piece of hard chalk scraped along a blackboard may cause a considerable amount of annoy-ance or distraction with very low sound levels while much higher levels are not considered annoying under normal circumstances when people are attending ball games, listening to music, etc.

ANNOYANCE AND DISTRACTION FACTORS. The degree of annoy-ance produced by a given noise is significantly influenced by many factors, including:

1. The personal relationship of the individual with the noise pro-ducing source. If the noise source is caused by or in some way for himself, the noise is less likely to be annoying than if it were created by a neighbor. If the noise is created by a neighbor, the amount of annoyance is often affected by the individual's personal relationship with the neighbor.[17-19]
2. Annoyance caused by a given noise is usually greater indoors than outdoors.[17-19]
3. Noises produced at night are usually more annoying than the same noises produced in daytime.[17-21]
4. Past exposure patterns influence reactions to specific noise ex-posures. An individual living in a highly industrialized area is less likely to be disturbed by noise than suburban area residents.[17]
5. Annoyance generally increases as either the level or frequency of the noise increases.
6. Noises that are intermittent and occur randomly in time are nor-

mally judged more annoying than those that are continuous or unchanging.

7. A noise source that moves is usually judged to be more annoying than a stationary source.

It is obvious that all noise exposure circumstances must be fully described in each case before meaningful noise specifications can be established. The many variables involved prevent the establishment of a generally applicable guideline; however, several indoor noise limit guidelines have been proposed for a number of specific locations having average conditions. Although these guidelines do not always hold accurately, they do provide useful and necessary guidelines for architects, engineers, and others in many cases (see Table VIII).

MEASUREMENT PROCEDURES. Most of the procedures proposed for describing annoyance or distraction effects of noise make use of tabulations of noise measures that are correlated with different levels of human response in the specific activity or space considered. There have been a large number of noise measures proposed for these subjective responses, some being better for specific purposes than others.[4–16]

Two of the most widely used noise measures in indoor noise criteria are SIL (or PSIL) and A-frequency weighting (dBA) measures.[5–10, 22, 23] Table VIII shows design goals that will provide acceptable indoor space environments in most instances. Maximum permissible levels may be 5 to 10 dB higher than the design goal values given under some circumstances where noises are continuous and broadband, and where communication distances are relatively small.

INTERFERENCE WITH WORK. Noise can influence work in many ways, both directly and indirectly. The amount of interference with work may vary from small distractions caused by very low noise levels to alterations in visual and tactile perception that result from higher levels.[18, 24–27] Interference with communication is obviously another important factor to be considered when measuring work output.

As is the case with annoyance caused by noise, work interference cannot be described by noise levels alone and generally applicable guidelines are not available because of the many vari-

TABLE VIII

DESIGN GOALS FOR NOISE IN INDOOR SPACES

Location	A-Weighted Sound Pressure Level in (dBA)*	PSIL in (dB)*
Residences		
Rural and suburban	25-30	20-25
Urban	25-35	20-30
Industrial	30-40	25-35
Offices		
Conference rooms	25-35	20-30
Large	25-30	20-25
Small	20-35	25-30
Executive offices	30-40	25-35
Closed office (wall to ceiling)	30-45	25-40
Open office (half-walls)	35-50	30-45
Halls and corridors	35-55	30-50
Churches and schools		
Libraries	30-40	25-35
Classrooms	30-40	25-35
Laboratories	35-45	30-40
Halls and corridors	35-55	30-50
Kitchens	45-55	40-50
Auditoriums		
Lecture halls	35-40	30-35
Concert halls	25-30	20-25
Movie theatres	35-45	30-40
Lobbies	40-50	35-45
Restaurants	40-50	35-45
Cafeterias	45-55	40-50
Stores	40-50	35-45
Hospitals		
Private rooms	30-40	25-35
Operating rooms	35-45	30-40
Laboratories	40-50	35-45
Lobbies	40-50	35-45
Halls and corridors	40-50	35-45
Manufacturing areas	As low as practical but in all cases less than: 85	80

* Noise levels measured while the spaces are not in use.

ables involved. Experiments have shown that the effect of noise is more likely to result in an increased rate of errors or accidents rather than decreased total work output.[24] Generally, these effects are increased as the noise level is increased, particularly if the level rises above about 90 dB in the central octave bands.

Some studies have shown that broadband masking noise or instrumental music can be used effectively to mask interrupted noises, or hushed conversations, and thus reduce distractions. However, there is evidence of significant intersubject variability and other factors that preclude the general applicability of these data.

REFERENCES

1. American Conference of Governmental Industrial Hygienists. Threshold Limit Values of Physical Agents Adopted by AC IH for 1970.
2. Safety and Health Standards for Federal Supply Contracts (Walsh-Healey Public Contracts Act). U. S. Department of Labor. *Federal Register, 34*:7948-49 (May 20, 1969).
3. Guidelines for Noise Exposure Control. *Am Ind Hyg Assoc J, 28*:418-424 (Sept.-Oct. 1967).
   ibid., *Arch Environ Health, 15*:674-678 (Nov. 1967).
   ibid., *J Occup Med, 9*:571-575 (Nov. 1967).
   ibid., *Am Assoc Ind Nurses J 16*:17-21 (May 1968).
4. French, N. R. and Steinberg, J. C.: Sound Control in Airplanes. *J Acoust Soc Am, 19*:90-119, 1947.
5. Beranek, L. L.: *Acoustics,* New York, McGraw-Hill, 1954.
6. Beranek, L. L.: Airplane Quieting II—Specification of Acceptable Noise Levels. *Trans. ASME 69*:96-100, 1947.
7. Beranek, L. L.: Criteria for office quieting based on questionnaire rating studies. *J Acoust Soc Am, 28*:833-852, 1956.
8. Beranek, L. L.: Revised criteria for noise in buildings. *Noise Control 3, 1*:19-27, 1957.
9. Beranek, L. L., Reynolds, J. L. and Wilson, K. E.: Apparatus and procedures for predicting ventilation system noise. *J Acoust Soc Am 25*:313-321, 1953.
10. Webster, J. C.: SIL—Past, present and future. *Sound and Vibration, 22*: 26 (Aug. 1969).
11. Young, R. W.: Don't forget the simple sound-level-meter. *Noise Control 4, 3*:42-43, 1958.
12. Kryter, K. D.: Concepts of perceived noisiness, their implementation and application. *J Acoust Soc Am, 43*:344-361, 1968.
13. Kryter, K. D. and Williams, C. E.: Masking of speech by aircraft noise. *J Acoust Soc Am, 39*:138-150, 1966.
14. Williams, C. E., Stevens, K. N., Hecker, M. H. L. and Pearson, K. S.: The speech interference effects of aircraft noise. Federal Aviation Administration Report DS-67-19, 1967.
15. Klumpp, R. G. and Webster, J. C.: Physical measurements of equally speech-interfering navy noises. *J Acoust Soc Am, 35*:1328-1338, 1963.

16. Kryter, K. D.: The meaning and measurement of perceived noise level. *Noise Control 6, 5*:12, 1960.
17. Fletcher, H.: Auditory patterns. *Rev Mod Phys, 12*:47-65, 1940.
18. Parrack, H.: Community Reaction Noise. Chapter 36, *Handbook of Noise Control*, C. M. Harris, Ed. New York, N. Y., McGraw-Hill Book Company (1957).
19. Cohen, A.: Noise effects on health, productivity and well-being. *Trans N Y Acad Sci, 30*:910-918 (May, 1968).
20. Wilson, A.: *Noise* (Chapter IV). London, England, Her Majesty's Stationers (1963).
21. Kryter, K. D.: Psychological reactions to aircraft noise. *Science, 151*:1346-1355, 1966.
22. Peterson, A. P. G. and Gross, E. E.: *Handbook of Noise Measurements*. General Radio Company, West Concord, Massachusetts (1963).
23. ASHRAE Guide and Data Book—Fundamentals and Equipment. Amer. Soc. of Heating and Refrig. and Air-Conditioning Engr's, New York, N. Y. (1970).
24. Broadbent, D. E.: Effects of Noise on Behavior. Chapter 10, *Handbook of Noise Control*, C. M. Harris, Ed. New York, N. Y., McGraw-Hill, (1957).
25. Carpenter, A.: How does noise affect the individual? *Impulse, 24*, 1964.
26. Broussard, I. G. et al.: The Influence of Noise on Visual Contrast Threshold. U. S. Army Med. Res. Lab. Rept. No. 101, Fort Knox, Kentucky (1952).
27. Loeb, M.: The Influence of Intense Noise on Performance of a Precise Fatiguing Task. Army Med. Res. Lab. Rept. No. 268, Fort Knox, Kentucky (1957).

Chapter 14

NOISE CONTROL

Vibrations of any solid object will produce pressure variations in air that may be perceived as sound or noise when the vibration amplitudes are sufficiently high and the vibration frequencies are in the audible range. Vibration amplitudes are directly related to the noise levels produced; thus, reduction of mechanical vibration amplitudes may be a very effective noise control measure.

If vibration of component parts of a machine cannot be reduced sufficiently to prevent noise problems from developing in surrounding areas, the noise levels must be controlled by enclosures, barriers, isolation procedures, or by the use of noise absorbing materials. Often it is necessary to make use of combinations of these noise control procedures in order to obtain the required noise reduction.

Reduction of Radiated Noise

The overall noise level radiated from a machine may be the product of a number of different individual noise sources within the machine and, in many cases, each individual noise source must be considered separately for the most efficient noise control measures. Because of the logarithmic nature of the individual noise source contribution, it is essential that any noise control measure be directed toward the individual sources in the order of their contributions to the overall noise level. Otherwise, much time, effort and money can be wasted. For example:

Consider a machine that produces an overall sound pressure level of 98 dB at a given location near the machine. If this machine has three

226

individual noise source components capable of producing levels of 86, 91 and 96 dB at the same location if operated singly, the 96 dB source should be treated first with attention being given to the 91 dB and 86 dB sources later in that order. If noise control measures were applied to the 86 dB source first, this source could be completely removed and the overall level would be reduced by only about 0.3 dB. However, if the 96 dB and 91 dB sources were reduced by 12 and 10 dB, respectively, the overall level would be reduced by more than 9 dB (see Physics of Sound chapter) .

Often it is impractical or impossible to determine the contribution of an individual noise source within a machine by an overall measurement of the noise because other noise-making parts are running at the same time. In these cases, the contributions of the individual sources can usually be determined from frequency analyses of the overall noise levels produced. Correlations can be made between the frequency bands having the highest levels and the running speeds of various machine components which might produce these noises. Another practical guide for pinpointing a noise source in a background of other noise sources is to correlate dimensions of the radiating source with the frequency spectra because only those vibrating parts having dimensions similar to, or larger than, a quarter wavelength (in air) are capable of radiating noise efficiently.

Once the principal noise-making components are located and action priorities established, the most effective noise control procedures must be selected. More than one control procedure may be required to reduce the levels radiated by some sources. Where two or more control procedures may be ineffective when used singly, together they may produce significant results.

COMPONENT SIZE, SHAPE AND MATERIAL. Where possible, machine component sizes should be held to dimensions that are small in comparison to the quarter wavelength (in air) of any vibrational energy that might be connected to the component so that noise will not be radiated efficiently. If it is not possible to hold the overall dimensions of a machine part to a small size, it may be possible to use two pieces instead of one in such a way that the second piece is isolated from the vibration source.

Any machine component should be made in a shape and size

to resist vibration and, in particular, to avoid resonances* which may cause high level noise radiation. Heavy, rigid parts are usually preferred in the design of quiet equipment; however, lightweight material can be used in many cases if properly supported and damped.

VIBRATION DAMPING. Materials used in the construction of machines have varying degrees of internal damping; however, the effect of internal damping is small in comparison with the damping effectiveness of specially developed damping materials that can be added. For example, lead and other materials have high internal damping characteristics but specially compounded damping materials with the same weight are generally much more effective wherever damping is required.

Vibration-damping materials normally are effective in just two cases: (1) where forced vibration frequencies correspond with the resonant frequencies in component parts of the attached equipment; or (2) where impact-type shocks are applied to relatively thin surfaces.

Resonant conditions can be detected by slowly increasing the operating speed of a machine from below to above its normal operating range. If a significant increase in loudness is heard, or if a tone suddenly becomes clearly audible at certain speeds, a resonant condition is indicated and a vibration damping treatment probably will be effective. If there is not a marked change in character or loudness of the noise radiated as the machine speed is increased, it is doubtful that a vibration damping treatment will be worthwhile. A gradual increase of loudness or pitch during an increase of operating speed does not indicate a resonant condition.

Metal panels often have many resonant frequencies that can be excited by either continued forced vibrations or a single blow. Examples of unwanted resonant panel noise may be found in many commonly used products ranging from automobile bodies

---

* Resonance of a component part exists when any change in the excitation frequency of forced vibration causes a decrease in the vibration amplitude of the component part.

to porch furniture. Damping treatments may often be used to reduce the overall levels produced by resonant panels and, in addition, the damping treatment normally results in a shift of noise
energy to lower frequencies where the ear is less sensitive.

In cases where damping treatment is indicated, the area of coverage is often critical. Complete coverage of a vibrating panel in-
sures good damping; however, it is not the most economical use
of the damping material, and it sometimes adds significantly to
the weight of the product. A single point application of a damping device or material is seldom effective; however, spot damping
treatments (small area coverage) can be effective if care is taken
to place the damping materials precisely on the areas having maximum vibration amplitude. Unfortunately, the spot treatment
procedure has the obvious disadvantage of requiring tedious vibration measurements to determine the areas where spot damping
must be applied.

The thickness (or weight per unit area) of a vibration damping material is also related to its effectiveness; however, the many
parameters involved in different applications make it impossible
to establish definite rules on the thickness required for a specific
problem.

A few general guides in the application of damping treatment
are as follows:

1. A given damping treatment is usually more effective for high than
   for low vibration frequencies.
2. A heavy piece of equipment will require a heavier damping treatment than a light piece.
3. The stamping of ribs in flat sheet metal panels will raise the natural
   resonant frequencies of a panel without increasing its mass, thereby
   making possible the advantages noted in Items 1 and 2.

TOLERANCES. Vibrational amplitudes of considerably less than
one-thousandth of an inch can produce high-level noise. Thus,
excessive tolerances or worn parts in moving systems often are
primary noise sources.

A first step in a tolerance-noise control procedure is to replace
all worn parts and to properly align all moving pieces. In many

cases, this maintenance of equipment provides the added advantage that a machine will run more efficiently and it will last longer. Noise is indeed wasted energy in many instances.

If proper maintenance of equipment does not provide enough noise reduction, it may be necessary to decrease the original tolerances between some of the moving parts or to select new materials for component parts. Reduced tolerances prevents excessive movement of parts and this procedure will normally lower noise levels; however, care must be taken not to reduce tolerances too much because the machine's operation may be impaired or the higher friction and the resulting heat may shorten the life of component parts. Similarly, materials with high internal damping or relatively soft surfaces will usually reduce the noise produced from shock or impact, but the operational life of these materials may be very short. Compromise between noise radiation, cost, and wearability will often determine whether the radiated noise can be controlled at the source or if noise control measures must be taken external to the source.

Vibration Isolation

Vibration of a machine may be transmitted to its supporting surface if rigidly mounted and these vibrations may in turn cause noise to be radiated from the floor, ceiling, walls, or other structures attached to the supporting surface. In these cases, one of the most effective noise control measures may be to mount the machine on vibration isolators.

Vibration isolators are made from a number of different materials and their designs take many different forms. Coil or leaf springs, gas or liquid filled devices, and pads made from rubber, cork, felt, or fiber glass are common forms of vibration isolators. The choice of the most effective vibration isolator depends upon such factors as the machine weight and size, the vibration frequency spectra, and the environmental conditions to which the isolator will be exposed. The proper isolator characteristics must be chosen for a particular job if it is to be effective and long lasting. In fact, the choice of the wrong mechanical characteristics of vibration isolators may not only be ineffective but they may amplify the forced vibrations transmitted to the supporting surface of the machine.

All connections to a vibrating machine other than mounting points must also be properly designed for vibration isolation; otherwise, benefits from the vibration isolating mounts may be lost. Electrical, fuel, control, ventilation, and other connections may all require different kinds of flexible connections in order to obtain maximum effectiveness. Here again, definite rules for the design of flexible connectors cannot be drawn because of the many parameters involved. Generally, the following guides can be used for the design of flexible couplers:

1. If possible, the connection to the machine should be made where the vibration amplitudes are at a minimum and the other end of the connection should be made on the most solid and massive support available.
2. A relatively rigid machine coupling can be tolerated if it is terminated on a solid and massive surface. However, a very flexible coupling may be necessary if the machine is coupled to a flexible and lightweight surface.
3. If connections are to be made with metal or non-metal tubing, long loops or coils should be used that are flexible in all directions.
4. Where non-metals cannot be used because of high temperature or solvent problems, special flexible metal tubes made of stainless steel, brass, copper, or Monel are available. Special flexible metal tubing normally cannot withstand high pressures and should be carefully chosen for a particular application.

A complete treatment of the problem of vibration isolators is beyond the scope of this text. More details on the theory and application of vibration isolation may be found in References 1-6.

Reduction of Noise Away from the Source

If sufficient noise reduction is not possible by direct treatment of the noise source or by mechanically isolating the source from surrounding structures, the next step is to use noise control measures in the surrounding areas. Two common noise control procedures that can be used singly or together to reduce radiated noise levels are (1) to partially or completely enclose the noise source with materials having high sound transmission loss characteristics, or (2) to absorb the noise with sound absorbing materials placed in selected locations.

Noise Barriers and Enclosures

The effectiveness of a material for use as a barrier to noise (transmission loss characteristic) is highly dependent upon its weight per unit area. Normally, the kind of material used for a noise barrier is relatively unimportant if the material is not porous and it is constructed so that the necessary weight per unit area is provided.

The transmission loss (TL) provided by a barrier normally is highly dependent on the frequency of sound with the loss at high frequencies being considerably greater than at low frequencies. The TL of most single-wall type barriers for randomly incident noise increases about 5 dB for each doubling of frequency.

The relationship of transmission loss provided by a single-wall type barrier to its weight per unit area is commonly expressed in terms of an average TL for frequencies between 125 and 2,000 Hz. This single number value is sufficiently accurate for most practical purposes since the 5 dB/doubling of frequency holds reasonably well for most single wall structures. Transmission losses for a large variety of single-wall barriers are available in the literature.[4-10]

Multiple wall construction with enclosed air spaces provides considerably more attenuation than the single-wall mass law would predict.[7-9] However, considerable care must be taken to avoid rigid connections between the multiple wall surfaces when they are constructed or any advantages in attenuation will be lost.[9, 10]

Noise leaks which may result from cracks, holes, windows, or doors in a noise barrier can severely limit noise reduction characteristics. In particular, care must be taken throughout construction to prevent acoustical leaks that may be caused by electrical outlets, plumbing connections, telephone lines, etc., in otherwise effective barriers. For example, a hole 1.5-inch square in a wall will transmit about the same amount of acoustical energy as 100 square feet of a wall area which has a TL of 40 dB.

The choice of a simple barrier, a partial enclosure, or a complete enclosure depends upon several factors including:

1. The position of the noise source or sources with respect to the exposure area.
2. The acoustical characteristics of the surrounding area.
3. The frequency spectrum of the noise.
4. The amount of noise reduction required.

A simple barrier may be effective if the positioning of the noise source or sources and the acoustical characteristics of the surrounding area are such that the major noise contribution is coming from one general direction. Also, it must be feasible to build a barrier whose smallest cross-sectional dimension is large compared to the wavelengths of the major noise spectrum components (see Physics of Sound chapter) in a location between the source and the exposure area.

If a single barrier does not provide adequate noise reduction because of multiple angles of incidence, or because of too much low frequency (large wavelengths) energy bends around the barrier, then additional wall or ceiling barriers are often effective. If the multiple barrier, or partial enclosure, structure is not effective, a complete enclosure may be necessary.

Any barrier or enclosure must be carefully isolated mechanically from the noise source. Otherwise forced vibrations may cause noise to be radiated from the barrier or enclosure and its quieting effects will be nullified. Connections through the enclosure to the machine are particularly important. Tubing, wiring, and other small connections should be passed through rubber grommets that are placed near corners or other stiffening members of the enclosure. If needed, ventilating air should be supplied through ducts lined with sound-absorbing material. In addition, all portions of the enclosure should be carefully designed to avoid dimensions having resonant frequencies corresponding to the spectra of principal noise components of the source.

When barriers or enclosures confine the radiated noise in a relatively small volume which has hard acoustically reflecting surfaces, the radiated noise will combine with the reflected energy so that the overall levels around the source are substantially increased. For this reason, an enclosure constructed with panels having a TL of 25 dB may provide only 5 dB noise reduction if the noise levels inside the enclosure are increased by 20 dB from the reflected energy buildup. In these cases, noise absorption materials must be used within the enclosure to minimize the reflected energy buildup.

NOISE ABSORPTION. Good sound absorbing materials are normally light in weight and porous in contrast to the massive and nonporous requirements for a good noise barrier. Thus, a good sound absorber is usually a poor sound barrier, and vice versa.

To be a good sound absorber, the sound waves must penetrate into the absorbing material where the sound is dissipated in the form of friction and heat. The amount of sound entering a porous material (and the amount of sound energy absorbed) is dependent upon the wavelength of the sound and its angle of incidence upon the absorbing material.

The ability of a material to absorb sound of a particular frequency is often described by a sound-absorption coefficient (a) which is the ratio of the sound energy absorbed by the material to the amount of energy incident upon it. A surface that absorbs all energy incident upon its surface is said to have an absorption coefficient of one, while a surface that reflects all energy has an absorption coefficient of zero. An average sound absorption coefficient, $\bar{a}$, in a room having several different surface materials is found for a given frequency by

$$\bar{a} = \frac{\alpha_1 S_1 + \alpha_2 S_2 + \alpha_3 S_3 + \cdots \alpha_n S_N}{S_1 + S_2 + S_3 + \cdots S_N},$$

where $a_1, a_2, a_3 \ldots a_n$ are the coefficients of absorption of the various surfaces of the room having corresponding areas $S_1, S_2, S_3 \ldots S_n$. The coefficients of absorption for most surface materials are readily available in the literature.[6, 11, 12]

The relationship between average sound-pressure level, L_p, power level, L_P, and single-frequency absorption coefficients for a given semi-reverberant room may be written as

$$L_p = L_P + 10 \log \left(\frac{Q}{4\pi r^2} \right) + 10.5 \text{ dB re } 0.00002 \text{ n/m}^2,$$

where r is the distance in feet from the measurement point to the source, Q is the directivity factor, and $R = aS/1 - \bar{a}$ is the room constant in square feet (see Physics of Sound chapter). In a highly reverberant field, the average sound-pressure level can be written as

$$L_p = L_P - 10 \log R + 16.6 \text{ dB re } 0.00002 \text{ n/m}^2.$$

A rule of thumb that may be used to determine the amount of noise reduction possible from the application of acoustically absorbent materials on room surfaces is

$$\text{dB reduction} = 10 \log \frac{\text{absorption units after treatment}}{\text{absorption units before treatment}}$$

where the absorption units are the sum of the products of surface areas and their respective noise absorption coefficients.

The overall noise-absorbing efficiency of acoustic materials is sometimes expressed by a single number known as the Noise Reduction Coefficient (NRC). The NRC is found arithmetically by averaging four absorption coefficients between 250 and 2,000 cps (usually 250, 500, 1,000 and 2,000 Hz). Small differences in NRC may not be detectable, so it is common practice to round off coefficients to the nearest 0.05.

Specifications for Purchasing Equipment

General principles of noise control are well known but unfortunately little effort has been expended toward applying this knowledge. The lack of progress in noise reduction can be attributed for the most part to the absence of a demand for quiet equipment. Quieting procedures normally will increase the cost of equipment and manufacturers will not jeopardize sales by increased cost in a competitive market unless the demand for quietness is made by the buyers. Thus, one of the most effective steps in controlling noise may be through comprehensive purchasing specifications that demand quiet products.

Another very strong reason for noise limits in purchasing specifications is that noise control procedures are usually much more effective and less expensive when taken during the design and development stages rather than after the equipment is in use. Many equipment manufacturers have the technical ability to produce quiet machinery and will welcome reasonable noise limits in purchasing specifications.

STANDARDS. Standard methods for measuring and reporting noise levels have been developed by several manufacturing groups or associations for use with their products. Organizations that have noise measurement and reporting specifications include the American Gear Manufacturers Association,[1] the American Society of Heating, Refrigeration, and Air-Conditioning Engineers,[2] the Air Moving and Conditioning Association,[3] the Institute of Electrical and Electronic Engineers,[4] the American Iron and Steel Institute,[5] and the National Electrical Manufacturers Association.[6] The American Iron and Steel Institute's Guidelines for Noise Control Specifications for Purchasing Equipment is shown in Appendix 1.

Unfortunately, many manufacturers do not belong to organizations that have standard methods of measuring and reporting noise characteristics, and the specifications set forth by other groups may not be applicable. A comparison of noise characteristics from competitive machines from different manufacturers may be meaningless unless the measurements are clearly defined and applicable for describing the noise made by the equipment.

NOISE CONTROL SPECIFICATIONS. Standard procedures that are best for specifying noise characteristics of one piece of equipment may not be best for another because of size, use, levels, etc. Therefore, only general guidelines can be given in setting up overall engineering specifications.[7, 8]

A major objective of any engineering specification is to make the equipment manufacturer aware of his responsibility for the noise produced by his equipment. If the manufacturer does not belong to a group that has their own noise measurement specifications which are acceptable, he should be guided by a reference in the purchasing specification to a pertinent standard procedure such as one of those referenced 1 to 5. Otherwise, a specific set of measurement and reporting instructions should be provided in the specification.

In any engineering specification for noise, the acceptable noise levels obviously must be listed but, in addition, the test signals, the instrumentation, the test procedures, and the test environment must also be carefully specified. The characteristics of acceptable noise levels should be specified in detail wherever possible; however, in some instances, it may not be possible to specify the levels precisely because of equipment size or unusual conditions of use. In these cases, a selection from available equipment can be made on the basis of the lowest noise levels produced.

TEST SIGNALS. Octave band sound pressure level measurements are usually adequate to describe the noise characteristics of a machine; however, more specific information in the form of narrow-band analyses may be desired when a large portion of the energy is contained in narrow frequency bands. In all cases linear and A-weighted overall measurements should be made before and after each series of octave- or narrow-band analyses.

TEST INSTRUMENTATION. All instruments used for noise measurements should meet the latest standards of the American National Standards Institute.[9, 10] Also, these instruments should be calibrated electrically and acoustically immediately before and after the measurements on each piece of equipment to be tested.

TEST PROCEDURES. Noise measurements are the vender's responsibility; however, to be sure that measurements are performed properly, the purchaser should reserve the right to send qualified representatives to vender's plant to observe or to conduct noise tests if necessary. General test requirements may include the following steps:

1. Noise measurements should be made when the equipment is operating at both normal and maximum running speeds. In all cases, the equipment should be mounted in the same manner as intended for permanent operation.
2. Noise measurement equipment should be located so that electric or magnetic fields, mechanical vibrations, wind, or other extraneous factors will not affect the accuracy of the data.
3. Measurements should be made at locations corresponding to positions where human ears may be located when the equipment is in its proposed permanent location. In addition, measurements should be made around the equipment at 30-degree intervals, 5 feet above the floor level at a horizontal distance of from 3 to 6 feet from the equipment. All measurement positions should be accurately recorded. A sample noise survey data sheet is shown in Figure 1.
4. Wherever mean noise levels vary by more than 6 dB during normal

operation, measurements should be repeated to describe each operational phase that produces different noise levels.

5. All sound pressure level measurements should be taken with the slow meter damping characteristics and average meter indications recorded when the range of meter deflections are less than 4 dB. When the meter deflections equal or exceed 4 dB, the range of meter deflections, and any other prominent level variation characteristics, should also be recorded.

6. Octave band, A-frequency weighted, and flat[9, 10] sound pressure level measurements should be made at each measurement location. When the noises produced contain pure-tone noise components, a narrow band analysis may be necessary (see Chapter 3).

7. Other noise measurement data that should be recorded includes: (1) the type, model, and serial numbers of all instruments used; (2) the microphone type and serial number; (3) the microphone mounting or cable length; (4) the microphone orientation; (5) calibration information; (6) the response speed of the indicating meter; and (7) any remarks covering any significant phase of the test procedure not covered elsewhere.

TEST LOCATION. The ideal test location for one noise maker may not be ideal for another because of differences in size, frequency or directional characteristics, and levels produced. For most relatively small noise sources, a free- or reverberant field for testing is best and this requires specially treated anechoic or reverbration chambers.

Size or noise-making devices may prevent testing in an anechoic room, reverbration chamber, or other carefully controlled or predictable test environment. However, meaningful measurements can often be made in other locations if the test environment can be described carefully in a simple manner, i.e. if there are no significant noise reflecting surfaces other than the inner surfaces of the test room, or if other reflecting surfaces can be described acoustically in simple terms. A test room description should include:

1. Complete elevation and floor plan sketches of the equipment location in the test room along with room dimensions. Positions and descriptions of other equipment in the test room should be included.

2. Materials used on the floor, walls and ceiling of the test room.

3. Floor supports used for the equipment under test; i.e., Is it bolted

down on concrete, on vibration mounts, etc.? The mounting should be the same as planned for the permanent operating position.

4. Ambient noise levels at the time of the test should be recorded for each frequency weighting, octave band, or narrow band used in the measurement procedure. Ambient levels should be more than 10 dB below any level recorded.

REQUIREMENTS. The Guidelines for Noise Exposure Control[13] may be used as a guide for establishing noise exposure limits. The total noise contributed by all noise sources should be less than the established limits.

It must be possible to use the noise measurement data supplied by the equipment manufacturer to determine the levels that will be produced in the work area. Calculations using sound power or sound pressure level can be made as described in Chapter 2 if adequate information is provided.

An alternate way of approaching this problem is to place the burden of performance upon the manufacturer of the equipment being purchased. The purchasing specification can require that the purchased equipment will not produce sound pressure levels greater than the specified level in the area where the equipment is to be used. This kind of specification has had only limited success because manufacturers are often unable or unwilling to estimate levels in a complex acoustical environment.

REFERENCES

1. *Fan Engineering*, 6th Edition, edited by Robert Jorgensen, Buffalo Forge Company, Buffalo, N. Y. (1961).
2. Den Hartog, J. P.: *Mechanical Vibrations*, McGraw-Hill, New York, 1947.
3. Crede, C. E.: *Vibration and Shock Isolation*, Wiley, New York, 1951.
4. Geiger, P. H.: *Noise-Reduction Manual*, Engineering Research Institute, University of Michigan (1953).
5. Harris, C. M.: *Handbook of Noise Control*, McGraw-Hill, New York, 1957.
6. Beranek, L. L.: *Noise Reduction*, McGraw-Hill, New York, 1960.
7. Sound Insulation of Walls and Floor Construction, National Bureau of Standards, U. S. Department of Commerce, Building Materials and Structure Report BMS 17 with 2 supplements.
8. Buckingham, E.: Theory and interpretation of experiments on transmission of sound through partition walls, *Scientific Papers of the Bureau of Standards*, 20:193-219, 1925.

9. Recommended Practice for Laboratory Measurement of Airborne Sound Transmission Loss of Building Floors and Walls, ASTME90-55, Philadelphia, Pa.

10. Bonvallet, G. L.: Retaining high sound transmission loss in industrial plants, *Noise Control*, 3.2:61-64, 1957.

11. Sound Absorption Coefficients of the More Common Acoustic Materials, National Bureau of Standards, U. S. Department of Commerce, Letter Circular LC870.

12. Sound Absorption Coefficients for Architectural Acoustical Materials, Acoustical Materials Association, New York, N. Y.

13. AGMA Standard 295.02-65, Specifications for Measurement of Sound on High Speed Helical and Herringbone Gear Units, American Gear Manufacturers Association, One Thomas Circle, Washington, D. C.

14. ASHRA Standard 36-62, Measurement of Sound Power Radiated from Heating, Refrigerating and Air Conditioning Equipment, American Society of Heating, Refrigerating and Air Conditioning Engineers, Incorporated, 345 East 47th Street, New York, New York.

15. AMCA Standard 300-67, Test Code for Sound Rating, Air Moving and Conditioning Association, Inc., 205 West Toughy Avenue, Park Ridge, Illinois.

16. Test Procedure for Air-Borne Noise Measurements on Rotating Electrical Machinery, Institute of Electrical and Electronic Engineers, Inc., 345 East 47th Street, New York, New York, 1965.

17. Guidelines for Noise Control Specifications for Purchasing Equipment, Iron and Steel Engineer, May 1970.

18. Standards Publication, Gas Turbine Sound and Its Reduction, Publication No. 33-1964, National Electrical Manufacturers Association, 155 East 44th Street, New York, New York.

19. Industrial Noise Manual, Second Edition, American Industrial Hygiene Association, Detroit, Michigan, 1966.

20. ISO Recommendation R-495, General Requirements for the Preparation of Test Codes for Measuring the Noise Emitted by Machines, International Organization for Standardization, Address request to American National Standards Institute, 335 East 45th Street, New York, New York 10017.

21. American National Standard Specification for Sound Level Meters, ANSI S1.4-1971, American National Standards Assn., New York, New York, 1971.

22. American National Standard Specification for Octave, Half-Octave, and Third Octave Band Filter Sets, ANSI S1.11-1966, American National Standards Assn., New York, New York, 1966.

23. American National Standard Method for Physical Measurement of Sound, ANSI S1.2-1962, American National Standards Institute, New York, New York, 1962.

24. Proposed American National Standard Method for Rating the Sound Power Spectra of Small Stationary Noise Sources, ANSI S3.17-197X (Third Draft Dec. 1971). American National Standard Institute.

25. Guidelines for Noise Exposure Control, Intersociety Committee on Guidelines for Noise Exposure Control, American Industrial Hygiene Assoc. J.

Chapter 15

NOISE CONTROL EXAMPLES

ENGINEERING PROCEDURES for the control of noise may take many forms. The most effective and economical means for achieving a reasonably quiet work environment is to use machines and equipment designed to produce a minimum amount of noise. Unfortunately, many long-lived and expensive machines, now in use, produce very high noise levels that must be controlled by engineering means. Some examples of machines and equipment that have been quieted by engineering means are listed below.

TABLE IX

SOUND ABSORPTION COEFFICIENTS OF MATERIALS[2]

The absorption coefficient (α) of a surface which is exposed to a sound field is the ratio of the sound energy absorbed by the surface to the sound energy incident upon the surface. For instance, if 55% of the incident sound energy is absorbed when it strikes the surface of a material, the α of that material would be 0.55. Since the α of a material varies according to many factors, such as frequency of the noise, density, type of mounting, surface conditions, etc., be sure to use the α for the exact conditions to be used and from performance data listings such as shown below. For a more comprehensive list of the absorption coefficients of acoustical materials, refer to the bulletin published yearly by the Acoustical Materials Association, 335 East 45th Street, New York, N. Y. 10017.

| Materials | Coefficients (Hz) | | | | | |
	125	250	500	1,000	2,000	4,000
Brick—glazed	.01	.01	.01	.01	.02	.02
Brick—unglazed	.03	.03	.03	.04	.05	.07
Brick—unglazed, painted	.01	.01	.02	.02	.02	.03
Carpet—heavy, on concrete	.02	.06	.14	.37	.60	.65
Same—on 40 oz. hairfelt or foam rubber (carpet has coarse backing)	.08	.24	.57	.69	.71	.73
Same—with impermeable latex backing on 40 oz. hairfelt or foam rubber	.08	.27	.39	.34	.48	.63
Concrete block—coarse	.36	.44	.31	.29	.39	.25
Concrete block—painted	.10	.05	.06	.07	.09	.08

242

Materials	Coefficients (Hz)					
	125	250	500	1,000	2,000	4,000
Concrete block—poured .... .01	.01	.02	.02	.02	.03
Fabrics						
Light velour—10 oz. per sq. yd. hung						
straight, in contact with wall ... .03	.04	.11	.17	.24	.35
Medium velour—14 oz. per sq. yd.						
draped to half area .... .07	.31	.49	.75	.70	.60
Heavy velour—18 oz. per sq. yd.						
draped. to half area .... .14	.35	.55	.72	.70	.65
Floors						
Concrete or terrazzo .... .01	.01	.015	.02	.02	.02
Linoleum, asphalt, rubber or cork						
tile on concrete .... .02	.03	.03	.03	.03	.02
Wood .... .15	.11	.10 -	.07	.06	.07
Wood parquet in asphalt on concrete .04	.04	.07	.06	.06	.07
Glass						
Large panes of heavy plate glass ... .18	.06	.04	.03	.02	.02
Ordinary window glass .... .35	.25	.18	.12	.07	.04
Glass Fiber—mounted with impervious						
backing—3 lb/cu ft, 1" thick ...... .14	.55	.67	.97	.90	.85
Glass Fiber—mounted with impervious						
backing—3 lb/cu ft, 2" thick ...... .39	.78	.94	.96	.85	.84
Glass Fiber—mounted with impervious						
backing—3 lb/cu ft, 3" thick ...... .43	.91	.99	.98	.95	.93
Gypsum Board—½" nailed to 2 × 4's,						
16" o.c. .... .29	.10	.05	.04	.07	.09
Marble .... .01	.01	.01	.01	.02	.02
Openings						
Stage, depending on furnishings			.25- .75			
Deep balcony, upholstered seats			.50-1.00			
Grills, ventilating			.15- .50			
Grills, ventilating to outside			1.00			
Plaster—gypsum or lime, smooth finish						
on tile or brick .... .013	.015	.02	.03	.04	.05
Plaster—gypsum or lime, rough finish						
on lath .... .14	.10	.06	.05	.04	.03
Same, with smooth finish .... .14	.10	.06	.04	.04	.03
Plywood paneling—⅜" thick .... .28	.22	.17	.09	.10	.11
Sand						
Dry—4" thick .... .15	.35	.40	.50	.55	.80
Dry—12" thick .... .20	.30	.40	.50	.60	.75
Wet—14 lb. water per cu. ft., 4" thick .05	.05	.05	.05	.05	.15
Steel						
Water .... .01	.01	.01	.01	.02	.02
As in a swimming pool .... .008	.008	.013	.015	.020	.025

1. Examples of Noise Absorption

Machines that use moving parts such as cams, gears, reciprocating pieces, and metal stops are often located in large, acoustically reverberant areas that reflect and build up noise levels in the room. A significant reduction of noise levels can be accomplished at times, in locations away from the noise sources, by use of absorption materials. The type, amount, configuration, and placement of absorption materials must be considered specifically for each application; however, the choice of absorbing materials can be guided by the absorption coefficients shown in Table IX.

> Example 1.1 The noise produced by ten wire cutting machines around the periphery of a 20 ft. × 60 ft. × 75 ft. reverberant room was reduced as shown below by the installation of absorption material above the machines.

Octave band center frequency (Hz) [1]	31.5	63	125	250	500	1,000	2,000	4,000	8,000
Noise reduction in dB	—	—	—	2	5	5	10	12	10

> Example 1.2 Several motor generator sets were producing excessive noise levels in a large reverberant room. Noise levels at significant distances away from the generators were reduced as shown below by hanging 6 lb/ft³ Fiberglas baffles in rows just above the level of lights on 3 ft centers. These baffles may be completely encased in a thin film of materials such as polyethylene or mylar without significantly reducing their effectiveness in many applications.

Octave band center frequency (Hz)	31.5	63	125	250	500	1,000	2,000	4,000	8,000
Noise reduction (dB)	—	4	7	9	10	7	8	8	3

> Example 1.3 The noise levels produced in a large reverberant textile mill weave room was reduced with Eloff Hanson Sonosorbers suspended above the lights as shown below.

Octave band center frequency (Hz)	31.5	63	125	250	500	1,000	2,000	4,000	8,000
Noise reduction (dB)	—	6	9	6	6	6	11	11	12

2. Examples Using Noise Barriers and Enclosures

The noise reduction (NR) that can be attained with barriers depends upon the characteristics of the noise source, the barrier configuration and materials used, and the acoustical environment on either side of the barrier. The material used for noise barriers may be described generally in terms of its transmission loss (TL) (see Table X), but all other factors must be considered for specific problems.

The noise reduction achieved by various configurations of specific barrier or enclosure materials may vary significantly. Gen-

TABLE X

SOUND TRANSMISSION LOSS OF GENERAL BUILDING MATERIALS AND STRUCTURES[2]

The sound attenuation provided by a barrier to airborne diffuse sound energy may be described in terms of its sound transmission loss (TL). TL is defined (in dB) as ten times the logarithm to the base 10 of the ratio of the acoustic energy transmitted through a barrier to the acoustic energy incident upon its opposite side. It is a physical property of the barrier material and not of the construction techniques used.

Material or Structure	125	175	250	350	500	700	1,000	2,000	4,000
A. Doors									
1. Heavy wooden door—special hardware; rubber gasket at top, sides and bottom; 2.5" thick; 12.5 lb/sq ft	30	30	30	29	24	25	26	37	36
2. Steel clad door—well-sealed at door casing and threshold	42	47	51	48	48	45	46	48	45
3. Flush—hollow core; well-sealed at door casing and threshold	14	21	27	24	25	25	26	29	31
4. Solid oak—with cracks as ordinarily hung; 1.75" thick	12		15		20		22	16	
5. Wooden door (30" × 84"), special soundproof construction—well-sealed at door casing and threshold; 3" thick; 7 lb/sq ft	31	27	32	30	33	31	29	37	41
B. Glass									
1. 0.125" thick; 1.5 lb/sq ft	27	29	30	31	33	34	34	34	42
2. 0.25" thick; 3 lb/sq ft	27	29	31	32	33	34	34	34	42
3. 0.5" thick; 6 lb/sq ft	17	20	22	23	24	27	29	34	24
4. 1" thick; 12 lb/sq ft	27	31	32	33	35	36	32	37	44
C. Walls—Homogeneous									
1. Steel sheet—fluted; 18 gage stiffened at edges by 2 × 4 wood strips; joints sealed; 4.4 lb/sq ft	30	20	20	21	22	17	30	29	31
2. Asbestos board—corrugated, stiffened horizontally by 2 × 8 in. wood beam; joints sealed; 7.0 lb/sq ft	33	29	31	34	33	33	33	42	39
3. Sheet steel—30 gage; 0.012" thick; 0.5 lb/sq ft	3	6		11		16		21	26
4. Sheet steel—16 gage; 0.598" thick; 2.5 lb/sq ft	13	18		23		28		33	38
5. Sheet steel—10 gage; 0.1345" thick; 5.625 lb/sq ft	18	23		28		33		38	43
6. Sheet steel—0.25" thick; 10 lb/sq ft	23	28	38	33	41	38	46	43	48
7. Sheet steel—0.375" thick; 15 lb/sq ft	26	31	39	36	42	41	47	41	51
8. Sheet steel—0.5" thick; 20 lb/sq ft	28	33		38		43		48	53
9. Sheet aluminum—16 gage; 0.051" thick; 0.734 lb/sq ft	5	8		13		18		23	28
10. Sheet aluminum—10 gage; 0.102" thick; 1.47 lb/sq ft	8	14		19		24		29	34

TABLE X (continued)

Material or Structure	125	175	250	350	500	700	1,000	2,000	4,000
11. Plywood—0.25" thick; 0.73 lb/sq ft		20		19		24		27	22
12. Plywood—0.5" thick; 1.5 lb/sq ft	8	14		19		24		29	34
13. Plywood—0.75" thick; 2.25 lb/sq ft	12	17		22		27		32	37
14. Sheet lead—0.0625" thick; 3.9 lb/sq ft			32		33		32	32	32
15. Sheet lead—0.125" thick; 8.2 lb/sq ft			31		27		37	44	33
16. Glass fiber board—6 lb/cu ft; 1" thick; 0.5 lb/sq ft	5	5	5	5	5	4	4	4	3
17. Laminated glass fiber (FRP); 0.375" thick			26		31		38	37	38
D. Walls—nonhomogeneous									
1. Gypsum wallboard—two 1/2" sheets cemented together, joints wood battened; 1" thick; 4.5 lb/sq ft	24	25	29	32	31	33	32	30	34
2. Gypsum wallboard—four 1/2" sheets cemented together; fastened together with sheet metal screws; dovetail-type joints paper taped; 2" thick; 8/9 lb/sq ft	28	35	32	37	34	36	40	38	49
3. 1/4" plywood glued to both sides of 1 × 3 studs, 16 in. o.c.; 3" thick; 2.5 lb/sq ft	16	16	18	20	26	27	28	37	33
4. Same as (3) above, but 1/2" gypsum wallboard nailed to each face; 4" thick; 6.6 lb/sq ft	26	34	33	40	39	44	46	50	50
5. 1/4" dense fiberboard on both sides of 2 × 4 wood studs, 16" o.c.; fiberboard joints at studs; 4/5" thick; 3.8 lb/sq ft	16	19	22	32	28	33	38	50	52
6. Soft-type fiberboard (3/4") on both sides of 2 × 4 wood studs, 16" o.c.; fiberboard joints at studs; 5" thick; 4.3 lb/sq ft	21	18	21	27	31	32	38	49	53
7. 1/2" gypsum wallboard on both sides of 2 × 4 wood studs, 16" o.c.; 4.5" thick; 5.9 lb/sq ft	20	22	27	35	37	39	43	48	43
8. Two 3/8" gypsum wallboard sheets glued together and applied to each side of 2 × 4 wood studs, 16" o.c.; 5" thick; 8.2 lb/sq ft	27	24	31	35	40	42	46	53	48
9. 2" glass fiber (3 lb/cu ft) + lead vinyl composite; 0.87 lb/sq ft			4		4		13	26	31
10. 3/8" steel + 2.375" polyurethane foam (2 lb/cu ft) + 1/16" steel			38		52		55	64	77
11. Same as (10) above, but 2.5" glass fiber (3 lb/cu ft) instead of foam			37		51		56	65	76
12. 1/4" steel + 1" polyurethane foam (2 lb/cu ft) + 0.055" lead vinyl composite; 1.0 lb/sq ft			38		45		57	56	67

TABLE X (continued)

Material or Structure	Aggregate	125	175	250	350	500	700	1,000	2,000	4,000
E. Masonry										
1. Reinforced concrete; 4" thick; 53 lb/sq ft		37	33	36	44	45	50	52	60	67
2. Brick—common; 12" thick; 121 lb/sq ft		45	49	44	52	53	54	59	60	61
3. 3-3/4 × 4-7/8 × 8 glass brick; 3.75" th.		30	36	35	39	40	45	49	49	43
4. Concrete block—4" hollow, no surface treatment		27	29	32	35	37	42	45	46	48
5. Concrete block—4" hollow, one coat resin—emulsion paint		30	33	34	36	41	45	50	55	53
6. Concrete block—4" hollow, one coat cement base paint	Cinder Aggregate	37	40	43	45	46	49	54	56	55
7. Concrete block—6" hollow, no surface treatment		28	34	36	41	45	48	51	52	47
8. Concrete block—8" hollow, no surface treatment		18	24	28	34	37	39	40	42	40
9. Concrete block—8" hollow, one coat cement base paint		30	36	40	44	46	48	51	50	41
10. Concrete block—8" hollow, filled with vermiculite insulators		20	29	33	36	38	38	40	45	47
11. Concrete block—4" hollow, no surface treatment		21	26	28	31	35	38	41	44	43
12. Concrete block—4" hollow, one coat resin-emulsion paint	Expanded Shale Aggregate	26	30	32	34	37	42	43	46	44
13. Concrete block—4" hollow, two coats resin-emulsion paint		24	31	33	35	38	42	44	47	44
14. Concrete block—4" hollow, one coat cement-base paint		23	30	35	38	42	43	44	48	43
15. Concrete block—4" hollow, two coats cement-base paint		34	38	40	42	45	47	49	51	46
16. Concrete block—6" hollow, no surface treatment		22	27	32	36	40	43	46	45	43
17. Concrete block—4" hollow, no surface treatment		30	36	39	41	43	44	47	54	50
18. Concrete block—4" hollow, one coat cement base paint on face	Dense Aggregate	30	36	39	41	43	44	47	54	49
19. Concrete block—6" hollow, no surface treatment		37	46	50	50	50	53	56	56	46
20. Concrete block—6" hollow, one coat resin-emulsion paint each face		37	50	54	52	53	55	57	56	46
21. Concrete block—8" hollow, no surface treatment		40	47	53	54	54	56	58	58	50
22. Concrete block—8" hollow, two coats resin-emulsion paint each face		38	50	54	54	55	58	60	38	49

erally, a single-wall barrier with no openings placed between the source and the person exposed might expect 2 to 5 dB reduction in the low frequencies and 10 to 15 dB in the high frequencies. Distance of the source and observer from the barrier is also a significant factor. If both the source and observer are close to the barrier, higher noise reduction values are possible. The effects of two- or three-sided barriers are difficult to predict on a general basis; however, well-designed partial enclosures may provide about 5 to 10 dB noise reduction in the low frequencies and about 20 to 25 dB in the high frequencies. Complete enclosures of practical designs may provide in excess of 10 to 15 dB noise reduction in the low frequencies and in excess of 30 dB in the high frequencies. Caution must be taken with any barrier or enclosure to

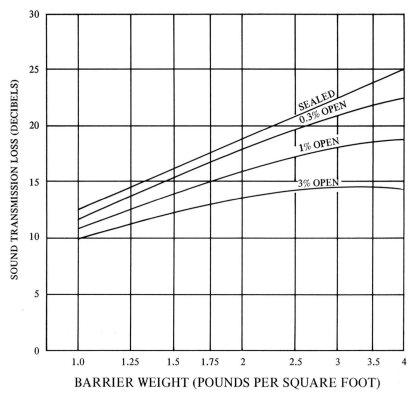

Figure 41. Average Sound Transmission Loss of a Single Sound Barrier as a Function of Barrier Mass and Percentage of Open Area.

HIGHWAY NOISE (dBA, L_{10}) AT VARIOUS DISTANCES FROM EDGE OF 4-LANE HIGHWAY
TRAFFIC: 5,000 VEHICLES PER HOURS, 5% TRUCKS, 53 MPH

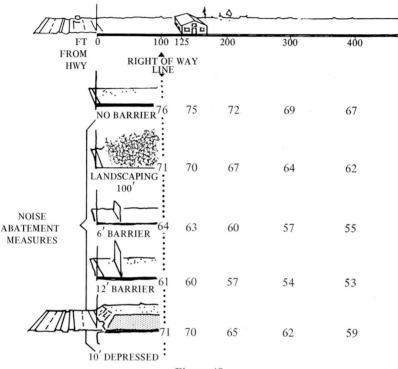

Figure 42.

be sure there are no unnecessary openings. Figure 41 shows the average transmission losses of a single barrier as a function of barrier mass and percentage of open area.

> Example 2.1   An operator positioned close to a punch press that uses compressed air jets to blow foreign particles from the die was exposed to excessive noise levels. A $\frac{1}{4}$-inch thick safety glass provided good visibility and access to the work position, and gave the following noise reduction at the operator's head position.

O.B. (Hz)	31.5	63	125	250	500	1,000	2,000	4,000	8,000
N.R. (dB)	—	—	1	2	3	9	14	20	22

> Example 2.2   Highway noise at various distances from the edge of a four-lane highway are plotted below with no barrier and with dif-

ferent barrier configurations.[3] The traffic density during these measurements averaged 5,000 vehicles per hour with five percent trucks.
The average vehicle speed was about 53 mph.

Example 2.3   A sheet metal belt guard was installed around a high
speed rubber-tooth drive belt. The noise reduction achieved is shown
below.

O.B. (Hz)	31.5	63	125	250	500	1,000	2,000	4,000	8,000
N.R. (dB)	—	—	—	—	—	—	7	9	19

Example 2.4   An electric motor-gear drive assembly was enclosed using
⅛-inch steel with welded joints which was lined with 1-inch Fiberglas (No. 615) board. Silencers for intake and exhaust ventilation
air were constructed of 12-inch parallel plates of 1-inch coated Fiberglas (No. 615) PF board spaced 1 inch apart. The noise reduction
achieved is shown below.

O.B. (Hz)	31.5	63	125	250	500	1,000	2,000	4,000	8,000
N.R. (dB)	—	5	6	12	14	25	35	24	23

Example 2.5   A complete enclosure was constructed to enclose large
sirens for production testing. The enclosure was made with sheet
steel lined with Fiberglas, the inner side of which in turn was
covered with an open-mesh protective surface. The noise reduction
is shown below.

O.B. (Hz)	31.5	63	125	250	500	1,000	2,000	4,000	8,000
N.R. (dB)	—	—	—	15	13	27	33	38	43

Example 2.6   An operator of a pneumatic system that included compressors and ducts for conveying pellets spent a large portion of his
time at a central location. An enclosure for the operator was designed using wood framing with ⅝-inch gypsum board inside and
out. The open spaces between the boards were filled with Fiberglas
and all joints in the gypsum board were sealed. Double-glazed windows were provided for observation of equipment on all sides. The
noise reduction is shown below.

O.B. (Hz)	31.5	63	125	250	500	1,000	2,000	4,000	8,000
N.R. (dB)	8	6	8	15	15	10	14	18	19

3. Examples Using Impact, Radiation, and Vibration Reduction

Example 3.1   A high speed film rewind machine (15 HP) produced
excessive noise from the metal-to-metal impacts between gear teeth.
Fiber gears were substituted for the metal ones and the gears were
flooded in oil. The noise reduction is shown below.

O.B. (Hz)	31.5	63	125	250	500	1,000	2,000	4,000	8,000
N.R. (dB)	—	10	6	5	5	8	20	16	14

Example 3.2   An eight-foot diameter hopper with an electric solenoid-
type vibrator coupled solidly to a bottom bin was causing excessive

noise. A live bottom bin by Vibra Screw was installed that required less vibratory power since only the cone is vibrated. Also, the new system had less radiation area and there was no metal-to-metal impacts. The noise reduction achieved is shown below.

O.B. (Hz)		31.5	63	125	250	500	1,000	2,000	4,000	8,000
N.R. (dB)		—	7	6	20	22	16	12	12	9

Example 3.3   Screw machine stock tubes constructed of solid steel usually make excessive noise because there is nearly continuous impact between the tube and the screw stock. New tubes, such as the Corlett Turner Silent Stock tube, constructed as a sandwich with an absorbent material between the outer steel tube and an inner helically wound liner, provide significantly lower noise levels. The noise reduction achieved with the new tube design operated at 4,000 rpm with $\frac{1}{2}$-inch hexagonal stock is shown below.

O.B. (Hz)		31.5	63	125	250	500	1,000	2,000	4,000	8,000
N.R. (dB)		—	12	15	15	14	20	29	34	30

4. Examples Using Acoustical Damping

Example 4.1   A metal enclosure around a rubber compounding mill vibrated freely, thus amplifying the motor, gear, and roll noises of the mill. An application of vibration damping material ($\frac{1}{4}$-inch Aquaplas F 102A) to the inner surface of the metal enclosure reduced the noise as shown below.

O.B. (Hz)		31.5	63	125	250	500	1,000	2,000	4,000	8,000
N.R. (dB)		10	9	9	13	9	7	8	10	11

Example 4.2   The guards and exhaust hoods of a ten-blade gang ripsaw was coated with MMM Underseal (EC-244). The noise reduction attained while the saw was idling is shown below.

O.B. (Hz)		31.5	63	125	250	500	1,000	2,000	4,000	8,000
N.R. (dB)		6	7	10	7	5	3	3	5	6

Example 4.3   A $\frac{3}{8}$-inch steel casing of a 2,000 HP extruder gear and its base were vibrating excessively causing unwanted noise. Accelerometer measurements showed the casing and the 1-inch steel base were vibrating at about the same level. The casing was damped with a $\frac{1}{4}$-inch felt (No. 11 Anchor Packing Co.) plus an outer covering of $\frac{1}{4}$-inch steel. The felt-steel sandwich was bolted together on 8-inch centers. The steel base had 9-inch deep ribs that made the felt-steel damping impractical so the base was damped by a thick cover of sand. The noise reduction attained is shown below.

O.B. (Hz)		31.5	63	125	250	500	1,000	2,000	4,000	8,000
N.R. (dB)		—	—	—	—	4	17	26	24	18

5. Examples Using Reduced Driving Force

Any noise produced by a repetitive force that is caused by an eccentricity or imbalance of a rotating member will increase with rotational speed. Obviously, one very important noise control procedure is to dynamically balance all rotating pieces. Also, these pieces should rotate concentrically. Proper maintenance of all bearing and other rotating contact surfaces is essential to keep equipment running quietly.

No machine should be operated at an unnecessarily high speed. In many instances, a significant reduction in noise can be achieved by using a larger machine that can do the same job while operating at lower speeds.

Reduction of driving force in almost any form is an effective noise control procedure. In many instances, a reduction of driving force will provide the additional advantage of reduced radiation area.

> Example 5.1   A blower exhaust system running at 705 rpm, 6-inch statis pressure, and 13,800 cfm was badly out of balance and bearings needed replacing. After new bearings were installed and the system was balanced, the following improvement was found.

O.B. (Hz)	31.5	63	125	250	500	1,000	2,000	4,000	8,000
N.R. (dB)	—	3	3	11	12	11	10	8	10

> Example 5.2   An oversized propeller-type fan (36-inch) mounted in the wall of a large reverberant room produced excessive noise when operated at 870 rpm. It was possible to get the significant noise reduction shown below, while at the same time providing sufficient ventilation, by reducing the fan speed from 870 to 690 rpm.

O.B. (Hz)	31.5	63	125	250	500	1,000	2,000	4,000	8,000
N.R. (dB)	—	3	7	8	12	9	8	6	4

> Example 5.3   Small metal parts were dropped several inches into a metal chute where they were moved by gravity onto another operation. The dropping distance and weight of the pieces could not be changed, so the chute surface was covered with a layer of 1/16-inch paperboard and this layer was in turn covered by 18-gage steel. The noise reduction of this sandwich covering is shown below.

O.B. (Hz)	31.5	63	125	250	500	1,000	2,000	4,000	8,000
N.R. (dB)	4	4	4	2	7	9	12	14	16

Example 5.4   Steel balls tumbling against the steel shell of a ball mill was producing excessive noise. The steel shell was lined with resilient material (rubber) to achieve the noise reduction shown below.

O.B. (Hz)	31.5	63	125	250	500	1,000	2,000	4,000	8,000
N.R. (dB)	—	3	4	6	7	11	12	15	19

6. Examples Using Mufflers and Air Noise Generation Control Means

Example 6.1   An air driven impact gun usually makes excessive noise. A simple means of reducing this noise is to pipe the exhausted air to a remote location by means of a rubber hose. Another noise reduction means is to use an internal muffler. The following noise reduction figures were achieved with an air gun running free.

O.B. (Hz)	31.5	63	125	250	500	1,000	2,000	4,000	8,000
N.R. (dB) Muffler	—	—	2	2	4	15	9	6	7
N.R. (dB) Rubber Hose	—	—	19	17	30	42	29	28	28

Example 6.2   The air intakes of reciprocating air compressors often create objectionable low frequency noise. An intake filter muffler, such as the Burgess Manning Model Delta P—SDF, can reduce the noise in the 63 cps octave band by as much as 23 dB.

Example 6.3   The discharge of a Gast Air Motor (Model 4 AM and 6 AM) created excessive noise. A Burgess Manning Delta P CA type muffler installed on the discharge outlet produced the following noise reduction.

O.B. (Hz)	31.5	63	125	250	500	1,000	2,000	4,000	8,000
N.R. (dB)	—	2	7	7	9	10	23	29	23

Example 6.4   The blower noise from the discharge of a pneumatic conveying system handling synthetic fiber fluff was excessive. An absorbing-type muffler was not desired because of the possibility of snagging and plugging. A resonant-type muffler supplied by Universal Silencer Corporation provided the noise reduction shown below.

O.B. (Hz)	31.5	63	125	250	500	1,000	2,000	4,000	8,000
N.R. (dB)	—	12	23	13	11	10	—	—	—

Example 6.5   An air intake of a 7,000 HP gas turbine operating at 5,800 rpm and 6,200 HP created excessive noise. A parallel baffle muffler consisting of six plates, each 3.5-inch wide, filled with Fiberglas and faced with 18-gage perforated sheet steel was attached to the intake and the baffle was in turn fed by an unlined 0.25-inch

duct made of steel plate. The cross-section of the duct was 7 feet ×
8 feet. The noise reduction achieved is shown below.

O.B. (Hz)	31.5	63	125	250	500	1,000	2,000	4,000	8,000
N.R. (dB)	—	—	10	16	22	33	35	27	26

Example 6.6 The noise produced by a tube reamer was reduced by
the following values by mounting a Wilson 8,500 muffler on the
exhaust.

O.B. (Hz)	31.5	63	125	250	500	1,000	2,000	4,000	8,000
N.R. (dB)	2	2	3	10	23	26	28	16	18

7. Examples Using Drive System Modifications

Example 7.1 A rubber-toothed belt used to drive a pump was replaced by a V-belt drive. The noise reduction achieved is shown
below.

O.B. (Hz)	31.5	63	125	250	500	1,000	2,000	4,000	8,000
N.R. (dB)	—	5	4	4	2	—	8	17	18

Example 7.2 An edger-planer for trimming foamed plastic created
noise levels as high as 102 dB in the 250 Hz octave band. The noise
was caused primarily by the cutter blades chopping the conveying
air stream. The clearance between the cutter blades and the casing
was increased from ³⁄₃₂-inch to 1-inch, thereby lowering the air
velocity and reducing the noise level to 84 dB in the 250 Hz band.

A single noise control procedure often may be ineffective by itself, but when coupled with one or more other procedures, it may
produce significant results. As an example, a typical noise source
having a frequency spectrum in which all octave band pressure
levels are essentially the same may have the following noise reduction values for the various noise control procedures shown below.

Noise Reduction Procedure	Noise Reduction (in dB) as a Function of Frequency (in Octave Bands)								
	31.5	63	125	250	500	1,000	2,000	4,000	8,000
1. Mounted on Vibration Isolators	11	7	3	—	—	—	—	—	—
2. Single Wall Barrier	—	—	3	5	6	6	6	6	7
3. Complete Enclosure of Absorbing Material	—	—	—	4	5	5	6	7	7
4. Complete Enclosure of Solid Material with No Absorption Inside	—	2	5	14	18	26	26	27	29
5. Complete Enclosure of Solid Material with No Absorption									

Inside Mounted on Vibration Isolators	11	8	7	16	21	29	34	35	40
6. Complete Enclosure of Solid Material with Absorption Inside Mounted on Vibration Isolators	11	11	13	25	32	38	40	42	45
7. Complete No. 6 Procedure Mounted on Vibration Isolators and Enclosed in Solid Material with Absorption Inside	20	17	22	44	50	57	57	59	64

Many of the examples of noise control in this chapter were taken from material prepared for the American Industrial Hygiene Association (AIHA) Noise Manual.[2] A more extensive listing of examples and a more complete general discussion of engineering noise control can be found in the AIHA Manual.

REFERENCES

1. Preferred Frequencies and Band Numbers for Acoustical Measurements, American National Standards Institute (ANSI) Standard S1.6-1967.
2. Industrial Noise Manual, 2nd Ed., American Industrial Hygiene Association, Detroit, Michigan, 1966.
3. Department of Transportation Noise Standards. *Federal Register, 37*(114): 94-95, 1972.

Chapter 16

THE HEARING CONSERVATION PROGRAM

WITH THE PASSAGE of the Occupational Noise Exposure Amendment of the Walsh Healey regulation in 1969 and the Occupational Safety and Health Act in 1971, management's decision to protect the hearing of employees is no longer voluntary. All industries in which noice levels exceed the limits described in Chapter 9 must reduce the levels, or start hearing conservation programs.

Industry today is safety-minded. Aside from the human tragedy involved, accidents are expensive to industry and most industries feel that money spent in prevention produces a very satisfactory return on the investment, both in dollars and in human satisfaction. Industrial medicine has demonstrated that excessive exposure to certain materials handled by workers can produce illness through their mechanical and toxic effects. Solvent and other toxic vapors, fumes or metallic particles, and silica dust must be reduced to safe levels to avoid injury. Recently, interest has been aroused in the possible injurious affects of the physical environment, and it has been found that too much heat, too much humidity, too much radiation, or too much noise can produce adverse physiologic effects, frank illness, loss of time, and loss of dollars.

We are concerned here with the effects upon the inner ear of excessive exposure to industrial noise. The medical profession has no satisfactory treatment presently available for hearing loss caused by noise.

Setting up a conservation-of-hearing program costs industry both time and money. The decision to invest that time and money is a management decision and is based upon a determination of whether or not a noise problem exists. For an answer to this question management must rely on the industrial physician and engineer and their colleagues, who are responsible for advising management on the control of industrial health hazards. Chapters 11 and 12 go into detail regarding the factors that must be considered to obtain accurate measurements. However, for a rough estimate, if a continuous noise makes even loud conversation difficult, it probably exceeds the safe level.

Once it has been established that a noice problem exists management is next concerned with the question, "What are the economic consequences of claims for industrial hearing loss, if they can be sustained in Compensation Court or at Common Law?"

Everyone who has an interest in the problem should acquaint himself with the situation in his own state, with federal legislation, and particularly with court decisions, legislative activities, and legal costs that bear on the problem. With this information and some idea of the risk of incurring claims, some estimate of the economic risk should be possible.

Benefits of Hearing Testing

Management is next concerned with the question, "What benefits can be gained by organizing an audiometric testing program?" First of all, an audiometric testing program is a protection against unjustified claims, to which the employer would be vulnerable unless he could produce evidence of previous hearing loss.

Using preemployment audiograms to establish a record of hearing acuity of all employees is very similar to the procedure often used in industry for protecting itself against unjustified claims by means of preemployment and routine chest x-rays. For example: Should a worker in a dusty area complain of pulmonary disability and a chest x-ray discloses tuberculosis, we may have *a priori* claim that this injury was caused by his current exposure, *unless* preemployment and subsequent x-rays demonstrate that his tuberculosis was preexisting and was not aggravated by his current exposure.

Similarly, in the case of a claim for deafness due to exposure to industrial noise, a preemployment audiogram on record showing a hearing loss upon employment and subsequent routine audiograms showing only those changes expected because of advancing age make it improbable to sustain a claim for hearing loss as a result of current employment. The value to the employer of an audiometric testing program in such a situation is obvious.

There is another aspect to an organized audiometric program, however, which is more appealing to the physician: Its value in preventive medicine. The usual occupational hearing loss follows a gradual process and develops slowly over months or years of exposure. Furthermore, there is generally a degree of recovery after exposure ceases. If the loss can be ascertained in its early phase, a considerable degree of recovery can be expected if the individual's exposure to noise is reduced or eliminated. Such remedial measures can be instituted when the need for them is revealed through the audiometric program.

Management will be in a position to reach a decision if the risk of incurring claims for industrial hearing loss can be estimated, if the economic consequences of claims for hearing loss are understood, and if the potential benefits of an organized audiometric testing program are fully appreciated. These benefits are twofold. They insure against unjustified claims, *and* they make possible a truly preventive medical program that can protect the worker against ever sustaining an occupational hearing loss.

Important though the contributions of an audiometric testing program may be, and even though its costs may be acceptable to management, hesitation to institute the program may arise from two considerations:

1. Would the initiation of a conservation-of-hearing program appear to be a confession of guilt on the part of a management and an acknowledgement that a noise hazard exists?
2. Would it invite claims for occupational hearing loss?

With respect to the first question, instituting an audiometric program is no more confession of guilt than instituting a program of routine chest x-rays, or blood counts, or any other routine medical examination. Its purpose is to gather information and to appraise the health status of the worker so that his health may be better protected. It also seems rather naive to assume today that workers are unaware of the fact that they are working in a noisy environment, or that there is such a thing as industrial hearing loss. As with all other industrial health situations it would seem better to face problems where they exist, evaluate them accurately, and institute all necessary control measures, rather than to hope they will solve themselves if left alone. It is the consensus of all authorities working in this field that a forthright approach is far more effective than procrastination.

As for the second question, a hearing loss is not created by its detection. It either exists, or it does not exist. If audiograms are taken correctly and show normal hearing, they protect the employer against unjustified claims. If they show impaired hearing, the door is open to a thorough investigation of the cause of the impairment, whether it be caused by disease or by occupational noise exposure; and the necessary measures can then be taken for prevention of further hearing loss and the maximum conservation of existing hearing.

It should be remembered that (1) hearing loss may increase with length of exposure to excessive noise, (2) there is often some recovery of hearing acuity when exposure to noise is reduced to safe levels, and (3) an organized audiometric testing program permits evaluation of both the existing hearing acuity and the efficiency of control measures. Therefore, it would seem that the advantages to be gained far outweigh the hypothetical disadvantages, where a hazardous noise exposure exists.

Another extremely important advantage of a conservation-of-hearing program is the detection of all employees with hearing losses that might be curable or might be prevented from getting worse. By making a careful otological diagnosis of all the hearing losses of employees in the plant, a good program will detect numerous individuals whose hearing can be cured by referring them to well-trained local specialists. For example, in one southern plant that instituted an excellent conservation-of-hearing program, twenty-seven individuals with marked hearing loss had their hearing restored by a local otologist whose surgical skill has become fully appreciated in his community. The industry itself has also benefited by a substantial improvement in its relations with labor and the community, and has become recognized as one sincerely interested in the health of its employees.

How To Sell Management Hearing Conservation

Some individual in the company or plant must recognize the need to determine whether a noise problem exists and to sell management on doing something about it. In large companies it is usually the Safety Engineer, the Plant Physician, or the Nurse, who after reading about occupational hearing loss or attending a lecture on the subject presents the problem to a superior, usually the Personnel Director or even a Vice-President. In a small plant there generally is no medical director and there may not even be a safety director or nurse. In such plants, management generally does not become aware of the problem until a federal or state inspector submits a warning, or until an employee files a claim for compensation (usually through a lawyer).

Until the Occupational Safety and Health Act was passed, most plants did very little about hearing conservation even after being apprised of their noise problems. Of course, a few major companies noted for their safety and health interests have been conducting effective programs for many years. Most notable are the Dupont Co., telephone companies, certain airplane companies, Firestone, Ingersoll-Rand, Ford Motor Co., Chicopee, Meade, Burlington Industries, and Cone Mills. But on the whole there has been more discussion than action in the practice of hearing conservation.

With the advent of federal and state regulations and the rigorous enforcement by the Department of Labor, many companies are beginning to comply with the regulations. It is the job of the Safety Engineer, Physician, and Nurse to convince management to meet regulations for medical and safety reasons as well as economic ones. Noisy plants will find it far more economical to prevent deafness than to pay compensation and engage in legal disputes.

The program must be sold first to top management and have its complete approval and cooperation. To achieve this, many plants will have to bring in an outside consultant who can impress top management with the important advantages of the program. In describing the need for a hearing program and how and who will run it, an estimate of the cost must be presented. Very few companies have enough competent personnel to implement the entire program by themselves. Most plants will have to seek the help of an acoustics consultant, safety engineer, and especially an otologist familiar with this work. The cost proposal should also include expenses for equipment and ear protectors. The cost of possible noise control measures should also be presented. It is essential to keep costs very low; and in the author's experiences most industries have done so unless they have embarked on programs without expert and experienced guidance. The more common reasons for costly mistakes by some companies have been purchasing the wrong audiometers, too expensive test rooms, impractical mobile trailers and the purchase of ineffective ear protectors that employees refuse to wear. Film strips and movies of an educational and motivational nature, along with personal presentations, should be shown to management and labor before distributing ear protectors. Such films are being used by the Ford Motor Co., Burlington and Cone Industries, and many others. The author (JS) has prepared a film applicable to management and labor.

What Is a Hearing Conservation Program

Once top management has approved the overall program and provided the funding, it becomes the responsibility of the plant physician and engineer to put it into action. The essential components of a hearing conservation program are:

1. Measurement of plant noise and determination of which employees are exposed to levels that could produce hearing damage.
2. Hearing testing—advisable for all employees, but essential for those in noisy jobs.

3. Obtaining otoscopic examination and histories of noise exposures and ear diseases on all employees, and correlating data with job noise.
4. Determining where noise control measures are feasible, and developing a good ear protection program.
5. Disposition of individual employees with hearing problems, as well as the diagnosis of all causes of hearing loss found throughout the plant.

If it is possible to reduce plant noise to a safe level then no further attention may be necessary. A Hearing Testing Program, however, may be of some help for reasons already cited, but especially to protect management from unwarranted claims and legal harassment. If noise levels cannot be brought down to within safe limits by noise control, then a full hearing program is advisable and essential.

Initiating and maintaining a conservation-of-hearing program is the responsibility of a team rather than of a single individual; it requires the cooperation of the industrial physician, safety engineer, hygienist, nurse, industrial-relations and personnel managers, and a consultant otologist, as well as others. The direct supervision of the overall program should be the responsibility of the industrial physician if available; since it is ultimately a medical problem. The team of specialists gathering and interpreting data should ideally center around the medical department. The plant physician, being aware of the handicaps produced by deafness, can generally be the chief motivating force in impressing management with the importance of instituting the audiometric program and noise-abatement measures.

The Role of the Safety Engineer and Industrial Hygienist

If a plant physician is not available, responsibility for the overall program falls to the safety or hygiene engineer. In any event, it is often the task of this engineer initially to recognize the need for a noise and hearing survey, and to help decide how extensive a conservation-of-hearing program need to be. He also frequently performs the noise survey and recommends noise control measures. If an outside consultant is retained to make the survey, he should work in close cooperation with the plant safety and hygiene engineers so they may follow through with his recommendations, continuing an active watch over the program and making necessary changes, particularly in an expanding plant.

The plant engineer also has the responsibility for evaluating ear protectors and deciding which are most suitable in the various noise areas. Chapter 17 serves as a guide to engineers making such decisions. Educating plant personnel to the importance of a conservation-of-hearing program is also the job of the safety engineer. He must help instruct employees in the proper use of ear protectors and assume responsibility for their being effectively used during working hours. The job foreman or superintendent is most helpful in making certain that personnel in noisy areas wear ear protectors. Impressing supervisors with the importance of a conservation-of-hearing program is an essential duty of the safety or hygiene engineer. A supervisory training course should be conducted on the conservation-of-hearing program that is to be established. Attendance should be mandatory for supervisors of departments in potentially hazardous noise areas. They should be informed on the reasons for developing a conservation-of-hearing program, the effects noise can have on individuals, the policy of the company toward harmful and injurious noises, and on what the supervisors are expected to contribute to the program. It is helpful to demonstrate the hearing distortion caused by damaging noises. Ear protectors and other protective equipment should be discussed and demonstrated. The use of an audiometer and the purpose of taking audiograms should be explained.

Some plants require all employees and visitors who enter a noisy area to wear ear protectors. An extra supply of various types and sizes of protectors should be available in noisy areas for special purposes, such as for use by visitors or inspectors.

The plant engineer can also be of great help in selecting a room suitable for performing hearing tests. If such a room is not readily available, the engineer must recommend adequate modifications of an existing room, or advise on the purchase of a commercial test booth.

Scheduling employees for audiometric tests is a joint function of the engineer and medical department. The engineer must have a thorough knowledge of each department to be tested in order to arrange the testing schedule with minimum interference with normal work. He must know in advance the amount of time each audiometric test will take, and the time required for each employee to teach the test room from his particular job. By staggering the flow of employees, the testing can be done without having the employees waiting in line to be tested or without overloading the tester. Consideration should always be given to temporary hearing loss when scheduling for audiometry. In most instances where effective ear protectors are used, it may be possible to test employees by scheduling routine follow-up tests about 5 minutes apart.

The plant engineer or foreman should try to have all employees who work in noisy areas report to the medical department for terminal stabilized hearing tests prior to their being discharged or transferred to another plant, or to a job of a different nature.

Whenever extraordinary manufacturing processes are introduced that produce more intense noise than the usual operations, they should be investigated by the safety engineer so that he may take precautionary measures to protect employees. A department head may not realize the increased danger to the hearing of exposed personnel.

The Role of the Industrial Nurse

The plant nurse is probably the most important person in a Hearing Conservation Program. Even if a plant physician is available a good nurse generally does the major portion of the work; and if a physician is not available, she often assumes many of his responsibilities.

Most important the nurse creates the image of the Hearing Conservation Program. She is the chief of Public Relations between management and employees. If she is enthusiastic and pleasant, and supports the program with sincerity and understanding, it will succeed. If not, the program will be mediocre or fail. Her attitude towards employees when she is doing audiometry is of paramount importance. Kindness, humor, and warmth must prevail to avoid alienating employees and stirring up trouble. It is the nurse who has the first and prolonged contact with the employee. She not only conducts the hearing test but occasionally she has to explain the results to the employee. She also fits the ear protectors and motivates employees to accept them, and she frequently checks to see they are being used effectively. She screens those employees to be seen by a physician. She keeps and assesses records and takes histories. She should be taught to uncover important information and also to examine the ear canal and eardrum with an otoscope. She does all this in addition to many other responsibilities in and out of Hearing Conservation. Therefore, the nurse is most important and has to be well trained. She should be certified in industrial hearing testing by taking the program described in Chapter 7 at the best facility available.

EXAMINING THE EAR

To provide the industrial nurse with a general background in the ear examination as the otologist performs it, and to show her how she can often be of greater assistance in many industrial problems involving the ear, we include the following information.

The industrial nurse should be able to examine the external auditory canal and the eardrum with an otoscope. She should be able to distinguish a normal from an abnormal eardrum. In some instances she may be called upon to remove wax from the external canals of employees who show no evidence of perforation of the eardrums. Such procedures should be done under the direction of the industrial physician.

When a patient complains of ear discomfort or a foreign body in his ear and a physician is not immediately available, it is proper for the nurse to undertake a preliminary examination. It is also in order for her to do so if an audiogram, just taken, reflects a marked hearing deterioration from the previous record, especially if she suspects that impacted cerumen might be the cause of the change in the hearing level. However it is essential that the examination be performed carefully and without discomfort to the employee.

Before inserting an otoscope tip into an ear canal, it is wise to shine the light of the otoscope (or that from a headlight) upon the outer ear and into the auditory canal, in order not to overlook a boil or cyst that might be situated at the very entrance, where it would otherwise be covered by the otoscope.

When the otologist does such an examination, he generally uses the largest otoscope tip that will fit into the canal. This permits the broadest view. In addition, a snug fit enables him to compress air in the canal with a rubber syringe if he wishes to test the mobility of the eardrum. This procedure is also useful to detect a possible perforation in the eardrum.

Ear Canal Findings

If wax or debris is present, it should be carefully removed so that the entire drum can be seen. Whenever possible the wax should be gently picked out in one piece with a dull ear curette. Irrigation should be reserved for those cases where the wax is impacted and difficult to pick or wipe out, and where there is no likelihood of a perforation being present. This procedure is preferably performed by a physician. Any debris, such as that due to external otitis or otitis media should be carefully wiped out with a thin cotton-tipped applicator, or a physician may remove it with a fine suction tip.

In the event that bony protrusions (exostoses) are present in the canal, care should be taken to avoid injuring the thin skin covering them, so as to prevent bleeding and infection. If a large tip on the otoscope makes it difficult to see the drum for any reason, a smaller one is used, but it should be inserted very gently.

The Eardrum

Much information can be derived from discerning scrutiny of the eardrum. In a normal eardrum, a cone of light is classically seen coming from the end of the handle of the malleus because of the manner in which the sloping drum reflects the light from the otoscope. In some eardrums the cone of light may not be seen, but this does not necessarily mean that a real abnormality exists. Absence of the cone of light may result from an unusual slope of the drum or a deviation in the angle of the external canal, or it may be due to a thickening of the eardrum, or senile changes that prevent reflection of the light.

An essential point is whether the drum is intact (Plates 1-5, Frontispiece). A hole in the eardrum is usually quite visible, but at times it is obscure. Occasionally, what appears to be a hole is really an old healed perforation covered with a thin, transparent film of epithelium. If there is a discharge that does not come from the external canal, or the discharge is mucoid, the perforation emitting the secretion must be located. A pinpoint perforation should be suspected when a patient complains that he hears air whistling in his ear whenever he blows his nose or sneezes.

It is clear from the mere mention of these difficulties and complications that the scope of the ear examination within the province of the industrial nurse is necessarily limited, and subject to confirmation or correction by an experienced physician.

There are several ways in which an otologist can detect a perforation in the eardrum. One is to move the drum back and forth with air pressure in the external canal. This is done with a Siegeloscope or the rubber bulb attached to some otoscopes. If the drum doesn't move, or moves only slightly, the perforation may become visible since the perforated area moves more sluggishly than the rest of the drum. If the location of the perforation is high in the drum (Shrapnell's area), it may still move fairly well.

Another technique used in detecting a perforation is to have the patient swallow, while a camphorated mist is forced into one nostril and the other is pinched closed. If the Eustachian tube is patent and there is a perforation in the drum, the mist will be seen issuing through the small perforation while the examiner looks into the external auditory canal. Sometimes spraying boric acid powder on the drum helps delineate the edges of the perforation. The same procedures can also be used to determine whether there is a transplant film over a healed perforation but gentleness and care are essential to avoid breaking the film.

Another important thing to look for is shadow formation behind the drum, particularly as caused by fluid in the middle ear. To accomplish this, we should try to look through the drum rather than merely at it. What seemed to be a simple surface will then resemble a map, with a dark shadow for the round window and a lighter area for the promontory, a pink area for the incus, and many other features.

Fluid in the Middle Ear

Fluid in the middle ear often eludes detection even though it causes hearing loss, thus leading to a mistaken diagnosis. For instance, a patient may have a 30 decibel conductive hearing loss with an eardrum that appears practically normal. A diagnosis of otosclerosis would be suggested and stapes surgery would seem to be indicated. When reflecting the eardrum during surgery, however, the otologic surgeon might encounter a thick mucoid gelatinous mass, especially around the oval and round windows, and the correct diagnosis would not be otosclerosis but secretory otitis media. The fluid was simply not detected preoperatively.

Fluid in the middle ears should be searched for diligently if bone conduction is slightly reduced in an otherwise classical picture of conductive hearing loss. There are several ways to detect fluid in the middle ear. If a well-defined fluid level is seen through the eardrum, the diagnosis is simple. However, we should bear in mind that strands of scar tissue in the drum and bands in the middle ear can simulate a fluid level.

It is helpful to determine whether the apparent fluid level maintains its position while the patient's head is bent forward and backward. If it is a fluid level, it will remain horizontal even if the head is bent forward, the same as the level in a partially filled glass of water will remain horizontal when the glass is tilted. However, if the apparent level moves with the head, it is a sign that it is attached to the eardrum, and is probably a fibrous strand in the drum.

With air pressure in the external canal, it is difficult to get free to-and-fro motion of the drum if there is much fluid behind it in the middle ear. In contrast, a normal drum is easily moved. Occasionally, bubbles can be seen in the fluid. This assures a diagnosis of fluid in the ear.

Politzerization

Politzerization is of great help in detecting fluid but should not be performed in the presence of an upper respiratory infection, particularly one affecting the nose. During the politzerization the fluid and bubbles can be briefly seen through the drum; then they usually disappear. The patient may also suddenly hear better. Whenever there is any doubt about the middle ear fluid being present, an otologist generally performs a myringotomy for diagnostic and therapeutic reasons. In adults, this is best done without local or general anesthesia by using a sharp knife to puncture the posterior portion of the drum. If fluid is present some will usually ooze out spontaneously, or it can be forced out by politzeration or suction through the myringotomy wound if it is done deftly. Manipulation involved in trying to produce some local anesthesia often prolong the procedure and cause discomfort.

The eardrum may reveal still other findings, such as scars and placques. These reflect previous infections and tissue changes in the eardrum. In themselves, they rarely cause any significant degree of hearing loss. Occasionally, an eardrum appears blue or purple. This may be due to blood in the middle ear, or to entrapped fluid, or it may just be a peculiar type of retracted ear drum. A reddish color is occasionally due to a tumor (glomus jugulare) extending into the middle ear. If there is any possibility that such a tumor may be present, exploration should be done with great circumspection.

Retracted Eardrum

This brings us to the retracted eardrum, another abnormal finding. It is easy to understand why one physician will look at a drum and say it is normal and another will say it is retracted. Eardrums vary in their appearance, and the concept of retraction is subject to these variations. This should make little difference in otology for even a moderate amount of retraction usually does not cause any substantial hearing loss. Only when the drum is markedly retracted, and especially when it is pulled into the promontory, is there a correlation between retraction and hearing. In such instances, politzerization can restore hearing by returning the drum to its original position. Occasionally the drum is overdistended during politzerization and it then appears flaccid and relaxed.

In all cases of retracted eardrum, the cause should be sought in the nasopharynx, sinuses and Eustachian tubes. Allergies and adenoid hypertrophy are the most common causes, but neoplasms must also be excluded, especially in unilateral cases. Aerotitis media may be another cause of a retracted eardrum. In some, politzerization is not possible, and a small Eustachian catheter has to be gently guided by a nasopharyngoscope positioned through the other nares. Then air can be carefully forced in until the tube is opened. By placing a listening tube in the patient's ear and the other end in the physician's ear the sound of air can be heard as it enters the middle ear.

Middle Ear Damage

Perhaps the most confusing otologic picture presents itself when the eardrum is largely eroded and the middle ear is discharging; a similar problem arises when some kind of ear surgery has deformed the normal landmarks. It is necessary in such cases to appraise the condition of the middle ear in order to decide upon the proper treatment, and to evaluate the chances of restoring hearing. In view of the extensive amount of otologic surgery that has been performed in recent years, it is always wise to look for scars of previous operations, both postauricular and endaural, the latter being situated just above the tragus. A postauricular scar usually indicates mastoid surgery. If the eardrum is practically normal it was in all likelihood a simple mastoidectomy and the hearing may be normal. If the eardrum is absent and the malleus and incus are also absent, a radical mastoidectomy was done, and the hearing level should be about 50 to 60 dB. Intermediate between the simple and the radical mastoidectomies are a variety of surgical procedures aimed at preserving as much hearing as possible while eradicating infection. These procedures are usually called modified radical mastoidectomies or tympanoplasties. Usually the drum or part of it is visible and some form of ossicular chain is present. A plastic tube may have been inserted to restore ossicular continuity; also a vein graft or skin graft may have been applied to replace the eardrum that had been removed previously. The endaural scar could also indicate a fenestration operation, in which case a bizarre looking eardrum will be visible. Quite often these cavities are covered with debris and require gentle cleaning to permit a clear view. Caution is necessary in cleaning such a cavity, to avoid inducing vertigo and nystagmus when working around the fenestrated area.

Ear Surgery

A large amount of stapes surgery is being performed; but usually this leaves no tell-tale scar, so it must be uncovered in the history. In such cases, the incision is made inside the external auditory canal on its posterior wall, and the drum is reflected forward upon itself, so that the surgeon can work in the middle ear. Healing is almost free of visible scars in the canal.

It is common to see eardrums of most peculiar appearance in which infection has played no part. In most cases, the unusual features are the result of myringoplasties with either skin fascia, vein or heart valve grafts. The drum may appear thick and flaccid or whitist, and it may show few landmarks. The patient can supply the pertinent information in such instances. Another strange appearance is the protrusion from the eardrum of a tiny piece of plastic tubing that has been inserted through a small perforation to prevent closure, and to allow drainage from the middle ear. This is usually done in cases of persistent secretory otitis media. In addition, chickenpox occasionally leaves a pock mark on the eardrum that may persist for many years.

With better understanding of the ear and the problems it presents in industry, the nurse can assume an important role in the ear examination and in cautious treatment of certain ear disorders. Her role in audiometry is, of utmost importance, of course, and leads naturally to a greater interest in otology.

Scheduling for Audiograms

The nurse and Safety Director must work together to schedule employees for hearing tests so that not much time will be lost from their jobs, and at a time when they will be free of tempo-rary hearing loss.

Lost time from productive work can be a serious financial con-cern to industry. If hundreds of employees lose a half-hour each from their jobs because they have to have their hearing tested, the cost to the company can be substantial. In most instances, hearing tests should be scheduled so effectively that an employee loses less than fifteen minutes from his work for routine audi-ometry, and slightly more time for the initial test which includes a history and ear examination.

At no time, however, should the accuracy of an audiogram be sacrificed for speed, but a well-trained tester who has been certi-fied and experienced should not take more than five minutes to get a satisfactory routine audiogram. Repeat audiograms on the same individual should be done in less time. With this in mind, employees should be scheduled so as to avoid a waiting line at the hearing testing area since a long line of non-working employees is not a happy sight to management. If for various reasons, an employee is difficult to test during a scheduled program, the em-ployee should be asked to return at another time when more at-tention can be given him without keeping others waiting.

Avoiding TTS in Audiometry

It is generally agreed that the hearing of new employees should be tested when there is no auditory fatigue present, that is, prior to exposure to industrial noise. Yet the most advantageous time to do succeeding tests is not so apparent. Should subsequent au-diograms on personnel who have already been exposed to intense noise be done after a weekend of rest (such as a Monday morn-ing); or should they be done immediately after exposure, or later at a specified time in order to avoid measuring temporary loss? One of the objectives of industrial hearing conservation pro-grams is to compare an employees' hearing thresholds before he begins work, with a stabilized hearing threshold after he has worked in a noisy environment for a given time, such as many months or years. This comparison serves to promptly detect any employee who is unusually sensitive to the specific noise and to require him to wear more effective ear protectors or shorten his exposure periods. It is not justifiable however to compare an initial auditory threshold that is free of temporary hearing loss with a subsequent one that demonstrates considerable temporary hearing loss, and conclude that an employee is more prone to permanent deafness. Only permanent thresholds are comparable for this purpose. Furthermore, there is no evidence that ears which sustain prolonged or exaggerated temporary hearing loss as now measured are more susceptible to permanent deafness. It may even be possible that some of these ears are more resistant to permanent hearing loss than those that show less fatigue.

It is difficult to be certain in all situations that no temporary hearing loss exists. Some authorities have suggested that temporary loss may exist for many weeks or even months after exposure to intense noise, but this latter has not been validated experimentally.

Evaluating Auditory Fatigue

It is not practical in a large industry to delay hearing tests until each employee has been free of industrial noise for 16 or even 12 hours. The testing of large numbers of employees can certainly not be completed on a Monday morning. By conducting minimal pilot experiments, such as described, it may be possible for each industry concerned with the problem of noise to determine if auditory fatigue is a factor in routine testing, and also to plan audiometry so that the resulting thresholds will have more medicolegal meaning.

In all areas where the noise level exceeds about 92 dBA select about five employees who have the best hearing in each area. Particularly try to select employees whose hearing is normal or almost normal. Do accurate audiograms on these employees early in the morning before they go to work and after they have had at least fifteen hours away from noise. Then take another audiogram after at least three hours of exposure with the requirement that the employee must have been exposed continuously for the hour immediately before the second audiogram. The employee should not be using ear protectors during this experimental test for three hours duration. The second audiogram should be taken within three to four minutes after exposure. Tests should be done by certified technicians using excellent technique and an adequately quiet room, and both audiograms should be done on the same audiometer. Measure accurately the noise level to which the employee is exposed during the three hours. Then determine if there is any substantial temporary hearing loss after three hours of exposure in any of the employees.

If there is more than 10 dB of TTS produced at any frequency in any noise area on individuals with normal hearing then audiograms have to be delayed some specific amount of time in order to avoid measuring TTS for routine testing. Further studies have to be performed to see exactly how long such TTS lasts. If no significant TTS develops within five minutes after exposure, then it is safe to do audiometry anytime after the employee leaves his job.

In studies conducted by one of the authors (JS), the following conclusions were found:

1. In a steady noise of 89-90 dBA, employees with essentially normal hearing sustain little TTS at any frequency when tested three minutes after three hours exposure. Since in most industries it takes more than five minutes after noise exposure for an employee to have his hearing tested, it appears that audiograms can be performed in such continuous noise levels after employees have been away from the noise at least five minutes. Since individuals with normal hearing are more susceptible to TTS than those with some degree of sensorineural hearing loss this guide would be even more applicable for employees with nerve deafness. Since intermittent noise is known to have less effect on hearing than steady noise, it seems reasonable to assume that intermittent noise exposure below 91dBA should not be a reason for deferring the taking of audiograms. This should not be interpreted to mean that employees in 89-90 dBA noise do not have to wear ear protectors. Just because there is no measureable TTS in these circumstances does not necessarily mean that no PTS can develop.

2. In continuous noise levels of 91-92 dBA threshold average shifts were around 10 dB in one or more high frequencies. From this experience we would recommend that employees working in such noise levels have their audiograms done at least fifteen minutes after leaving their work.

3. In continuous noise levels of 93-95 dBA the TTS becomes very measureable when employees do not wear ear protectors. Audiograms in such instances have to be done only after at least an hour or more absence from noise.

4. One temporary solution to the problem of scheduling hearing tests without increasing costs and slowing production is to be certain that employees scheduled for hearing testing wear ear protection prior to the time of test. In continuous noise levels up to about 100 dB it is practical to do audiograms free of TTS on employees who use ear protectors effectively after they have been away from noise five minutes. The emphasis is on effective use of ear protection.

These findings in our study can serve as a reasonable guideline for scheduling audiometric tests in industries with noise levels below 100 dBA.

By conducting similar pilot studies each industry can establish the best time to do audiograms on individuals employed in noisy areas. With the growing effectiveness of ear protectors and careful instruction in their use, it appears likely that hearing tests can be done within five or ten minutes after exposure to less than 100 dB of noise, if it is certain that an employee has been using ear protectors effectively during his work period. In noise levels above 100 dB it is wise to run experiments to determine whether audiograms taken in the morning before exposure and those taken after a workday of exposure show any significant difference in the thresholds.

The Role of the Industrial Physician and Otologist

Industrial physicians in noisy plants should receive intensive training in occupational hearing loss. The authors have been conducting such a training course for the past twenty years. This book contains the contents of a one-week course which provides a complete perspective of occupational hearing loss, as well as practical instruction in how to initiate and conduct hearing conservation programs in industry. The course is geared for industrial physicians, otologists, safety engineers, hygienists, nurses, lawyers, technicians, and representatives of management and labor. Many more training courses are needed throughout the country, consequently the contents of this book are summarized to serve as a guide for establishing new courses. The course should be basic and presented with the assumption that few of the participants have had previous experience in hearing conservation.

A description of the substance of the course follows:

1. *Orientation. Physiology and Functional Anatomy*
   The manner in which the ear functions. . . . Anatomy emphasized only in relation to transmission of sound or as it may be a factor in the auditory pathology. Anatomy in the cochlea emphasized. . . . The role of the middle ear and Eustachian tube. . . . Clarification of transmission of sound energy by bone conduction, so that limitations of ear protectors as attenuators may be better appreciated.

2. *Overall Problems of Industrial Deafness*
   Why conservation of hearing in industry is an important problem from the medical as well as the medicolegal viewpoint. . . . How roughly to determine if a plant has a noise problem. . . . How to obtain a noise survey. . . . How to obtain audiometric tests on employees. . . . Who are the industrial personnel responsible for correlating the noise and hearing surveys. . . . How to determine if a noise is hazardous to hearing. . . . What preventative measures need be taken. . . . The economics of an industrial conservation-of-hearing program. . . . Industrial relations and educational procedures necessary in such a program.

3. *Physics of Sound*
   Elementary physics of sound as applied to the measurement of noise and hearing. . . . The nature of sound—how it reaches the ear. . . . Frequency characteristics of the ear. . . . Ultrasonics. . . . How speed of sound is affected by various media. . . . Pure tones. . . . Frequency and intensity. . . . Octaves. . . . Wave length. . . . Standing wave. . . . Measuring sound intensity. . . . Microbar. . . . Sensitivity range of the ear for intensity. . . . The decibel and its logarithmic character. . . . dBA measurements. . . . Reference levels for noise measurement and hearing loss. . . . Reason for using the decibel changes. . . . Examples of common noisy occupations in terms of decibels.

4. *Psycho-Acoustics*
   The field of psycho-acoustics as it concerns hearing testing, and the evaluation of results of noise and hearing surveys. . . . Clarification of such terms as pitch, frequency, loudness, and intensity. . . . The phenomenon of hearing. . . . The difficulties involved in measuring hearing. . . . The importance of a response mechanism in hearing testing. . . . Types of responses. . . . Disadvantages in

industrial situations. . . . What is threshold. . . . The type of threshold obtained in industrial hearing tests—how it differs from research testing. . . . The reference level, or average normal hearing, on the audiometers—how this is obtained. . . . What the audiometer measures. . . . What it does not measure. . . . The limitations of threshold testing in interpretations of audiograms. . . . Speech hearing tests. . . . Threshold for speech. . . . Discrimination testing above threshold. . . . Relation of speech and hearing noise. . . . The psychological effects of intense noise. . . . Effect of noise on efficiency, performance, and the human body. . . . Auditory fatigue and its relation to permanent deafness. . . . Status of susceptibility tests for deafness. . . . Ambient noise, and the effect of masking in hearing testing.

5. *Seminar*

   Movies are shown that demonstrate the function of the middle and inner ear, the fundamentals of the physics of sound, the damaging effects of industrial deafness, the elements of noise control, and methods of auditory rehabilitation.

6. *Measurement of Hearing Loss*

   Why conversational and whispered voice tests do not meet needs of industrial testing. . . . Techniques and limitations of screening tests. . . . Self-recording audiometry and objective audiometry. . . . Description of technique for pure-tone individual audiometry in industrial situations. . . . Who should perform audiometry. . . . How to select a room for audiometric testing. . . . What is an audiometer. . . . How should one be selected. . . . Calibration of an audiometer. . . . Importance of valid and reliable audiograms. . . . The importance of the initial audiogram. . . . Instructions to the subject prior to performing an audiogram. . . . How the subject should be seated. . . . How to perform a routine audiogram. . . . How to expedite testing in certain situations. . . . How to record an audiogram with serial forms for industrial purposes. . . . What a tester should tell the subject. . . . Review of the common errors of audiometry.

7. *Audiometry Laboratory*

   Under the critical eye of instructors students practice performing audiometric tests on subjects, using various types of standard audiometers. At the end of each laboratory session instructors emphasize the errors most commonly made, and restate the reasons for requiring uniform procedures in audiometric testing. By using different types of commercially available audiometers students can determine which is most suitable for their particular needs. Caution is taken that instructors do not influence students by their own preferences. Throughout the period of the course the audiometers remain available for further use by students who may wish, or need, further practice in performing hearing testing.

8. *Sound Levels; Frequency Analysis*

All commonly used equipment for making noise measurements is demonstrated and explained. Each student is supervised as he makes noise level measurements and frequency analyses of an intense steady-state noise recorded on tape. Instruction is given in how to care for the equipment, how to calibrate it, what to do if it needs repair, what equipment costs; how to make sound level measurements of steady-state noise and what additional measures are needed for impact noise; how to determine if measurements are reliable, how to hold and use the microphone and how to correct for extension cables; how to test for microphonics and vibrations, how to make frequency analyses in octave bands and how to check reliability of results in each band with the overall level; where to make measurements in various types of plants, how to determine sources of error, how to record noise measurements and how to analyze data obtained.

9. *Malingering*

The types of malingering encountered. . . . Reasons for malingering. . . . Methods of detection. . . . What tester should do when he suspects malingering. . . . Description of the manner by which the otologist established a reliable threshold for malingering subjects. . . . How to reduce the incidence of malingering in conservation-of-hearing programs.

10. *Records*

Data that must be obtained and recorded during hearing testing program. . . . Otological examination and history. . . . Data to be recorded on audiogram, such as subject's duration of exposure to noise, period of rest prior to audiogram, etc. . . . Various methods of keeping records for industrial and research purposes.

11. *Acoustics, Ear Protectors, Etc.*

Acoustics and noise control. . . . Damage risk criteria. . . . Suggestions for evaluating noises in plants represented by students. . . . Recording and plotting a noise survey. . . . Demonstration of types of commercially available ear protectors. . . . Advantages and disadvantages. . . . Suggested educational program in preparing plant employees for hearing testing program. . . . How to indoctrinate employees in the use of ear protectors. . . . How to adapt a room for industrial hearing testing. . . . Commercially available testing booths. . . . Ventilation problems. . . . Brief description of bandwidths and masking.

12. *Field Work*

Students visit a noisy plant and conduct a hearing and noise survey. Through the plant's safety engineer, with whom arrangements have been made in advance, employees are available for hearing testing, and test rooms set up with audiometers. Each student has the opportunity to perform and record a complete noise survey under instruction, evaluate the suitability of the test room, calibrate the audiometer, and test a representative number of employees who have recently been exposed to the intense noise being measured. Data collected are analyzed at a seminar later in the day.

13. *Medicolegal Panel*

Formal presentation of medicolegal aspects of industrial deafness, by an experienced attorney or other qualified individual. . . . Panel discussion follows in which all students and faculty members participate, with all important and pertinent phases of this matter discussed: compensation law, development of interest in Federal legislation and in key states, correlating pure-tone hearing loss and hearing handicap for speech, what industries can do to obviate unjust medicolegal entanglements resulting from industrial deafness, how to prepare records for legal purposes, etc.

14. *Interpretation of Audiograms; Pathology of Hearing*

Responsibility for interpreting audiograms and making diagnosis exclusively that of the otologist. . . . Pitfalls in making diagnosis solely on the basis of an audiogram. . . . Nature of the examination the otologist needs to make in order to reach a valid diagnosis. . . . Understanding the otologist's report. . . . Description of various types of hearing disorders and how closely some of them resemble industrial deafness in the audiometric picture. . . . How noise produces deafness. . . . Difficulties of bone conduction testing. . . . Value of speech hearing tests to determine handicapping nature of loss. . . . Recruitment and its clinical effects. . . . Psychological effects of hearing loss, with particular emphasis on industrial deafness. How to make management aware of these factors. . . . Auditory rehabilitation and value of hearing aids in certain types of deafness. . . . Responsibilities of an otologist as a consultant to an industry with noise problems.

15. *Establishing a Conservation of Hearing Program*

How to determine if a noise is causing deafness in exposed personnel. . . . Who should perform the noise measurement. . . . How to evaluate results of the noise survey and institute a hearing testing program. . . . How to train a tester to obtain reliable audiograms. . . . The responsibilities of the safety engineer, the hygienist, the industrial physician. . . . Responsibilities of manage-

ment and labor in the overall program. . . . How often to repeat
routine audiograms. . . . The criteria for hiring new employees in
specific noisy industries. . . . Criteria for referring employees with
hearing loss to otologists. . . . How to integrate into a "team" those
persons who are vital to a successful conservation-of-hearing
program.

16. *Review*

Each faculty member sums up his foregoing lectures in order that
the students may be left with an integrated concept of a proper
conservation-of-hearing program, and with full awareness of how
they can initiate and conduct such a program in their own industries.

While the course is being given, pertinent reprints from the literature and bibliographic material are made available to the students. The keystone of the entire program is the experienced faculty, which presents the information in such a manner that it is
readily absorbed, understood, and retained, even by students who
have had no previous experience in any phase of industrial deafness.

Now let us consider the problems that confront an industrial
physician when he concerns himself with occupational hearing
loss in his plant.

Does the Plant Have a Noise Problem?

If the plant has a safety engineer, and a sound level meter, the
industrial physician should ask him to perform a noise survey
and locate all areas in the plant where noise levels exceed 90
dBA. If the plant does not have a safety engineer or does not
have the necessary equipment, it is practical to hire a consultant
to perform this survey. The experienced consultant will generally
provide much information that will be of great assistance to the
plant. After obtaining the noise survey the industrial physician
is then able to decide whether or not employees are exposed in a
noisy area for sufficient duration to sustain hearing damage. The
guide provided in Chapter 9 should be used for this decision.
The industrial physician must consult with industrial personnel
superintendents, and foremen, to determine how long each employee is actually exposed to excessive noise levels. The physician
must then discuss with Management the feasibility of noise re-

duction, and the need for a hearing-conservation-program. One of the prime responsibilities of the physician is to make decisions concerning the effects of noise upon individual employees, and to decide whether or not an employee is to be hired or (if hired) permitted to work at a noisy job. To make such decisions, the physician must rely on an accurate hearing testing program.

Hearing Testing Program

Setting up and maintaining an accurate hearing testing program is the industrial physician's responsibility. He must be assured of excellent hearing testing at all times. This is especially true because of the legal aspects of occupational deafness. Physical noise measurements alone are of little value if an employee enters a claim for occupational hearing loss unless accurate pre-employment and routine follow-up testing have been accomplished. Even though the physician himself generally does not do the hearing testing, he is responsible for its *accuracy*. The testing itself may be done by an industrial nurse or any other well-trained individual. However, it is often better to do no hearing testing at the plant than to perform audiometry in an inaccurate manner. The physician must continually audit the accuracy of the audiograms and the technique being used. For instance, the physician must recognize that if a series of audiograms show excessive low frequency threshold losses with few if any normals, some cause must be sought other than in the employee's hearing. It may be due to a high ambient noise level in the test room, or a defective audiometer, or perhaps even to poor testing techniques.

If the physician has a number of outlying small plants of only 20 or 50 employees, it is hardly justifiable to purchase an audiometer and test booth and to set up a hearing testing facility in each plant. Rather, a satisfactory solution is to arrange for a local otologist or audiologist to do the hearing tests. The otologist can also perform a sufficient number of other examinations so that he may include in his report the cause of every case of hearing loss encountered among the employees. The industrial physician should have copies of all the audiograms performed in the small outlying plants. Often it may be more practical for the industrial physician to send his nurse with a portable audiometer to the various outlying plants to perform routine audiometry, or to hire a company that can provide this service. Pre-employment audiometry can also be accomplished by special arrangement with such a company.

Who Should Have Hearing Tests?

Occasionally one encounters the comment that performing hearing tests on only a few men in a plant would stir up a hornet's nest and incite action among the other employees. For this reason, many managements feel that hearing testing should be done on large groups, or on the entire complement of employees, rather than on a selected few supposedly exposed to noise. The economics of the situation and the experience of the industrial Personnel Director are factors influencing a decision. We believe that since hearing conservation is a medical problem dedicated not only to prevent noise deafness but to detect and possibly cure all types of hearing loss, every person in the plant should have his hearing tested and his audiogram evaluated for diagnosis and care.

The Director of a most effective Hearing-Conservation Program in a large textile company presented the following reasons to his Management to convince them of the need for such a program:

1. Recent policy changes regarding transfers tend to increase departmental transfers. Therefore, employees should have a threshold audiogram, whether being transferred from or to a high decibel area.
2. Present employees could have hearing deficiencies caused by many factors, such as previous employment, sickness, exposure to loud noises, injuries, etc. We should have a record showing these deficiencies.
3. We should have an audiogram on *all* terminating employees, and this would be difficult to obtain unless we already had on record a threshold audiogram.
4. With all of our present employees tested and all new employees being tested, there would never be any concern about *when* to test.
5. Change of equipment in low-level noise areas could change the dBA reading, and National Standards may also be changed.

6. Part of an employee's education on our hearing-conservation program could begin before it becomes necessary to fit him with protective equipment.

7. The philosophy of a hearing-conservation program should be Management's concern for *all* employees. To single out only those employees that are exposed to hazardous noise could bring accusations of employer self-interest, and might have some affect on the effectiveness of the company's program.

8. Audiogram results can be very beneficial when they indicate a condition that may be correctable.

9. All employees have seen the video tape presentation of our Companies Program.

10. There have been many requests from employees (hourly and salaried) to have their hearing checked.

Therefore, I recommend that we give audiometric tests and establish threshold levels for all employees in those plants that now have hearing-conservation programs.

Pre-Employment and Pre-Placement Audiograms

An employee's pre-employment audiogram establishes his hearing status before he is exposed to noise in his new job. This audiogram forms a baseline and is probably the most important test audiogram to be done. Special care is needed to obtain accurate thresholds. Since it has been estimated that over 20 percent of applicants for noisy industrial jobs already have some hearing loss at the time they present themselves for employment, the importance of securing an accurate initial hearing threshold record is obvious. Unfortunately, the author's (JS) experience as a consultant in examining the adequacy of hearing-testing programs in industrial plants, shows that accuracy in such testing is sometimes taken for granted.

When the author checked what was being done in one of these plants, he found that the audiometry had been done by an inadequately trained technician, unfamiliar with the pitfalls of industrial audiometry. It was discovered that a substantial number of employees whose initial audiograms showed them to have normal hearing, in reality had hearing losses of long duration quite unrelated to their present employment.

The production and recording of audiograms with a false appearance of accuracy by testers inadequately trained in the art of industrial audiometry is by no means uncommon, particularly in instances where subjects had accumulated previous experience with audiometric testing in the Armed Services and the Veterans Administration.

Instances are certain to arise in which so many new employees are hired in one day that it is impossible to test them all before they report for work. For this and other reasons it may be advisable to do pre-placement audiometry in addition to pre-employment testing. This means that initial tests are performed on employees when they are assigned to a job that has been classified as potentially hazardous to hearing.

The importance of the initial pre-employment or pre-placement audiogram as a document of legal importance should be considered carefully. Several thresholds at each frequency should be recorded to provide a base line with which future comparisons can be made reliably.

Hiring Personnel With Nerve Deafness

It is also essential for industries to perform employment hearing tests to decide whether or not an applicant should be hired. The physician and Personnel Director must determine the criteria for guidance but provide flexibility in individual cases.

From a practical aspect, American industry is hardly in a position to set very conservative and rigid standards for hiring applicants with nerve deafness. A tight labor market militates against this. Furthermore, it would screen out our most experienced and skilled individuals from noisy jobs. If an applicant applies for a chipping job inside turbines, for example, and professes to have had experience, and his audiogram shows normal hearing either he has most unusual ears or there is some question as to the extent of his previous experience. The decision to hire or not to hire an applicant rests not exclusively with the physician, but also with the Personnel Director.

If the plant decides it is advantageous to hire an individual with nerve deafness for a very noisy job, accurate histories of previous noise exposure and careful audiograms are most essential. Such an employee should be tested every few months for about six months, and then if no definite changes occur a schedule of testing every six months or annually can be followed. This type of employee should be compelled to wear ear protectors at all times during noise exposure.

It is difficult for Management to remove an employee from a job. For this reason Management may hesitate to hire an applicant with some nerve deafness if there is a likelihood of having to remove him after several months because of deterioration in his hearing. There is, of course, no clear cut general solution to such a situation. The problem has to be solved by both Labor and Management in individual industries, so that neither the employee nor his employer is compelled to overlook the serious problem of deafness. Management should feel free to hire employees with hearing handicaps, and if subsequent tests indicate that an employee's hearing is getting worse due to noise exposure despite all preventative measures, Management must be permitted to protect the employee by moving him to another job or by releasing him if necessary (within the regulation of any existing contract). To prevent industry from being liable for a handicapping hearing loss which was present prior to employment, and newly sustained losses which did not result from noise, legislation and compensation laws should be written to be equitable for both Management and Labor.

The threat of creating a new large group of hearing-handicapped, non-hirable employees (especially veterans with gunfire exposure) is a serious problem. American industry should not be compelled to discriminate against these citizens, but rather encouraged to continue helping them find suitable jobs.

An important related problem is the susceptibility of the ear already nerve deafened to noise. There is no valid evidence to show that employees with nerve deafness are more susceptible to noise damage than are those with normal hearing. It may even be that nerve deafened ears are less susceptible.

Since individuals with nerve deafness have not been shown to be more sensitive to further noise damage, we may feel free to hire such people if we bear in mind the following concepts:

1. Industry should be able to assure itself and the applicant that if he uses adequate ear protection provided by the company, his hearing will not sustain any substantial additional damage due to the environmental noise at his job.
2. Legislation and regulations, local, state, and federal, should protect the employer from liability for hearing loss not caused on the job.
3. The applicant's hearing level should meet the demands of his job, and he should not create a safety hazard as a result of impaired hearing, or as a result of attenuation of hearing with ear protectors.
4. Applicants diagnosed as having progressive hereditary nerve deafness should not be hired to work in noisy jobs.

There is no doubt that industry must continue to hire applicants with some degree of nerve deafness for noisy jobs, but every possible effort must be made to protect employees from high noise levels, and the employer from unwarranted liability. Only in such an atmosphere can a full and equitable solution to the problem be attained.

Personnel With Conductive Hearing Loss

Now, let us turn to a related problem. We have taken for granted that, if an applicant's hearing loss is diagnosed as conductive, he has built-in ear protection and can be hired safely. This may be true if we narrow our concern solely to noise-induced hearing loss; but certainly our concern is not limited to noise alone. We are interested in the health of the entire individual. Routine hiring of applicants with conductive hearing loss may not be advisable. Many of them with active ear infections may turn out to be over-burdening problems in the dispensary, requiring care and time off from work. More important, however, is the fact that most people with conductive hearing loss can have their hearing improved by proper medical or surgical care.

Industry's job should be to seek out such individuals already in their employ, and urge them to obtain proper care, thus perhaps having their hearing restored so they may live better lives socially and vocationally. New applicants should be referred to their own physician prior to being employed. The serious psychologic effects that deafness can have upon the personality make it imperative for industry to concern itself with the prevention and care of all types of deafness, not only that caused by noise.

Physician's Responsibility for Ear Protectors

The industrial physician is responsible for the distribution and fitting of ear protectors. He should have a list of all the areas in his plant with excessive noise levels. For each job classification the physician should have available two or three different ear protectors which the Safety Engineer has established as being satisfactory for employees.

When the employee is assigned to such a job, he should be permitted to try these various ear protectors and select the type he feels most suitable. The physician must be certain that the employee is properly fitted; even the muff type protector on occasion will not fit certain head configurations. If insert protectors are chosen, the employee must be shown how to insert and remove them. Training in the proper care of all types of protectors is essential, as is an ongoing educational program reminding all personnel of the importance of wearing their protectors effectively.

Occasionally employees will be allergic to the material in the protectors or the liquid used to clean them. Changing the brand of protector or the method of cleaning and careful follow-up procedures usually rectifies this problem. If the ear protector recommended is the individually molded type, the impression of the ears should be made by a trained person after careful examination of the ear canal. A record should be kept of the make and size of ear protectors selected for each employee, so that replacements can be made readily.

The Consultant Otologist

The industrial physician should expect a consultant otologist to perform all tests necessary to establish an accurate diagnosis on patients referred to him. The otologist should also be willing to express a reasonable opinion as to the cause of deafness, and he should be available to testify as an expert witness in medicolegal situations.

When the olotogist sends a report to the industrial physician, it must include not only the otologist's conclusion but the results of all tests performed, since the report may be the focal point of a claim for compensation.

When legal situations arise, the otologist must testify and restrict his authoritative opinion to otological problems. He must not endeavor to speak with equal authority on the compensation aspects of the matter, unless he is qualified to do so. The otologist should remain as critically objective as possible in diagnosing the cause of a hearing loss.

The effectiveness of the industrial physician's entire conservation-of-hearing program is likely to be dependent upon the co-operative relationship he is able to establish with his consulting otologist. Without the otologist's helpful and specialized advice, the physician is very likely to discover, to his regret, that he has overlooked important aspects which should have been given careful consideration. While the otologist's advice and his important diagnosis of referred cases are vital to the industrial physician, it is the industrial physician who has full responsibility for the coordination of the program.

In small or large plants where there is no industrial physician available, it is advisable to have a consulting otologist (trained in industrial audiometry and conservation-of-hearing) help establish the program, and review every audiogram performed. This can be done even if the audiograms are mailed to the physician. He can supply reasonable advice concerning further tests necessary to establish a diagnosis and recommend what disposition should be made of the individual problem.

WHEN TO REFER AN EMPLOYEE FOR OTOLOGIC STUDY

Unless special arrangements are made with an otologist trained in industrial conservation-of-hearing, it is financially impractical to refer all employees in a plant to the otologic office for examination. The medical costs, and the cost of lost time from work would be excessive. However, it is advisable to refer all employees who have reactions from the use of ear protectors or whose hearing is getting progressively worse even though they use ear protectors properly. Certainly all potential legal problems should be evaluated by an otologist, as well as other special problems such as accidents and unusual ear symptoms.

How Frequently Should Audiograms Be Done?

Industrial employees who work in noise levels below 90 dBA should have an audiogram about every two years. Employees already in a job classified as potentially hazardous should have a follow-up audiogram in about six months, and then either annually or every six months thereafter depending on the intensity of the noise and whether or not the audiogram shows any substantial change. If the tests indicate that no permanent change in hearing has occurred, it is safe thereafter to test such an employee annually. Routine audiometry is the best and only sure way of being certain that an employee's hearing is being properly protected. Routine audiometry also monitors the effective use of ear protectors. It is a well-known fact that many employees use ear protectors that provide little or no protection chiefly because they are not properly inserted. Another benefit of audiometry is realized in the case of an individual whose hearing continues to deteriorate despite the effective use of ear protectors. An excellent otologist can determine whether the deafness is really due to noise exposure or to some other cause. It is difficult for an industrial physician to request that an employee be transferred from a noisy job to a non-noisy job merely because the individual's hearing is deteriorating. It is much better to provide more effective ear protectors than to transfer an individual to another position. Seniority and union contracts often make it difficult for transfers to be made even though the employee's hearing may be involved. The industrial physician will also want to make it a rule to have terminal audiograms performed, particularly on all personnel who have been working in noisy areas.

In concluding this chapter we should highlight briefly the most crucial part of every Hearing Conservation Program. Unless every employee exposed to hazardous noise levels is using ear protectors effectively, Hearing Conservation is not being practiced and we are not satisfying the intent of any standards or regulations. We should not mislead ourselves into believing (as some industries are doing) that taking noise measurements and even doing audiograms fulfills our obligation to hearing conservation. Neither of these steps serves to prevent occupational deafness unless an effective ear protection program is compulsory and constantly in force. It is here that the most concerted efforts must be exerted by the entire team. The results are rewarding for with comparatively little cost it is possible to prevent further occupational deafness from developing in over 98 percent of our industrial population. Surely no satisfactory reason is available to prevent a plant from achieving this urgent objective as soon as possible.

RECOMMENDED READINGS

Glorig, Aram: *Noise and Your Ear,* New York, Grune and Stratton, 1958.

Guide for Conservation of Hearing in Noise. AAOO Subcommittee on Noise Research Center, 3819 Marple Ave., Dallas, Texas, Revised 1964.

Guild, Elizabeth: Ears can be protected, *Noise Control, 4*(9), 1958.

Industrial Noise Manual, American Industrial Hygiene Association, Detroit 27, Michigan, 2nd Edition, 1965.

Maas, Roger: Ear protection—why? . . . how? . . . *Supervision, 4* (9) , 1958.

Maas, Roger: Hearing protection in industry, *Nursing Outlook, 9*(5), 1961.

Maas, Roger: Hearing protection programs can succeed, *National Safety News,* March 1970.

Sataloff, J., et al:

 Incidence of hearing loss among job applicants, *Arch Environ Health, 12*(2), 1966.

 The environment in relation to otologic disease, *Arch Environ Health, 10*(3), 1965.

 Audiometric reliability in industry, *Arch Environ Health, 22*(1), 1971.

 Hiring employees with nerve deafness, *J Occup Med,* June 1969.

 Hearing Conservation—Industry's Responsibility, Environmental Control and Safety Management.

 How To Sell Top Management Hearing Conservation.

Chapter 17

PERSONAL PROTECTIVE DEVICES AND HEARING CONSERVATION PROGRAMS

THE BEST WAY to reduce noise exposures is to prevent noise generation. When it is not possible to reduce noise levels by treatment of the source, the problem may sometimes be solved by covering surrounding surfaces with acoustically absorbent materials, or by the use of noise barriers. Another obvious means of reducing noise exposures is to move either the offending noise source

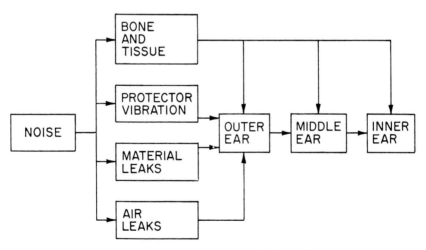

Figure 43. Noise Pathways to the Inner Ear.

291

or the persons exposed to another location. In situations where it is impractical to attain enough noise reduction by these means, personal protective devices must be used.

An effective personal protective device serves as a barrier between the noise and the inner ear where noise-induced damage to hearing may occur. Ear protector devices usually take the form of ear muffs which are worn over the external ear and provide an acoustical seal against the head, or ear plugs which provide an acoustical seal at the entrance to the external ear canal.

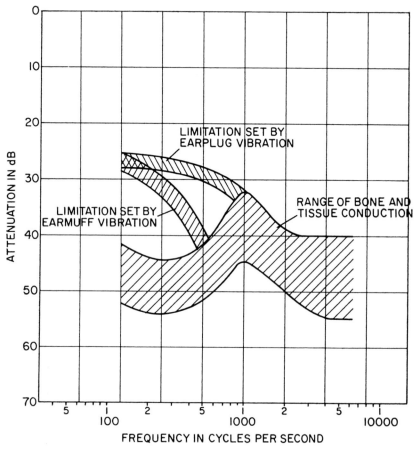

Figure 44. Practical Protection Limits for Plugs and Muffs.

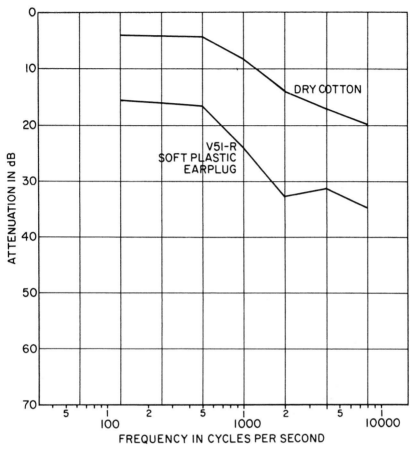

Figure 45. Mean Attenuation Characteristics of a Well-Fitted, Imperforate Earplug and an Earplug Made of Dry Cotton.

Protector Performance Characteristics and Limitations

The protection afforded by an ear protector depends upon its design and upon several physiological and physical characteristics of the wearer.[1] Sound energy may reach the inner ears of persons wearing protectors by four different pathways: (1) by passing through bone and tissue around the protector; (2) by causing vibration of the protector which in turn generates sound into the external ear canal; (3) by passing through leaks in the protector;

and (4) by passing through leaks around the protector. These pathways are illustrated in Figure 43.

Even if the protector should have no acoustical leaks through or around it, some noise will reach the inner ear by one or both of the first two pathways if the levels are sufficiently high. The practical limits set by the bone and tissue conduction threshold and the vibration of the protector vary considerably with the design of the protector and with the wearer's physical make-up but approximate limits for plugs and muffs are shown in Figure 44.[2, 3]

If ear protectors are to provide noise reductions approaching the practical limits shown in Figure 44, acoustical leaks through and around the protectors must be minimized. Figure 45 shows that the mean attenuation values of a well-fitted, imperforate, plastic earplug are considerably greater than those of a dry cotton plug which is porous. Figure 4 illustrates the effects of leaks around a poorly-fitted imperforate earplug and of a leak through a small orifice in the center of a well-fitted earplug.

The following rules should be followed to minimize losses due to acoustical leaks:

1. Ear protectors should be made of imperforate materials. If it is possible for air to pass freely through a material, noise will also be able to pass with little attenuation.
2. The protector should be designed to conform readily to the head or ear canal configuration so that an efficient acoustic seal can be achieved and the protector can be worn with reasonable comfort.
3. The protector should have a support means or a seal compliance that will minimize protector vibration.
4. Muff-type protectors should not be worn over long hair, poorly fitted eyeglass temples, or other obstacles.

Protector Types

Ears and Earplugs

Ear canals differ widely in size, shape, and position among individuals, and even between ears of the same individual. Therefore, earplugs must be chosen which are adaptable to a wide variety of ear canal configurations.

Ear canals vary in cross-section from about 3 mm to 14 mm, but a large majority fall in the range from 5 to 11 mm. Most ear

canals are elliptically shaped but some are round, and many have
only a small slit-like opening. Some ear canals are directed in a
straight line toward the center of the head, but most bend in various ways and are directed toward the front of the head.

In many cases, there is only a small space available to accommo-
date an earplug, but almost all entrances to ear canals can be
opened and straightened by pulling the external ear directly out
from the head (see Figure 47) so that an earplug can be seated
securely. For comfort and plug retention, the canals must return
to their approximate normal configuration once the protector is
seated.

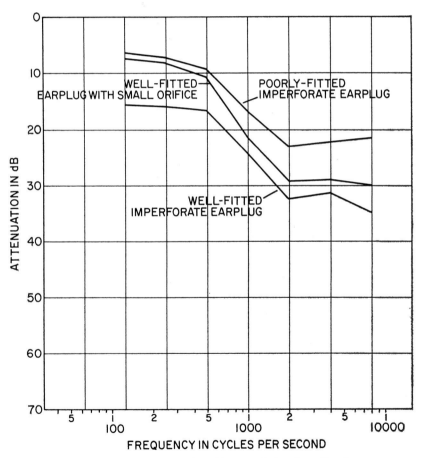

Figure 46. Mean Attenuation Characteristics of an Earplug.

Sized Earplugs

No single-sized molded earplug has proven to be very effective in attenuating noise when used in the large range of ear canal sizes and shapes. Most of the more widely accepted molded earplugs[4-16] come in three to five different sizes. In addition, the best sized earplugs are made of a soft and flexible material that will conform readily to the many different ear canal shapes so that a snug, airtight, and comfortable fit is possible.

Earplugs must be non-toxic and should have smooth surfaces that are easily cleaned with soap and water. Most earplugs are made of materials that will retain their size and flexibility over long periods of time; however, some ear waxes may cause changes in size and flexibility of protectors after extended size.

Of the many types of sized earplugs available, the assymmetrically-shaped V-51R shown in Figures 46 and 48 remains the most versatile in that it will provide a better seal in more ear canals than earplugs that are round and straight. This is not to

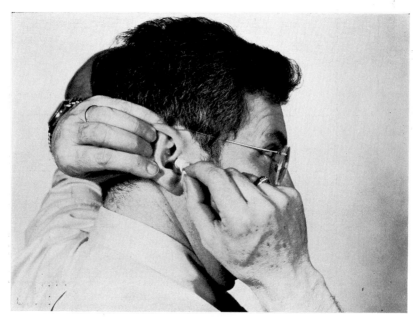

Figure 47. Recommended Method for Inserting Earplugs.

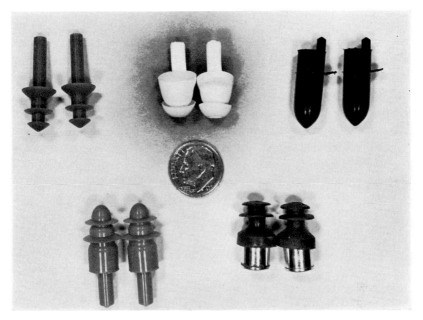

Figure 48. Examples of Sized Molded Earplugs.

say that the V-51R will provide the best protection in all ear canals. Some of the round and straight earplugs shown in Figure 48 may provide better attenuation values than the V-51R plug when they are worn in round and straight ear canals; however, the round and straight earplugs generally do not adapt well to sharply bending or slit-shaped canals.

Because of the distinct advantages in performance and fit for the symmetrical and asymmetrical earplug types, it is often advisable to keep both types in stock. It might be estimated that 50 percent V-51R and 50 percent symmetrical-type earplugs would be a reasonable selection for the beginning of a hearing conservation program *if* sized-earplugs are to be used. Offering a choice of protectors wherever possible often has an additional advantage in program acceptance.

As an aid for purchasing sized earplugs, the distribution of sizes in a large male population will be approximately as follows: 5 percent extra small, 15 percent small, 30 percent medium,

30 percent large, 15 percent extra large, and 5 percent larger than supplied by most earplug manufacturers. This size range, showing an equal percentage of wearers for medium and large sizes, is selected to provide the best fit for reasonable comfort and maximum attenuation. If an individual is permitted to fit himself, he will pay more attention to comfort in most cases and the size distribution will shift toward smaller sizes.

Some ear canals apparently increase in size with the regular use of earplugs; therefore, if a given ear falls between sizes, it is advisable to choose the larger of the two. It also is a good practice to check the fitting of earplugs periodically for this reason.

A common and often valid complaint is that the case costs more than the earplugs. However, a good case keeps the earplugs clean, in good condition, and readily available when needed, so the expense is often justified. Also, the total cost of sized plugs and container is generally below the price of one set of replacement cushions for earmuffs, and a good quality earplug container should outlast several pairs of earplugs.

Malleable Earplugs

Malleable earplugs are made of materials such as cotton, paper, wax, glass wool, and mixtures of these and other substances (see Figure 49). Typically, a small cone of this material is hand-formed and the apex of the cone is inserted into the ear canal with sufficient force so that the material conforms to the shape of the canal and holds itself in position.

The protection provided by the malleable earplugs varies according to the material used and how firmly the plug is seated. Cotton, by itself, is quite porous and generally provides very little protection (see Figure 45); however, mixtures of cotton, paper and wax, or glass wool can provide good protection if properly inserted.

In general, malleable plugs made of the non-porous and easily formed materials are capable of providing attenuation values equivalent to those provided by the best sized-type molded earplugs. Obviously, the plugs must be carefully formed and firmly inserted to obtain this high level of performance.

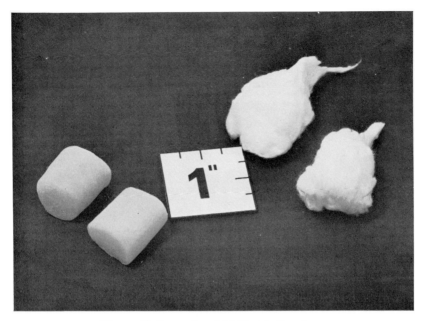

Figure 49. Examples of Malleable Earplugs.

Malleable earplugs should be formed and inserted with clean hands because any dirt or foreign objects inserted into the ear may cause irritation or infection. This means that malleable plugs should be carefully inserted at the beginning of a work shift, and they should not be removed and reinserted during the work period unless the hands are cleaned. Therefore, malleable plugs (and to a somewhat lesser extent, all earplugs) are a poor choice for use in dirty areas having intermittent high noise levels, or in other locations where it may be desirable to remove and reinsert protective devices during the work period.

Malleable plugs have the obvious advantage of universal fit over sized plugs; however, because they are used for only one, two, or perhaps three times, they are usually more expensive to use.

Head and Earmuffs

Most muff-type protectors[4, 7, 8, 14–18] now have similar designs as shown in Figure 50. Seal materials placed against the skin are

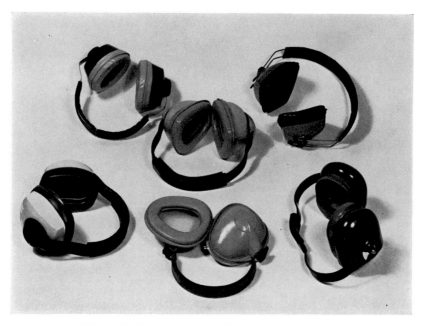

Figure 50. Examples of Muff-Type Ear Protectors.

non-toxic for the most part and fit, comfort factors, and general performance of comparable models do not vary widely.

If maximum protection is required, the protector earcups must be formed of a rigid, dense, imperforate material. Generally, the size of the enclosed volume within the muff shell is directly related to the low frequency attenuation. The ear seals should have a small circumference so that the acoustic seal takes place over the smallest possible irregularities in head contour. A small seal circumference also minimizes leaks caused by jaw and neck measurements.

The inside of each earcup should be partially filled with an open-cell material to absorb high frequency resonant noises. The material placed inside the cup should not contact the external ear; otherwise discomfort to the wearer and soil to the lining may result.

Earmuff cushions are generally made of a smooth plastic envelope filled with a foam or fluid material. Skin oil and perspiration have adverse effects on cushion materials, so that after extended use, the soft and compliant cushions may tend to become stiff and sometimes shrink. Fluid-filled cushions occasionally have the additional problem of leakage. For these reasons, most earmuffs are equipped with easily replaceable seals.

The acoustic seal materials used on earmuffs will provide maximum protection when placed on relatively smooth surfaces; therefore, less protection should be expected when muffs are worn over long hair, glasses, or other objects. Glasses with close-fitting, average-sized, plastic templets will cause about five to ten decibel reductions in attenuation in most cases, but this loss of protection can be reduced substantially if smaller, close-fitting, wire templets are used. Acoustic seal covers that are sometimes provided to absorb perspiration also reduce attenuation by several decibels because noise leaks through the porous material.

Obviously, the loss of protection is directly proportional to the size of the obstruction under the seal and every effort should be made to minimize these obstructions. If long hair or other obstructions cannot be avoided, it must be realized that the claimed attenuations will not be provided by muffs and it may be advisable to use other types of personal protective devices.

The force applied by the muff suspension is another factor directly related to the amount of protection provided. A compromise must be made in choosing the suspension force on the basis of performance versus comfort. Suspensions should never be deliberately sprung to reduce the applied force if maximum protection is desired.

Concha-Seated Ear Protectors

Protectors which cannot be strictly classified as insert- or muff-types include individually molded ear pieces and others that provide an acoustic seal in the concha or at the entrance to the ear canal. Individually molded ear pieces that are held in position by the external ear as shown in Figure 51 have been available for several years, but these devices have not been widely used because of their high cost and relatively poor performance. Recently, new materials[19, 20] have made this type of protector competitive in

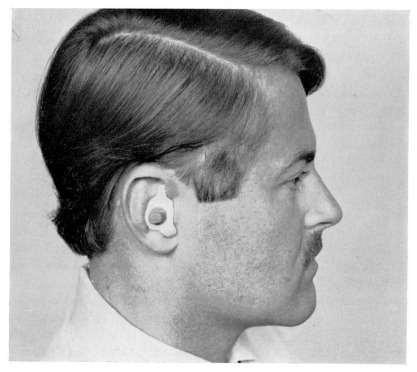

Figure 51. Individually Molded Ear Protectors.

price and its performance is quite good *if* the devices are molded carefully according to the manufacturers' instructions.

Another protector design in this class makes use of a narrow headband to press two soft plastic conical caps against the entrance to the external ear canal.[21]

Amount of Protection Provided in Practice

A comparison of the noise analysis of a particular noise exposure and the levels specified by the chosen hearing conservation criterion should be used to determine the amount of noise reduction required. When the hearing conservation criteria are expressed in octave bands, the amount of noise reduction required can be determined by subtracting the sound pressure levels (in decibels) specified by the criteria from the exposure levels (in decibels) measured in corresponding octave bands. When ear protectors are to be used to provide the necessary noise reduction, the attenuation that is provided within each of these bands must equal or exceed the noise reduction requirements (in decibels).

Hearing conservation criteria based on the A-frequency weighting may be used following the procedure described below:

Step 1: Take sound level measurements in octave bands at the point of exposure.

Step 2: Subtract from the octave-band levels (in decibels) obtained in Step 1 the center-frequency adjustment values for the A-frequency weighting shown in Table I.

Step 3: Subtract from the A-weighted octave bands calculated in Step

TABLE XI

A-FREQUENCY WEIGHTING ADJUSTMENTS[30]

f(Hz)	*Correction*
25	− 44.7
32	− 39.4
40	− 34.6
50	− 30.2
63	− 26.2
80	− 22.5
100	− 19.1
125	− 16.1
160	− 13.4
200	− 10.9
250	− 8.6
315	− 6.6
400	− 4.8
500	− 3.2
630	− 1.9
800	− 0.8
1,000	0.0
1,250	+ 0.6
1,600	+ 1.0
2,000	+ 1.2
2,500	+ 1.3
3,150	+ 1.2
4,000	+ 1.0
5,000	+ 0.5
6,300	− 0.1
8,000	− 1.1
10,000	− 2.5
12,500	− 4.3
16,000	− 6.6
20,000	− 9.3

TABLE XII

TABLE FOR COMBINING DECIBEL LEVELS OF NOISES WITH RANDOM FREQUENCY CHARACTERISTICS

Numerical Difference Between Levels L_1 and L_2	Sum (L_R) of dB Levels L_1 and L_2 L_3: Amount to Be Added to the Higher of L_1 or L_2	
0.0 to 0.1	3.0	Step 1: Determine the
0.2 to 0.3	2.9	difference between
0.4 to 0.5	2.8	the two levels to
0.6 to 0.7	2.7	be added (L_1 and L_2).
0.8 to 0.9	2.6	
1.0 to 1.2	2.5	Step 2: Find the number
1.3 to 1.4	2.4	(L_3) corresponding to
1.5 to 1.6	2.3	this difference in the
1.7 to 1.9	2.2	Table.
2.0 to 2.1	2.1	
2.2 to 2.4	2.0	Step 3: Add the number
2.5 to 2.7	1.9	(L_3) to the highest of
2.8 to 3.0	1.8	L_1 and L_2 to obtain
3.1 to 3.3	1.7	the resultant level
3.4 to 3.6	1.6	($L_R = L_1 + L_2$).
3.7 to 4.0	1.5	
4.1 to 4.3	1.4	
4.4 to 4.7	1.3	
4.8 to 5.1	1.2	
5.2 to 5.6	1.1	
5.7 to 6.1	1.0	
6.2 to 6.6	0.9	
6.7 to 7.2	0.8	
7.3 to 7.9	0.7	
8.0 to 8.6	0.6	
8.7 to 9.6	0.5	
9.7 to 10.7	0.4	
10.8 to 12.2	0.3	
12.3 to 14.5	0.2	
14.6 to 19.3	0.1	
19.4 to ∞	0.0	

2 the attenuation values provided by the protector for each corresponding octave band to obtain the A-weighted octave-band levels reaching the ear while wearing the ear protector.

Step 4: Calculate the equivalent A-weighted noise level reaching the ear while wearing the ear protector by adding the octave-band levels as shown in Table II. An alternate method for adding decibels is as follows:

$$\text{Equivalent dBA} = 10 \log_{10} (\text{antilog}_{11} \frac{L_{125}}{10}$$

$$+ \text{antilog}_{10} \frac{L_{250}}{10} + \ldots \text{antilog}_{10} \frac{L_{8,000}}{10}),$$

where L_{125} is the sound pressure level of the A-weighted octave band centered at 125 Hz; L_{250} the A-weighted octave-band level at 250 Hz; etc.

Example: The first and second columns in Table XIII contain octave-band sound pressure level data measured in a textile mill weaving room. The third column shows the same octave band data, but with an A-frequency weighting (using Table XI). The mean and mean minus one standard deviation attenuation values for a good muff-type ear protector (see Figure 52) are listed under (1) and (2) of the fourth column heading. By definition, 50 percent of the persons wearing this ear protector can be expected to have less than the mean attenuation values and about 14 percent can be expected to have less than the mean minus one standard deviation. Octave band levels reaching the ear canal while wearing the ear protector are listed for mean and mean minus one standard deviation attenuation values under the last column heading. The octave-band exposure levels listed in each of the last two columns may be added (using Table XII) to determine the dB (A) exposure levels while wearing ear protectors. In this example, the exposure level for those receiving the mean attenuation values from the protector would be 66 dB (A), and for those receiving mean minus one standard deviation values, the exposure level would be 71 dB (A). Either exposure level while wearing ear protectors is obviously well below the 90 dB (A) limit specified in the Walsh-Healey Act for eight-hour per day exposures.

Two factors must be carefully considered when selecting ear protectors to meet the noise reduction requirements.

1. The ear protector attenuation values determined according to the present ANSI standard[22, 29] are for single frequencies located at center of each octave band. These values are not always an accurate representation of the noise reduction capability of the protector throughout the octave band. In addition, the noise exposure spectrum may not be flat throughout the band.
2. The protection provided by ear protectors varies considerably among wearers and among the ways the protectors are worn on individuals. There are also significant differences in performance among some protectors of the same model. Standard deviations of 3 to 7 dB are commonly found in subjective measurements of pro-

TABLE XIII

PROTECTION PROVIDED BY EAR PROTECTORS WORN IN A WEAVING ROOM NOISE ENVIRONMENT

Octave Band Center Frequency in Hz	Weaving Room Spectra in dB	Weaving Room Spectrum with A-Weighting in dB	Muff-Type Protector Attenuation in dB (1)	(2)	Resultant Exposure to Inner Ear in dB (1)	(2)
125	90	(less 16 =) 74	16	9	58	65
250	92	(less 9 =) 83	21	15	62	68
500	94	(less 3 =) 91	31	23	60	68
1,000	95	(less 0 =) 95	42	30	53	65
2,000	97	(plus 1 =) 98	43	32	55	66
4,000	95	(plus 1 =) 96	45	35	51	61
8,000	91	(less 1 =) 90	34	22	56	68
Overall	103 dB	102 dB(A)			66	75 dB(A)

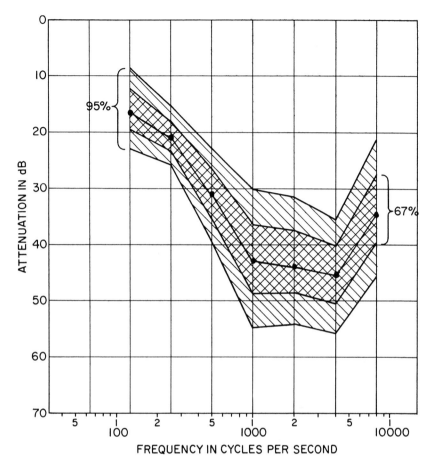

Figure 52. Mean Attenuation Characteristics of a Good Muff-Type Protector Plotted with One and Two Standard Deviation Shaded Areas (67 and 95 Percent Confidence Levels). Attenuation Values Determined According to the ANSI Specifications Using Pure-Tone Threshold Shift Techniques.[4]

tector attenuation at any test frequency; therefore, attenuation values may have a range of ± 6 to ± 14 dB for 95 percent confidence limits. Obviously, the variability in the amounts of protection provided must be considered along with the mean attenuation values when selecting an ear protector for a particular application.

It is always desirable to set confidence limits so that all persons will be protected 100 percent of the time; however, the spread of attenuation values is so great for a few individuals that very high level confidence limits are impractical. A practical choice would appear to be the mean attenuation minus one standard deviation which would provide confidence limits at about the 86 percent level. This confidence limit would be very similar to the limits set by most of the present rules and regulations concerning noise exposure levels which also have been limited due to practical considerations.

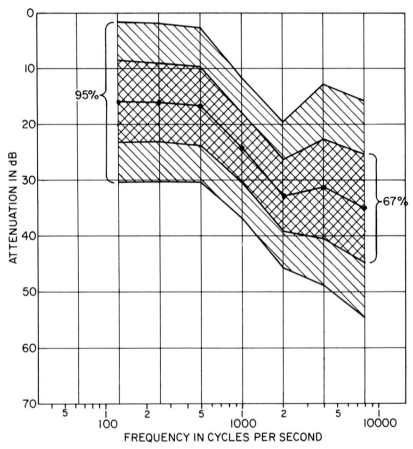

Figure 53. Mean attenuation characteristics plotted with one and two standard deviation shaded areas for a well-fitted imperforate earplug. Attenuation values determined according to the ANSI specifications using puretone threshold shift techniques.

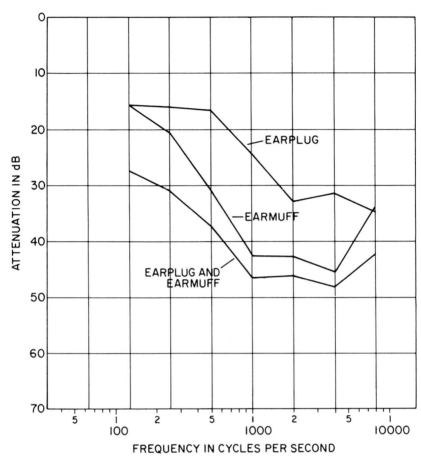

Figure 54. Mean attenuation characteristics of a muff and an earplug worn separately and together.

Because the effective protection provided by a given set of ear protectors can only be approximated in most field applications, a hearing monitoring program is strongly recommended for all persons wearing ear protector equipment wherever the margin of protection is small. Fortunately, a very large majority of noise exposures are at relatively low levels and the proper use of good ear protectors (see Figures 52 and 53) can provide adequate protection for a large majority of persons exposed to these noises.

If adequate protection cannot be provided by a single muff or earplug protector, both types can be worn at the same time to provide additional protection as shown in Figure 54. The combined attenuation of any two protectors cannot be predicted accurately due to complex coupling factors; however, the resultant attenuation from two good protectors might be estimated to average about six decibels greater attenuation than the higher of the two individual values at most test frequencies.

In summary, the use of a good ear protector can provide sufficient protection in a large majority of work environments where engineering control measures cannot be used successfully. For those relatively few persons exposed over long periods of time to noise levels in excess of 115 dBA, special care should be taken to be sure that the best protectors are used properly and hearing thresholds should be monitored regularly. For higher exposure levels over extended time periods, it may be necessary to use a combination of insert- and muff-type protectors and/or limit the time of exposure. Ear protectors will provide adequate protection for only a small percentage of wearers when worn in levels greater than 125 dBA over long periods of time.

Methods for Evaluating Protectors

Obviously, the only certain means for evaluating the effectiveness of personal protectors is to measure periodically the hearing thresholds of all persons exposed to noise. If no hearing losses are observed beyond those expected due to the aging process, the program may be considered to be successful. However, a hearing monitoring program may take years to be meaningful and a practical short-term guideline using protector attenuation values must be used to develop an effective program.

The present ANSI Method for the Measurement of the Real-Ear Attenuation of Ear Protectors at Threshold[22] specifies means to determine the differences between binaural pure-tone threshold levels with and without a protector in place at nine or more test frequencies. Because of the variations in attenuation values found between subjects and between measurements on the same subject, the present ANSI Method requires three replications of threshold measurements for each test tone with and without the protector in place on ten normal-hearing subjects. Obviously, this method has many limitations including the following:

1. The protectors are evaluated with low test tone levels which may not be meaningful when the protectors are used in high level noise.
2. The pure-tone signals provide limited information which may not always be representative of the attenuation provided for the frequency bands being considered.
3. The protectors are evaluated with sound approaching only from the direction the subject is facing. Attenuations measured with sound approaching from other directions may vary by more than 10 dB in some cases.
4. The time required for these measurements is excessively long and the test room requirements are strict.

Almost all of the available data on ear protector performance are based on the present ANSI standard, so it is important to recognize these limitations. This ANSI standard is being revised and many of these difficulties may be overcome; however, it will be some time before the revised standard is published and new data on the various protectors will become widely available.

Audible signals supplied by audiometer earphones or loudspeakers are used by some individuals to check the relative fit of different sizes of the same type of earplugs. These techniques are often helpful for this purpose; however, these methods should not be relied upon to provide absolute values of protection provided, nor can they be used to compare the effectiveness of different insert-type protectors.

Noise Reduction and Communication

Workers must be able to communicate with each other and to hear warning signals in many different high noise environments where both the noise and the wearing of ear protectors can influence communication. The effect of noise on communication depends to a large extent upon the spectrum of the noise, and is most significant when the noise has high level components in the speech frequency range from about 400 to 3,000 Hz. A review of speech interference studies[23, 24] shows that conversational speech begins to be difficult when the speaker and listener are separated by about two feet in noise levels of about 88 dBA. It is obvious that many such areas exist in work environments and the additional complication of ear protectors is often imposed at higher levels.

Communication While Wearing Protectors

Wearing ear protective devices obviously interferes with speech communication in quiet environments; however, wearing a conventional set of earplug- or muff-type protectors in noise levels above about 90 dB in octave bands (or about 97 dBA for flat spectra) should not interfere, and indeed may improve speech intelligibility for normal-hearing ears.[25, 26] Wearing ear protectors in high level noise can improve communication for normal ears because speech to noise ratios are kept nearly constant and the protected ear does not distort from overdriving caused by the high speech and noise levels. Research studies on this subject have been restricted to normal-hearing ears; thus, the effect of wearing ear protectors on intelligibility scores of persons with hearing impairments is not known.

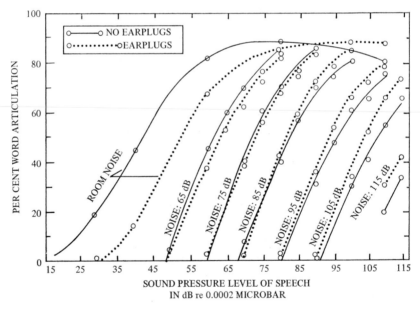

Figure 55. Showing the relationship between articulation and speech level with noise level as the parameter.[25]

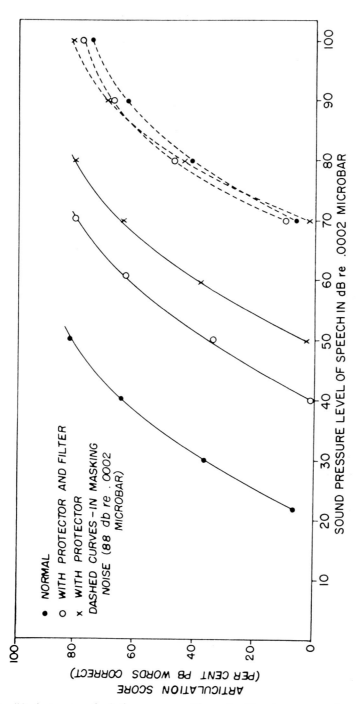

Figure 56. Average articulation curves with and without protector in quiet and with thermal masking noise (88 dB re 0.0002 Microbar).

The concept of blocking the ear in order to communicate better in noise is sometimes different for a worker to accept and he is likely to resist wearing protectors because of anticipated difficulties in communication. This opinion may be enforced if he tries the protector first in a quiet environment. Often, a worker will be attracted to ear protectors advertised as providing a "filter" that allows the low frequencies in the speech range to pass, but at the same time, blocks the noise. Some of these filter-type devices do provide better communication scores in quiet environments and they may be a good choice for use in relatively quiet areas where there are intermittent exposures to moderately high noises. However, in steady-state (constant) noise levels greater than about 90 dB in octave bands, the conventional insert- or muff-type protector provides communication scores that are at least as good as the filter type[26] (see Figures 55 and 56) and, in addition, the conventional protector provides better overall protection.

Communication Through Radio Headsets

The wearing of protectors may also help to improve the clarity of speech over electronic communication systems when used in high level noise environments (i.e. where insert-type protectors are worn under muff-type communication headsets). The improved perception of the speaker's own voice allows him to modulate his voice better and to avoid much of the distortion that often accompanies loud speech and shouting. Also, the listener can adjust his electronic gain control to obtain the level of undistorted speech that will give him the best reception. An exception may be found in very high levels, above about 130 dB overall, where speech perception is not always improved by the use of earplugs under communication headsets.

In high noise levels where communication must be accomplished with electronic systems, it is often desirable to improve the signal-to-noise ratio at the microphone as well as at the receiver. One common method for increasing the signal-to-noise ratio at the microphone is to use noise cancellation principles. A noise cancelling microphone picks up ambient noise through two aperatures, one on either side of its sensing element, and a portion of the low frequency noise is cancelled. The microphone sensing element is so oriented that the speech signal enters mainly through one aperature when the microphone is held close to the mouth so that speech is not cancelled.

An electronic noise-cancelling technique has also been used with limited success to increase intelligibility in noise environments.[27, 28] In these systems, the noise picked up by a microphone has its phase changed 180 degrees electronically and the phase adjusted signal is fed back into the headset.

In noise fields above about 120 dB re 0.0002 microbar overall, noise may be attenuated at the microphone by noise shields encasing the sensing element. Efficient noise attenuating shields tightly held around the mouth may be used with microphone systems to transmit intelligible communication in wide-band noise levels exceeding 140 dB.

Guides for the Selection of Protector Types

Both insert- and muff-type protectors have distinct advantages and disadvantages. Some of the features of each type are listed below:

Insert-Type Protectors

Advantages
1. They are small and are carried easily.
2. They can be worn conveniently and effectively with other personally worn items such as glasses, headgear, or hair styles.
3. They are relatively comfortable to wear in hot environments.
4. They are convenient to wear where the head must be maneuvered in close quarters.
5. The cost of sized earplugs is significantly less than muffs; however, hand-formed and personally molded protectors may be as much or more than muffs.

Disadvantages
1. Sized and molded insert protectors require more time and effort for fitting than for muffs.
2. The amount of protection provided by a good earplug is generally less and more variable between wearers than that provided by a good muff protector.

3. Dirt may be inserted into the ear canal if an earplug is removed and reinserted with dirty hands.
4. Earplugs are difficult to see in the ear from a distance; hence, it is difficult to monitor groups wearing these devices.
5. Earplugs can be worn only in healthy ear canals and, even in some healthy canals, a period of time is necessary for acceptance.

Muff-Type Protectors

Advantages
1. The protection provided by a good muff-type protector is generally greater and less variable between wearers than that of good earplugs.
2. A single size of earmuffs fits a large percentage of heads.
3. The relatively large muff size can be seen readily at a distance; thus, the wearing of these protectors is easily monitored.
4. Muffs are usually accepted more readily at the beginning of a hearing conservation program than earplugs.
5. Muffs can be worn even with many minor ear infections.
6. Muffs are not misplaced or lost as easily as are earplugs.

Disadvantages
1. Muffs are uncomfortable in hot environments.
2. Muffs are not as easily carried nor stored as earplugs.
3. Muffs are not as compatible with other personally worn items such as glasses and headgear as are earplugs.
4. Muff suspension forces may be reduced by usage, or by deliberate bending, so that the protection provided may be substantially less than expected.
5. The relatively large muff size may not be acceptable where the head must be maneuvered in close quarters.
6. Muffs are more expensive than most insert-type protectors.

It is doubtful that either the insert- or the muff-type protector alone can satisfy all needs in any organization. The obvious advantages of each should be used wherever possible to make a hearing conservation program more acceptable.

Requirements of an Effective Hearing Conservation Program

An effective hearing conservation program is not assured simply by making good ear protectors available to those persons exposed to high level noise. Top management and medical, industrial hygiene, and safety personnel, as well as those persons exposed to high noise levels, must all be made aware of the problem, and they all must support the hearing conservation program if it is to be effective. In addition, a responsible person must be designated as a coordinator to initiate the program and follow it through, sustaining his management's support.

The coordinator must determine the noise exposure patterns for all persons under his responsibility. He must evaluate other environmental factors such as temperature, humidity, the ease and importance of communication, and the need for other personal protective equipment including hard hats, safety glasses, welding helmets, and bulky gloves. With this information and by personally experimenting with different types of protectors in the various environments, he will be able to determine the type of protection to specify. After the program is underway, it is important that the coordinator maintain a close relationship with both management and employees in order to be aware of reactions to various phases of the program. In this way, any problem will become evident early and corrective measures can be taken before serious damage to the program results.

REFERENCES

1. von Gierke, H. E. and Warren, D. R.: *Protection of the Ear from Noise: Limiting Factors.* Benox Report, Univ. of Chicago: 47-60 (Dec. 1, 1953).
2. Nixon, C. W. and von Gierke, H. E.: Experiments on the bone-conduction threshold in a free sound field. *J Acoust Soc Am, 31*:1121-1125 (Aug. 1959).
3. Unpublished work by Paul L. Michael at The Pennsylvania State University.
4. American Optical Company, Safety Products Division, Southbridge, Massachusetts 01550.
5. Flents Products Company, 103 Park Avenue, New York, N. Y. 10017.
6. Frontier Industrial Products, 3521 Sunset Boulevard, Los Angeles, California 90026.
7. Glendale Optical Company, 130 Crossways Park Drive, Woodbury, New York 11797.
8. Mine Safety Appliances Company, Safety Products Division, 201 North Braddock Avenue, Pittsburgh, Pennsylvania 15230.
9. Billesholm products distributed by Rockford I. C. Webb, Inc., Rockford, Illinois 61110.
10. Safety Ear Protector Company, 5356 West Pico Boulevard, Los Angeles, California 90019.

11. Sigma Engineering Company, 11320 Burbank Boulevard, North Hollywood, California 91601.
12. Stayrite, Inc., 22-19 37th Avenue, Long Island City, New York 11101.
13. Surgical Mechanical Research, 1901-5 Beverly Boulevard, Los Angeles, California 90057.
14. Welsh Manufacturing Company, 9 Magnolia Street, Providence, Rhode Island 02909.
15. Willson Products Division, ESB, 2nd and Washington Streets, P. O. Box 622, Reading, Pennsylvania 19603.
16. United States Safety Service Company, 1535 Walnut Street, Kansas City, Missouri 64108.
17. Bausch and Lomb, Department 8992, Box 478, Rochester, New York 14602.
18. David Clark Company, Ear Protector Department, P. O. Box 555, Worchester, Massachusetts 01601.
19. General Electric Company, Medical Development Operation, River Road, Schenectady, New York 12305.
20. Sound Master Defenders, 1520 Broadway, Oakland, California 94612.
21. H. E. Douglass Engineering Sales Company, 3400 W. Burbank Boulevard, Burbank, California 91505.
22. American National Standard Method for the Measurement of the Real-Ear Attenuation of Ear Protectors at Threshold, Z24.22/427, American National Standards Institute, New York, N. Y. (1957).
23. Webster, John C.: Updating and interpreting the speech interference level (SIL). *J Audio Engrg Soc, 18*:114-118 (April, 1970).
24. Pollack, I. and Pickett, J. M.: Making of speech by noise at high sound levels. *J Acoust Soc Am, 30*:127-130 (Feb. 1958).
25. Kryter, K. D.: Effects of ear protective devices on the intelligibility of speech in noise. *J Acoust Soc Am, 18*:413-417 (Oct. 1946).
26. Michael, Paul L.: Ear protectors—their usefulness and limitations. *Arch Environ Health, 10*:612-618 (April 1965).
27. Meeker, W. F.: Active Ear Defender Systems: Component Considerations and Theory. WADC TR 57-368 (I) (1958).
28. Meeker, W. F.: Active Ear Defender Systems: Development of a Laboratory Model. WADC TR 57-368 (II) (1959).
29. Michael, Paul L. and Bolka, David F.: Personal ear protection evaluation —present and future. *Amer Industrial Hygiene Assoc J, 32*:753-756 (Nov. 1971).
30. American National Standard Specification for Sound Level Meters, S1.4-1971, American National Standards Institute, New York, N. Y. (1971).

Chapter 18

COMMUNITY NOISE

Introduction

THE EVER-INCREASING number of high level noise sources produce annoyance effects in almost all phases of our lives today.
The need for regulation and reduction of noise annoyance effects is found in the home, at the work place, in recreation areas
and in the community.

Although the need for guidelines or standards for limiting or
regulating the annoyance effects of noise has been apparent for
many years, a widely accepted national standard has yet to be established. Concentrated efforts have been made by individuals
and standards writing groups to develop a widely applicable
guideline or standard but none have been successful. Problems
encountered in the development of relationships between noise
and annoyance are complicated by many psychological, physiological, and physical factors. Such variables as (1) the attitude
of the listener toward the noise source, (2) the history of individual noise exposures, (3) the activities of and stresses upon the
listener during noise exposures, (4) the hearing sensitivities of
the listeners, and (5) other factors related to individual variability cause wide differences in noise reactions.

NUISANCE-TYPE REGULATIONS. Many local noise annoyance
rules and regulations have been enacted[1] but most are very inadequate. Older laws have been based, for the most part, on nuisance factors which often take the form "there shall be no unnecessary nor disturbing noise. . . ." These nuisance laws have the
obvious weakness that they cannot specify all conditions of how,
when, and to whom noise is unnecessary or disturbing; thus, in-

319

numerable arguments result in the interpretation of these laws when an attempt is made to enforce them.

More recently, zoning codes have been established which specify maximum noise levels for various zones. These so-called *performance* zoning codes are more objective and easier to enforce than the *nuisance* laws, but even so, many problems must be considered individually for the widely different conditions of noise exposures in individual communities.

PERFORMANCE-TYPE REGULATIONS. Writing groups under pressure to provide practical state-of-the-art recommendations, standards, regulations, or guidelines for exposures to noise levels below the level of physiological damage have found it necessary to consider "community response" rather than "annoyance" reactions to noise. This decision has been made because the group statistics involved in describing "community responses" to noise avoids many of the variables that are extremely difficult to account for in individual annoyance reaction situations. Some performance-type documents developed on the basis of community response have provided reasonably good predictions of response to noise for particular exposure situations; however, these rules or regulations have been based for the most part on specific exposures such as those from aircraft or from ground transportation and caution must be used in applying these results to other kinds of noise exposures.

Most of the new performance-type noise codes specify limits of sound pressure level that are based upon (1) a selected frequency weighting or noise analysis procedure, (2) the pattern of exposure times for various noise levels, (3) the ambient noise levels that would be expected in the particular kind of community without the offending noise source or sources, being present, and (4) a land-use zoning of the area.

Frequency-Weighting or Analysis of Community Noise

A large number of frequency weighting and analysis procedures have been proposed for use in estimating community reaction to noise. In recent years, single sound-pressure levels with A- and D-frequency weightings, and more complete analyses using octave, one-third octave, and narrower bands have been used in noise reaction measurement procedures.

The single readings using the A- or D-frequency weighting of sound-pressure level have the obvious advantages of short measurement times and overall simplicity in data manipulation. The A-frequency weighting, which is provided on most sound level meters, has been given considerable prominence in hearing conservation criteria[2, 3, 4] and for speech interference measurements[5, 6] as well as in procedures for estimating community reaction to noise.[7-13] The readily available A-frequency weighting is considered by many investigators to be one of the most practical noise measuring means available at this time for estimating community response to general wide-band noises.

AIRCRAFT NOISE. Exposures to aircraft noise are often unique for such factors as spectral and level characteristics and for listener's attitudes toward the source. These factors, plus the considerable work that has resulted from the strong pressure for control guidelines, have brought forth several reasonably good community reaction measuring procedures designed specifically for aircraft noise exposures.

A "D" frequency weighting[9] of sound-pressure level has been proposed for use in procedures to estimate community reaction to jet aircraft noise. The single reading with a "D" frequency weighting has been used in several European countries and it is being considered by the International Electrotechnical Commission (IEC) for use in their reports related to community noise.

Other, more sophisticated noise analysis techniques include:

1. Perceived Noise Level (PNL) measured in Perceived Noise Decibels (PN dB).
2. Effective Perceived Noise Levels (EPNL) measured in Effective Perceived Noise Decibels (EPN dB).
3. Noise Exposure Forecast (NEF) using EPN dB as the basic unit.

PNL is defined as an instantaneous measure of the noise produced at a given location based upon octave or third-octave sound pressure levels.[14, 15] EPNL values are derived from PNL instantaneous levels with added adjustments for high level pure-tone content and for flyover duration.[14, 15] NEF values are derived from EPNL levels with adjustments added for aircraft type, mix of aircraft, number of operations, runway utilization, flight path, operating procedures, and time of day.[14, 15]

Although the PNL, EPNL, and NEF procedures have been shown to be more accurate than single frequency weightings for the prediction of community reaction to aircraft noise for which they are designed, their relatively high degree of complexity cannot be justified for many other uses. Differences between aircraft and non-aircraft noise exposure factors such as noise characteristics, attitudes of listeners toward the source, and community compositions are significant in many situations. Thus, the complex measuring and data manipulation procedures of the PNL, EPNL, and NEF methods will not be covered in this text. Complete details on the use of these aircraft noise measures can be found in Department of Transportation Reports,[16] Environmental Protection Agency documents,[13, 15] and from other sources.[10, 11, 17–22]

NON-AIRCRAFT NOISE. At this time, the A-weighted sound levels are the most commonly used and the most practical means for measuring non-aircraft noise reactions. Certainly, instrumentation with A-weightings are more readily available and there is less chance for errors in measurement and data manipulation using this relatively simple procedure than with other more complicated methods. The simplicity of measurement, coupled with the lack of evidence to show that there are better overall measuring means, supports the choice of the A-weighting for non-aircraft noises at this time.

Measurement Equipment

A-weighted frequency response characteristics are included on most sound level meters. The choice of the sound level meter is not a major consideration except that it should meet the American National Standard Specification for Sound Level Meters, ANSI S1.4-1971 (Type 2),[23] to assure accurate and legally acceptable measurement data. Accessory equipment, such as tape or graphic level recorders, to be used with sound level meters should also conform with the sound level meter specifications.

Measurement Locations and Procedures

Sound pressure level measurements or recordings must be made at the place and time of annoyance. Outdoor measurements should be made at about four to five feet above the ground and, wherever possible, at least 10 feet from any solid structure that reflects sound. Complete descriptions of all measurement positions should be recorded and particular attention must be given to conditions that might influence measurements (see Noise Measurement Chapter). Care should be taken to operate the measuring equipment as specified by the manufacturer and to prevent the measurements from being influenced by such factors as wind over the microphone, noise from extraneous sources, or electromagnetic energy. Extremes in climatic conditions may cause significant differences in measured levels, so measurements should be made under normal conditions and a range of noise level variations should be obtained for extreme conditions.

STEADY AND FLUCTUATING NOISE LEVEL MEASUREMENTS. A number of different noise measurement procedures may be followed in making community noise measurements. If the noise is continuous with little variation in level, almost any measuring procedure using a simple sound level meter will be satisfactory. However, if the levels vary widely in a complex manner, it may be necessary to record the noise over a long period of time and perform complicated statistical analyses on the data to obtain an accurate determination of average values. The complicated procedures for determining average values of widely varying noise levels are not justified in many cases because community reactions to these widely varying levels may be different than the reactions to the same average values taken from noises with relatively constant levels on which the community noise level criteria are based. One relatively simple procedure for community noise measurement proposed as a standard by an American National Standards Institute writing group[24] is as follows:

1. Observe the A-level reading on the sound level meter (slow meter damping) for five (5) seconds and record (a) the best estimate of central tendency and (b) the range of the meter deflections, during that 5-second period, in decibels.

2. Repeat the observations of step (1) until the number of central-tendency readings equals or exceeds the total range (in decibels) of all the readings.
3. Find the arithmetic average of all the central-tendency readings in (1) and (2) above, and call this estimate the community noise level for this particular measuring time and location.

MULTIPLE NOISE SOURCES. In some cases, there will be several noise sources contributing to the A-weighted levels measured and it may be desirable to determine the contributions of each source for purposes of noise control or for assessing the responsibility for the noise. The simplest way to obtain the contribution of each source is to measure the weighted levels produced by each individual source when the other sources are not operating. If it is not possible to obtain measures of the individual source contributions directly, it may be necessary to analyze the overall noise levels in narrow frequency bands, generally one-third octave band or narrower, and correlate the characteristics of the overall levels with known characteristics of the individual noise sources.

Analysis procedures are time-consuming and not always very meaningful, so if at all possible, it is desirable to arrange for direct measurement of the individual sources. It may be possible to get these measurements at night, between work shifts, between process changes, or by special arrangements with supervisory personnel in charge of operation at one or more of the noise source locations.

INDOOR MEASUREMENTS. Indoor measurements should be made at locations at least three feet from walls or other reflecting surfaces. If regions of high and low levels are found close together (standing waves), three or four measurements about one foot apart should be averaged arithmetically.

Measurements should be taken with the room in the normal condition of use. If the windows may be opened or closed, measurements should be made under both conditions. If the noise levels are not steady, the time-level patterns of exposure must be determined.

IMPULSE NOISE MEASUREMENTS. Noise exposure criteria based on A-weighted sound pressure levels usually hold only for steady-state noises. The inertia in meter movements of conventional sound level meters prevent accurate readings of levels that change significantly in less than 0.2 seconds. To obtain accurate peak factor readings for single pressure pulses having level changes more than five dB in less than 0.2 seconds, a peak reading instrument or an oscilloscope must be used.

A conventional sound level meter can be used in most cases when there are more than 10 impulses per second because the peaks do not have time to drop significantly before the next peak comes along. Thus, the average of the saw-tooth-like meter deflections produced by the closely spaced pulses can be used for most purposes.

An important point to clarify before effort is expended in impulse measurements is the use to be made of the information. Only a few rules and regulations have provisions for impulsive noise and most of these documents simply specify a given adjustment to be made to the conventional sound level meter reading for "impulsive or hammering noises."

A Guide for Community Noise Criteria

Acceptable noise levels will vary from one community to another depending upon the kind of community and other variables. Ideally, noise codes are tailored to the individual community's character and requirements. If a community noise code has not been developed, the following guidelines might be used.[25]

BASIC LEVEL FOR A NOISE CODE. The basic steady-state noise criterion for outdoor, daytime exposures in rural residential, hospital, or other quiet areas is normally selected in the range of 35 to 45 dB (A). The particular value of this base level is selected with regard to the living habits, present and past, of the people in the particular area. For example, a young neighborhood which has several children may tolerate more noise than an older neighborhood composed mostly of retired people. When the base level is properly selected, there will be no observable reaction of the community to noises at or below this level.

The low level selected for the base criterion under the restricted conditions specified above are completely impractical for other kinds of communities where special adjustments must be made. It is impossible to provide the necessary adjustments for all situations in a reasonably sized document, but a large number of situations can be covered for various classes of exposures if adjustments for the following factors are considered.

1. The kind of community; i.e. rural; surburban; urban; urban with some work places, businesses, or main roads; city with heavy business and traffic; and heavy industry noise.
2. The duration and time pattern of exposures.
   (a) Steady-state constant exposure.
   (b) Non-uniform or intermittent steady-state exposure.
   (c) Impulsive noise exposures.
   (d) Pure-tone or whine characteristics in exposure.
3. Time of day; i.e. daytime, evening, night.
4. Indoors or outdoors.
5. Climatic conditions.
   (a) Wind.
   (b) Precipitation.
   (c) Temperature.
6. Special conditions for the district.

KIND OF COMMUNITY. The basic noise criterion set for quiet rural communities may be adjusted for various classes of noisier communities as shown in Table XIV. The definitions of the kinds of communities are broad and, in some cases, there will be difficulty in establishing the proper classification. In these questionable cases, careful individual consideration must be given to all factors involved before a limiting level is established. On the basis of a relatively small sample, it would appear that about 25 percent of all community noise complaints may be legitimate as

TABLE XIV

ADJUSTMENTS TO BE ADDED TO A BASIC
NOISE CRITERION FOR COMMUNITY TYPES

Type of Community	Adjustment in dB(A)
Rural residential	0
Suburban residential	+ 5
Urban residential	+10
Urban with work places, businesses, or main roads	+15
City with heavy business and traffic	+20
Heavy industry areas	+25

TABLE XV

ADJUSTMENTS TO BE ADDED TO A BASIC
NOISE CRITERION FOR NOISE DURATION

Noise Exposure Time (Percentage)	*Adjustments in dB(A)*
Between: 100 and 56	0
55 and 18	+ 5
17 and 6	+10
5 and 1.8	+15
1.7 and 0.6	+20
0.5 and 0.2	+25
Less than 0.2	+30

viewed by well-balanced individuals, about 50 percent may be due to people who are exceptionally sensitive to noise or who have a bad relationship with the noise source, and about 25 percent may be profit-motivated (i.e. wants the company to buy their house). In any case, if there are a large number of complaints that can be considered to be legitimate, the next lower classification should be considered.

DURATION AND TIME PATTERN OF EXPOSURES. The basic noise criteria discussed in the above text is concerned with steady, uninterrupted noise without impulsive character or audible tones. If the noise is interrupted by quiet periods, adjustment should be made in the criterion as shown in Table XV.

Noises with an impulsive character, such as those produced by hammering or riveting, are generally considered to be more annoying than steady noise and adjustments should be made to the basic criterion accordingly. When there are 10 or more of these impulses per second, a conventional sound level meter can generally be used to measure these sounds. For these rapidly repeated impulsive sounds, the basic criterion should be adjusted by −5 dB.

If there are less than 10 impulses of noise per second, an impulse-measuring instrument or an oscilloscope must be used to measure the sound. In addition, a different noise criterion must be developed for the particular noise characteristics and exposure conditions.

Noises that contain audible tone components such as whines, screeches, or hums are also more annoying than noises without

TABLE XVI

ADJUSTMENTS TO BE ADDED TO A BASIC NOISE CRITERION
FOR DIFFERENT TIMES DURING A 24-HOUR PERIOD

Time of Day	*Adjustment in dB(A)*
Daytime	0
Evening	− 5
Nighttime	−10

these characteristics. The base criterion should be adjusted by −5 dB when these audible tone components are present.

TIME OF DAY. Community noise exposures of a given level are normally considered to be more annoying during the night and evening hours than during the day. Adjustments to the basic criterion for different times of day are given in Table XVI.

The time limits for day, evening, and night may vary in different communities but might be considered generally to be as follows:

Day   0700 until 1800
Evening 1800 until 2300
Night   2300 until 0700

SUMMARY. The estimated community response to the noise criteria proposed above might be summarized as shown in Table XVII.

In some cases, the proposed criterion will not accurately predict the reaction of a community to specific noise and exposures. Special adjustments may have to be made to this criterion for these cases. Of particular importance is the background noise to which

TABLE XVII

ESTIMATED COMMUNITY RESPONSE TO NOISE
AS COMPARED TO THE PROPOSED CRITERIA

Difference Between Measured Noise and Adjusted Noise Criterion in dB(A)	*Estimated Community Response*
+ 0	No observed reaction
+ 5	Occasional complaints
+10	Widespread complaints
+15	Threats of community action
+20	Vigorous community action

the community has been exposed before the offending source or sources began to operate. In cases where communities have historically tolerated high background noise, the background noise levels may serve as the exposure limit criteria when new noise sources are considered. Additional reference materials on community noise may be found in References 25 to 49.

REFERENCES

1. Compilation of State and Local Ordinances on Noise Control, Congressional Record, pp. E9031-9112, October 29, 1969.
2. Walsh-Healey Public Contracts Act, Federal Register, Vol. 34, No. 96, Tuesday, May 20, 1969.
3. Threshold Limit Values of Physical Agents, Adopted by American Conference of Governmental Industrial Hygienists, 1014 Broadway, Cincinnati, Ohio 45202 (1969).
4. Occupational Safety and Health Act of 1970, Public Law 91-596, 91st Congress, S. 2193, December 29, 1970.
5. American National Standard Methods for the Calculation of the Articulation Index, ANSI S3.5-1969, American National Standards Institute, Inc.
6. Kryter, K. D.: Speech Communication in Noise, AFCRC-TR-54-52, Air Force Cambridge Research Center, Air Research and Development Command, Bolling Air Force Base, Washington, D. C., May 1955.
7. Draft ISO Recommendation: Noise Assessment with Respect to Community Response, No. 1996, November 1969.
8. Young, R. W. and Peterson, A.: On Estimating Noisiness of Aircraft Sounds, *J Acoust Soc Amer 45*:834-838, 1969.
9. Procedure for Describing Aircraft Noise Around an Airport, ISO Recommendation R507, International Organization for Standardization, June 1970.
10. Young, R. W.: Measurement of Noise Level and Exposure, *Transportion Noises,* University of Washington Press, 1970, p. 45.
11. Webster, J. C.: SIL—Past, present and future, *Sound and Vibration Magazine,* August 1969.
12. Congressional Record—Extension of Remarks—Compilation of State and Local Ordinances on Noise Control, E 9031-9112 (October 1969).
13. Laws and Regulatory Schemes for Noise Abatement, Environmental Protection Agency NTID 300.4 (December 31, 1971).
14. Kryter, Karl D.: Perceived Noisiness (Annoyance), *The Effects of Noise on Man,* Academic Press, 1970, p. 269.
15. Community Noise, Environmental Protection Agency NTID 300.3 (December 31, 1971).
16. A Study of the Magnitude of Transportation Noise Generation and

Potential Abatement, Vol. III, Report OST-ONA-71-1, Department of Transportation, Office of Noise Abatement, Washington, D. C. (November 1970).

17. Galloway, W. J. and Pietrasanta, A. C.: Land Use Planning Relating to Aircraft Noise, Technical Report No. 821, Bolt Beranek and Newman, Inc., published by the FAA, October 1964. Also published by the Department of Defense as AFM 86-5, TM 5-365, NAVDOCKS P-98, Land Use Planning with Respect to Aircraft Noise.

18. Galloway, W. J. and Bishop, D. E.: Noise Exposure Forecasts: Evolution, Evaluation, Extensions, and Land Use Interpretations, FAA-NO-70-9, August 1970.

19. Wyle Laboratories Research Staff, Supporting Information for the Adopted Noise Regulations for California Airports, WCR 70-3(R) Final Report to the California Department of Aeronautics, January 1971.

20. The Adopted Noise Regulations for California Airports, TITLE 4, Register 70, No. 48-11-28-70. Subchapter 6. Noise Standards.

21. Community Reaction to Airport Noise—Final Report, Volume 1, Tracor Document No. T-70-AU-7454-U, September 1970.

22. Ollerhead, J. B.: An Evaluation of Methods for Scaling Aircraft Noise Perception, Wyle Laboratories Research Staff Report WR70-17, Contract NAS1-9527, May 1971.

23. American National Standard Specification for Sound Level Meters, ANSI S1.4-1971, American National Standards Institute, Inc.

24. Method for Measurement of Community Noise, Draft No. 3, February 17, 1969, revised May 27, 1969, editorial changes added November 11, 1969. American National Standards Institute, New York.

25. Report to the President and Congress on Noise, U. S. Environmental Protection Agency, December 31, 1971.

26. Federal Aviation Regulations, Part 36, Noise Standards: Aircraft Type Certification, November 1969.

27. Mills, C. H. G. and Robinson, D. W.: The Subjective Rating of Motor Vehicle Noise, Appendix IX, *NOISE,* presented to Parliament by the Lord President of the Council and Minister for Science by Committee on the Problem of Noise, July 1963; Her Majesty's Stationery Office, Reprinted 1966.

28. Selection of a Unit for Specification of Motor Vehicle Noise, Appendix A, *Urban Highway Noise: Measurement, Simulation and Mixed Reactions,* Bolt Beranek and Newman Report 1505, April 1967.

29. Rosenblith, W. A., Stevens, K. N. and the Staff of Bolt Beranek and Newman, Inc.: Handbook of Acoustic Noise Control, Vol. 2, Noise and Man, WADC TR-52-204, Wright-Patterson Air Force Base, Ohio: Wright Air Development Center, 1953.

30. Stevens, K. N., Rosenblith, W. A. and Bolt, R. H.: Community Noise and City Planning, *Handbook of Noise Control,* Chapter 35, McGraw-Hill, 1957.

31. Parrack, H. O.: Community Reaction to Noise, *Handbook of Noise Control,* Chapter 36, McGraw-Hill, 1957.

32. Stevens, K. N. and Pietrasanta, A. C. and the Staff of Bolt Beranek and Newman, Inc.: Procedures for Estimating Noise Exposure and Resulting Community Reactions from Air Base Operations, WADC TN-57-10, Wright-Patterson Air Force Base, Ohio: Wright Air Development Center, 1957.

33. Bonvallet, G. L.: Levels and spectra of traffic, industrial and residential area noise, *J Acoust Soc Amer, 23*:435-439, July 1951.

34. Stevens, K. N.: A survey of background and aircraft noise in communities near airports, NACA Technical Note 3379, December 1954.

35. Donley, Ray: Community noise regulation, *Sound and Vibration Magazine,* February 1969.

36. Simpson, Myles and Biship, Dwight: Community Noise Measurements in Los Angeles, Detroit and Boston, Bolt Beranek and Newman Report No. 2078, June 1971.

37. Noise in Towns, *NOISE,* Chapter IV, 22-31, presented to Parliament by the Lord President of the Council and Minister for Science by Committee on the Problem of Noise, July 1963; Her Majesty's Stationery Office, reprinted 1966.

38. Olson, N.: Statistical Study of Traffic Noise, APS-476, Division of Physics, National Research Council of Canada, Ottawa, 1970.

39. Griffiths, I. D. and Langdon, F. J.: *J Sound and Vib, 8*:16, 1968.

40. Wyle Laboratories Research Staff, Noise from Transportation Systems, Recreation Vehicles and Devices Powered by Small Internal Combustion Engines, WR71-17, Office of Noise Abatement and Control, Environmental Protection Agency, Washington, D. C., November 1971.

41. Social Survey in the Vicinity of London (Heathrow) Airport, Appendix XI, *Noise,* presented to Parliament by the Lord President of the Council and Minister for Science by Committee on the Problem of Noise, July 1963; Her Majesty's Stationery Office, reprinted 1966.

42. Borsky, P. N.: Community Reactions to Air Force Noise, WADD Technical Report 60-689, Parts 1 and 2, Wright-Patterson AFB, Ohio, March 1961.

43. Galloway, W. J. and Von Gierke, H. E.: Individual and Community Reaction to Aircraft Noise: Present Status and Standardization Efforts, International Conference on the Reduction of Noise and Disturbance Caused by Civil Aircraft, London, November 1966.

44. Robinson, D. W.: The Concept of Noise Pollution Level, National

Physical Laboratory, Aerodynamics Division, NPL Aero Report Ac 38, March 1969.

45. Robinson, D. W.: Towards a Unified System of Noise Assessment, *J Sound and Vib, 14*(3):279-298, 1971.

46. Bottom, C. G. and Waters, D. M.: A Social Survey Into Annoyance Caused by the Interaction of Aircraft Noise and Traffic Noise, Department of Transport Technology TT-7102, Loughborough University of Technology.

47. A Study of the Magnitude of Transportation Noise Generation and Potential Abatement, Vols. I—VII, Department of Transportation, Office of Noise Abatement, Washington, D. C., November 1970.

48. Noise and Vibration Characteristics of High Speed Transit Vehicles, Technical Report OST-ONA-71-7, Department of Transportation, Office of Noise Abatement, Washington, D. C., June 1971.

49. Cohen, A.: Noise and Psychological State Proceedings of National Conference on Noise as a Public Health Hazard, American Speech and Hearing Association, Report No. 4, 89-98, February 1969.

Chapter 19

COMMON QUESTIONS AND ANSWERS

THIS CHAPTER CONTAINS a series of questions for self-teaching and self-auditing. Some of the questions provide multiple choice answers, others provide references in books, and some questions leave the reader to search for the answer in this book.

The questions have been accumulated from many sources to which the authors are indebted, but especially to the following: Industrial Hygiene Noise Manual, Lawrence A. Vassallo, Dr. M. Fox, Dr. Roger Maas, United States Department of Labor, and participants in our Occupational Hearing Loss institute generally held at Colby College, Waterville, Maine.

NOISE AND MEASUREMENT

1. The decibel is used to describe sound pressure levels because:
   1. it has physical units of pressure and closely follows the frequency characteristics of the human ear.
   2. it provides a convenient compressed scale to express the very wide range of sound pressures that are commonly found in industry.[1]
   3. it has physical units of pressure and it is referenced to 0.0002 microbar, the threshold of audibility.
   4. it provides a convenient way to add the pressures from different sound sources and to convert this total pressure to intensity units.
   5. it always expresses the sound pressure in levels that have frequency characteristics weighted in a logarithmic manner similar to that of the human ear.

333

2. When a sound source is located in a large room that has wall, ceiling, and floor surfaces that reflect a high percentage of the acoustic energy it may be expected that reverberant conditions exist. In a reverberant sound field the sound pressure created by a broad frequency band source will:
    1. decrease inversely with the distance from the source.
    2. decrease inversely with the square of the distance from the source.
    3. remain essentially constant throughout the reverberant room.[2]
    4. decrease with the square root of the distance from the source.
    5. be highly variable due to standing waves.

3. When sound pressures are measured at various distances from a pitched or pure tone sound source located in a small, highly reverberant room, it might be expected that:
    1. the sound pressure will decrease inversely with the distance from the source.
    2. the sound pressure will increase directly with the distance from the source.
    3. the sound pressure will decrease inversely with the square of the distance from the source.
    4. the sound intensity will decrease inversely with the distance from the source.
    5. the sound pressure will have pronounced maxima and minima but will not vary appreciably in overall level with distance.[3]

4. The American Standards Association specifications for sound level meters specifies that a sound level meter should have A, B, and C weighting networks. These networks serve to:
    1. provide a means for measuring the sound pressures of narrow bands of noise over the complete audio spectrum.
    2. provide an accurate means for measuring octave bands of noise over the complete audio spectrum.
    3. provide a means for measuring sound pressures using frequency weighting characteristics similar to those of the human ear at three different equal loudness contours.[4]

    4. provide a means of calibrating the sound level meter at three different frequencies.

    5. provide a means for directly measuring sound power using three different standard frequency weighting networks.

5. It is well known that excessive exposure to noise will cause a loss of hearing. In appraising a potential noise hazard, it is necessary to know that:

    1. damage always occurs slowly, and, if control measures are initiated immediately when noise-induced pain is experienced, loss of hearing can be prevented.

    2. damage occurs rapidly but loss to hearing can be completely prevented if control measures are initiated immediately when pain is experienced from excessive noise exposure.

    3. damage may occur very slowly and it may occur without pain being experienced.[5]

    4. the ear is most sensitive to the very high frequencies above 10 kcps and it is these frequencies that are responsible for most hearing losses.

    5. even a small noise-induced hearing loss will be obvious to the employee, and, if he is instructed to report this loss, preventative measures can be taken in time to prevent serious impairment.

6. A Rochelle Salt crystal microphone is commonly supplied with many pieces of sound measuring equipment. It is:

    1. particularly useful because it may be used in any environment regardless of extremes of temperature and humidity.

    2. very sensitive and relatively inexpensive, but it must not be used for prolonged periods in extremes of temperature and humidity.[6]

    3. chosen primarily because it can be used directly with extremely long cables without temperature corrections.

    4. chosen primarily because it can be used to measure sound pressure levels ranging from 40 to 200 db re 0.0002 microbar.

    5. often used as a standard microphone for calibration purposes because of its very flat frequency response from 20 cps to 20 kcps.

7. Dynamic microphones have been used in sound measurements for many years. Primarily, they are used in cases where:
   1. high level electrical and magnetic fields might be expected.
   2. very long cables are necessary.[7]
   3. flat frequency characteristics are needed between 20 cps and 20 kcps.
   4. sound pressures greater than 180 db re 0.0002 microbar are to be measured.
   5. polarizing voltages are available.
8. Condenser microphones are often used as accessory equipment for sound level meters. They are:
   1. used primarily in instances where an inexpensive transducer is required for narrow band measurements.
   2. often used as calibration standards because of their stability and their excellent wide range frequency characteristics.[8]
   3. often used because no polarizing voltage supplies are required.
   4. very stable and have excellent frequency characteristics, but they cannot be used to measure sound pressure levels above 120 db re 0.0002 microbar.
   5. preferred to the Rochelle Salt microphone because of their excellent stability; however, generally their frequency responses are not as good as those of Rochelle Salt microphones.
9. The primary function of a peak reading or impact noise analyzer is to:
   1. measure the sound power of the highest frequencies in a broad band noise.
   2. measure the sound pressure level of the highest frequencies in a broad band noise.
   3. measure the sound pressure level of broad band noises in terms of a peak to peak value.
   4. measure the peak amplitude of the sound pressure and its duration, or decay time.[9]

5. determine the highest frequency in the band being measured.

10. To get reliable sound level measurement data in areas where there is wind:

    1. it is necessary to use a crystal microphone because they are constructed so that wind cannot affect their operation.

    2. it is necessary to use a heavy wind screen that will provide an air-tight barrier completely around the microphone.

    3. a suitable wind screen should be used; it may be constructed of cloth offering moderate resistance to airflow such as sheer silk or nylon stretched completely around the microphone.[10]

    4. measurements are made as usual for there is no need for corrections or screening because the wind creates a direct pressure and the sound pressure of the noise being measured is an alternating pressure.

    5. a fixed correction factor must be added that is proportional to the wind velocity since the attenuation caused by the wind will cause the sound level meter to read low.

11. An octave band analyzer is used with a sound level meter to determine:

    1. The sound pressure levels in frequency bands, the highest frequencies of which are twice that of the lowest frequencies.[11]

    2. the sound pressure levels in frequency bands, the lowest frequencies of which are equal to the square root of the highest frequencies.

    3. the sound pressure levels in 1,000 cps frequency bands.

    4. the sound power levels in 1,000 cps frequency bands.

    5. the sound power levels in frequency bands, the lowest frequencies of which are equal to the square root of the highest frequencies.

12. Some analyzers used with sound level meters are adjustable to half octave bands; these bands:

    1. have the highest frequencies equal to twice the lowest frequencies in each band.

   2. have the lowest frequencies equal to the square root of the highest frequencies in each band.

   3. are all 500 cps in width.

   4. have the highest frequencies equal to 1.5 times the lowest frequencies in each band.

   5. have the highest frequencies equal to $\sqrt{2}$ times the lowest frequencies in each band.[12]

13. One-third octave band analyzers are used with sound level meters to measure:

   1. the sound pressure levels in frequency bands, the highest frequencies of which are equal to three times that of the lowest frequencies.

   2. the sound power levels in 333 cps band widths.

   3. the sound pressure levels in frequency bands, the lowest frequencies of which are the cube root of the highest frequencies.

   4. the sound pressure levels in frequency bands, the highest frequencies of which are $\sqrt[3]{2}$ times the lowest frequencies in each band.[13]

   5. The sound pressure levels in frequency bands, the highest frequencies of which are $\sqrt{3}$ times the lowest frequencies in each band.

14. In areas where there are broad band noise sources producing overall sound pressure levels of about 110 db re 0.0002 microbar, the use of the best, well-fitted, ear protective devices can be expected to:

   1. provide complete protection against noise induced hearing loss, but to reduce speech communication scores.

   2. cut the annoyance problem, but not to provide complete protection against noise induced hearing loss.

   3. provide complete protection against noise induced hearing loss, and to improve speech communication scores.[14]

   4. improve speech communication scores, but not to give complete protection against noise induced hearing loss.

   5. be necessary even if the individual works in these areas for long periods of time.

15. It is possible in some cases to select damage risk criteria that

can be used in determining which areas require noise control measures. These damage risk criteria:

1. provide very accurate dividing lines between safe and unsafe conditions for all kinds of noise exposures.
2. provide very accurate dividing lines between safe and unsafe conditions for all steady state noise exposures.
3. provide very accurate dividing lines between safe and unsafe conditions for all transient noise exposures.
4. have broad dividing lines between safe and unsafe exposure levels for most steady state noises but are generally not applicable for intermittent noises.[15]
5. have broad dividing lines between safe and unsafe exposure levels for most intermittent noises but are generally not applicable for steady state noises.

16. Sound level meters provide readings in terms of sound pressure levels which are:
    1. expressed in decibels by 20 times the logarithm to the base 10 of the ratio of the measured effective sound pressure of the sound to a reference effective sound pressure.[16]
    2. expressed in microbars by 20 times the logarithm to the base e of the measured effective sound pressure of the sound to a reference effective sound pressure.
    3. expressed in decibels by 20 times the logarithm to the base e of the ratio of the measured effective sound pressure of the sound to a reference effective sound pressure.
    4. expressed in decibels by 10 times the logarithm to the base 10 of the measured effective sound pressure of the sound to a reference effective sound pressure.
    5. expressed in microbars by 10 times the logarithm to the base e of the measured effective sound pressure of the sound to a reference effective sound pressure.

17. The pressure most commonly used as a reference for sound pressure levels in air is:
    1. 0.0001 microbar.
    2. 85 decibels.
    3. 0.002 microbar.
    4. 0.0002 microbar.[17]
    5. 0.001 microbar.

AUDIOMETRY

1. Why must all audiograms report the standard of the audiometer used?
2. Why is it important to record the serial number of the audiometer on each audiogram?
3. What should be done if a mistake is made in recording information on the audiogram?
4. Is it standard practice to record audiometric threshold not in 5 dB steps, such as 12, 19, 4, 6?
5. What are the advantages of a serial audiogram as compared to a graph audiogram?
6. How do you record a threshold if a subject fails to respond to the maximum intensity of a test tone on the audiometer?
7. How long should hearing records be retained?
8. Why is it important to record the time interval since the last noise exposure?
9. Why is it important to record the noise level and length of daily exposure in which the employee works?
10. Who is ultimately responsible for all records?
11. What is a shadow curve of hearing?
12. Why is it necessary to record the serial number of the audiometer on biological calibration sheets?
13. What other calibration data should be kept along with biological readings?
14. Is a newly-calibrated audiometer necessarily in calibration if it has been shipped in the mails?
15. What is the purpose of a biological calibration?
16. How often should biological calibration be performed and on whom?
17. Why is it proper to use more than two subjects to serve as biological standards?
18. Is it good practice for a technician to perform hearing testing on his own ears?
19. What is cross talk and how do you check for it?
20. Why is it important for an audiometer to be free of static, click and hum prior to testing?

21. If earphones are damaged, can they be replaced without complete electronic check of the audiometer?
22. What appendices of the earphones can be replaced without disturbing calibration?
23. Does placing the right earphone cord in the left earphone circuit upset the calibration of the right earphone?
24. Why is it important to handle earphones with extreme care?
25. Can an audiometer be calibrated without its earphones?
26. What happens if earphones are clapped together?
27. What is the proper tension to have on the earphone headband?
28. Is it good practice to turn the audiometer off after each hearing test?
29. What is the most common source of failure to get a signal in the earphones?
30. What happens to the intensity of the signal if a jack is not seated properly?
31. Is it necessary to keep the audiometer shipping carton?
32. If it has to be mailed, what mailing service appears to be very reliable in not damaging the equipment?
33. How often should an audiometer be checked by electronic calibration?
34. How can you tell if the calibration facility is really qualified to do the work completely and properly?
35. What information should you insist the service facility supply you when an audiometer is calibrated?
36. Is it good practice to obtain this information on a newly-purchased audiometer?
37. When a calibration facility supplies only partial information as to the readings obtained on your equipment, what does this indicate?
38. Are there certain criteria by which an audiometer must be calibrated?
39. What prior arrangements should be made with the audiometer supplier before purchasing his equipment?
40. How many audiometric zero reference standards are in use today?

41. Which is the newest?
42. What are the most common complaints regarding audiometer failure?
43. Is an acoustical calibration the same as an electronic calibration?
44. What is the limit of knowledge obtained with an acoustical calibration?
45. Name at least three dimensions checked for in an electronic calibration.
46. In daily biological calibration what is considered significant in regards to changes in readings on the same individual?
47. What should be done when this degree of change is noted?
48. Are earphone enclosures accepted for use by the Standards Bureau?
49. If you are not able to obtain normal thresholds on anyone at 500 and 1,000 Hz, is the audiometer necessarily out of calibration?
50. What would be another cause?
51. Are audiometer salesmen generally qualified to perform field maintenance on your equipment?

The answers to all the foregoing questions are found in Chapters 6 and 7 in this book.

GENERAL QUESTIONS

1. Does the technician require training if he is going to use a self-recording audiometer?

    A. Yes. He should be certified.

2. Does malingering occur with the use of a self-recording audiometer?

    A. Yes. In some instances much more frequently than with a manual type audiometer.

3. Should personnel with nerve deafness be hired for noisy jobs?

    A. See Chapter 16.

4. Is 8,000 cycles an important frequency to test with audiometer?

    A. It is very important to test for 8,000 cycles.
       See Chapter 8.

5. When do you refer an employee to an otologist for consultation?

    A. See Chapter 16.

6. How do you test an employee who complains of ringing in his ears during audiometry?

    A. See Chapter 8.

7. What does the United States Department of Labor expect in the area of enforcing and implementing the noise control regulation?

    A. They expect the technology which has been developed over the past 15 to 20 years to now be applied at work sites to protect workers from being exposed and suffering hearing losses. They expect designers and manufacturers to start reducing the noise levels generated by their products or to provide means for operators to be protected from the excessive noise levels. They expect better and more effective personal protective equipment and devices to be developed and made available. They expect some of the old, outmoded and obsolete noisy processes to be replaced with more modern, efficient and quieter processes. They expect the increased demand for expertise in this field to result in more students studying the subject and getting workers in environmental control as a career. They expect more consultants and consulting firms to provice services in this subject, and of course, expect fewer workers to end up with needless hearing disabilities.

8. What is a company expected to do to meet the federal standards or noise regulations?

    A. When employees are subjected to sound levels exceeding those listed in the regulations, feasible administrative or engineering controls shall be initiated and utilized. If such controls fail to reduce sound levels to within the prescribed levels. A continuing effective hearing conservation program shall be administered.

9. Can a company which does not have "A" scale sound level meters but has octave band analyzers use this equipment to record their noise levels?

    A. Yes. In the Walsh-Healey regulations is a chart graph on

which octave band sound pressure levels may be converted to the equivalent A-weighted sound level corresponding to the highest penetration into the sound level contours.

10. How will "feasible administrative or engineering controls" be interpreted? Will high cost or economic factors of control be considered?

A. There was much discussion over whether to state that "economically feasible" controls should be determined and implemented. It was finally decided the word "feasible" should be interpreted in the broadest possible sense and that economic factors should certainly be one of the major considerations—but not the only factor or the controlling factor. Economics may be considered in determining the time limits allowed to an employer in which to come into full compliance with the law.

11. What is required in a "continuing effective hearing conservation program"?

A. Where noise levels in the working environment exceed those allowable, a program is necessary to assure that the personal protective equipment provided and used is effective in preventing deterioration of a worker's hearing. The most desirable program would include pre-employment hearing examinations and periodic and regular audiometric tests and evaluations. Audiometry and the use and application of personal protective devices should be under medical supervision or be done by a nurse, audiologist or trained technician under medical direction.

12. What should be done if workers refuse to use personal protection?

A. It is management's prerogative and duty to see that all means and measures are taken to assure that work is conducted in a safe and healthful manner. This will require good education and training techniques and effective and forceful supervision. The standards state that personal protection shall be provided and used. This puts a burden on the worker to cooperate and use what management provides. The U. S. Department of Labor will cooperate with the employers, whenever and however appropriate, to assure the cooperation of employees. However, the Federal government cannot become directly involved in labor-management relations of this sort.

13. Does the Labor Department expect to provide some help to small companies who do not have full time safety staffs and may not have access to all the standards adopted by reference?

 A. An inspection survey guide is being developed for use by Department field personnel to guide them as to the situations to look for while making plant surveys and which will be keyed to the standards applicable to each situation. These survey guides will be available to public contractors as a "do-it-yourself" inspection guide so that a continuing inspection program can be set up by any small contractor within his own organization to assure his meeting the requirements of the law.

14. How often should noise-exposed individuals be tested?

 A. See Chapter 16.

15. What is the best procedure to remove ear wax prior to hearing testing?

 A. See Chapter 3 and 16.

16. How often should audiometric equipment be recalibrated— factory or laboratory?

 A. See Chapter 6.

17. What percentage of hearing loss should be allowed for normal presbycusis?

 A. See Chapter 9.

18. What is the proper method of disinfecting audiometer earphones?

 A. See Chapter 8.

19. How soon after hazardous noise exposure may an accurate hearing test be made?

 A. See Chapter 16.

20. What is the best method of "selling" the importance of ear protection program?

 A. See Chapter 16.

21. What is the best approach toward a compulsory ear protection program?
    A. See Chapter 17.

22. What ear protectors should be recommended in the event of chronic discharge from ears?
    A. See Chapter 17.

23. What is the answer to the mechanic who claims that ear protectors hinder his ability to detect mechanical failure with his machine?
    A. See Chapter 17.

24. How often should sound pressure level readings be made in a noisy plant?
    A. See Chapter 11.

25. What is the most generally accepted method of computing "equivalent exposure time" of individuals with intermittent exposure?
    A. See Chapter 9.

26. To what extent does the frequency component of a hazardous noise affect corresponding frequency in a person's hearing range?
    A. See Chapter 16.

27. When can it be definitely established that a certain individual is sufficiently susceptible to noise trauma to require moving him to another job in a quieter environment?
    A. See Chapter 16.

28. What visual aids such as films, literature, signs, slogans, etc. are available?
    A. See Chapter 16.

29. How important is ear protection to a person in the later stages of nerve deafness?
    A. See Chapter 16.

30. Should cooperation be sought from labor unions and employee's organizations?
    A. See Chapter 16.

31. What procedure should be followed in the event of an employee refusing (on religious or other grounds) to have hearing test or ears cleaned when needed?
    A. See Chapter 16.

32. What data should be obtained during pre-employment exam-
    ination regarding: (a) previous noise exposure, (b) history
    of other pathological causes, etc.
    A. See Chapter 7.
33. What information should be included with ear audiogram
    to substantiate its authenticity in court?
    A. See Chapter 7.
34. What ear protection should be required of a man showing
    a severe conductive loss?
    A. See Chapter 7.
35. What procedure should be followed when malingering is
    suspected?
    A. See Chapters 7 and 16.
36. What is a handicapping hearing loss?
    A. Chapter 1.
37. When are hearing aids helpful?
    A. When the average hearing loss in the speech frequencies
       exceeds about 35 dB (ANSI).
38. Is there a specific test for an individual's sensitivity to noise?
    A. Chapter 5.
39. What is occupational hearing loss?
    A. Chapter 5.
40. What is acoustic trauma?
    A. Chapter 4.
41. Are ultrasonic sounds dangerous to hearing?
    A. Chapter 9.
42. Do fluctuating thresholds of 10 or 15 dB mean malingering?
    A. Chapter 8.
43. Are sounds of high or low frequency more damaging to hear-
    ing?
    A. Chapter 9.
44. Is continuous or intermittent noise more damaging to hear-
    ing?
    A. Chapter 9.
45. Should all employees in a plant have hearing tests or only
    those in noise?
    A. Chapter 16.

46. Should audiograms be filed in the medical folders?
    A. Chapter 16.
47. What frequencies should be tested during audiometry?
    A. Chapter 7.
48. Must all audiograms be done after 10 hours post exposure?
    A. Chapter 16.
49. What kind of tuning fork should be used?
    A. Chapter 7.
50. Should industry do bone conduction testing?
    A. Chapter 16.
51. Does appearance of tympanic membrane predict hearing loss?
    A. No.
52. Can noise cause mental illness?
    A. This has not been established but certainly not occupational noise.

EAR PROTECTION

1. Is there a maximum amount of attenuation that ear protectors can provide?
   A. The maximum amount of attenuation provided by a well fitting head worn protector is about 55 dB. Limitations are set by bone and tissue conduction of the sound and the compliance of the protector.
2. In general what kind of protector gives the most attenuation?
   A. Well fitting head-worn protector generally provides more attenuation capability at most frequencies compared to the insert type protector.
3. Is it necessary to provide maximum attenuation capability in all noise areas?
   A. It is not necessary to provide maximum attenuation in all noise areas. The data from the octave band analysis can be used as a guide to determine what protector will provide the needed attenuation at the particular frequency bands.
4. What are some of the problems of "over protecting"?
   A. If a heavy head-worn protector is used in areas not requiring maximum protection, and the area is hot and/or

humid the device will be rejected on the basis of discomfort alone. In addition it may interfere with verbal communication, the hearing of warning signals, or the ability to detect equipment malfunctions. A lighter head-worn device or inset protector might solve all the problems mentioned and still provide the required attenuation.

5. Do ear muffs have to be fitted?

   A. Common fallacy is that head-worn protectors need not be "fitted." Head bands should be adjustable to allow for highly varying head sizes. The cushion bracket should have freedom to rotate to allow for differences in head shapes. Also the size of the cup should be checked to ascertain comfortable acceptance of the external ear. The final fit should be a good seal around the ear, proper tension of the cups against the head, and comfort.

6. In fitting insert protectors, does each ear of an individual have to be sized and fitted?

   A. Just as heads vary in size and shape, so do ear canals. Frequently individual canals on the same person will vary in size and shape. For this reason each ear should be fitted independently.

7. Why is providing only one type of protector not a good policy?

   A. Experience has shown that programs having only one type protector to offer employees have high failure rates. The psychological factor of "having a choice" is no small matter in successful programs. Attenuation needs, comfort and environmental conditions also point to misinformation of those advocating a "one-type-only" protection program.

8. Are all ear canals basically the same?

   A. Human ear canals have many differences. They can be round, oval, straight, convoluted, tinny or cavernous. There are even differences between the ear canals in each person.

9. Will a particular kind of ear insert fit all ear canals satisfactorily?

A. No. That is why ear insert protectors are manufactured in various shapes, and sizes.

10. What is the general configuration of a universal type plug?

A. Some insert protectors are made in what is commonly known as a universal type configuration. These are generally straight shafts with two or three discs varying in diameter placed along the shafts in a "Christmas tree" effect. The idea being that one of the discs will be large enough to seal against the walls of the canal. "Universal" type plugs are now being made with a series of discs; small but varying in size, medium, and the large discs, also varying in size.

11. What is the principle of operation of ear protectors and how do they achieve their effects?

A. The purpose of ear protection is to reduce the intensity of the changes in air pressure reaching the eardrum (attenuate). The ear protector serves as a partial road block to these pressure changes.

12. What are comments expressed by employees after wearing ear protection?

A. Comments from employees wearing ear protectors will vary as much as human natures. Complaints will focus on "pain, pressure, cause sweating and ear infection; headaches, tinnitus, vertigo, backaches, and hangnails." More rewarding comments will concentrate on "less ear fullness, hear better, better understanding, don't turn TV up so much, ear noise less, less tense, and less tired, to name a few."

13. Are voluntary programs as regards wearing of ear protection generally successful?

A. Just as the "one-type-only" program has a high failure rate, the voluntary program is usually doomed to a similar fate.

14. Why should complaints be considered as real problems and handled accordingly?

A. When an employee has complaints concerning his protectors it should be handled as his personal and real problem. The personal attention given him in offering another type protector, or making adjustments on the one he is presently using shows a genuine interest in his health and well-being and will lead to his acceptance of the device.

15. What procedure is most successful in handling a complaint of discomfort?

  A. If the complaint is one of discomfort with the insert type the ear canal should be inspected for trauma, infection, impacted wax, pimples or cysts. These should receive medical attention. During the medical therapy program another type protector should be issued if permitted by the attending physician. Permanent permission to go without ear protection in an area needing it is not acceptable. Other adjustments to limit this noise exposure will have to be made.

  If there are no physical signs to account for the discomfort the size and shape of the protector should be rechecked. Convoluted canals generally will not comfortably accept "bullet-shaped" or universal type devices.

  Inserts that have been worn for sometime should be examined to ascertain normal pliability of the material. Reaction to ear wax and perspiration sometimes hardens, cracks, or causes sharp edges of the once soft, smooth, composition of the insert.

  Employees also have been known to swap inserts with fellow workers or to buy plugs from a local druggist or sporting goods store. Neither of these should be tolerated. The first because of obvious hygienic reasons; and the second because all controls over the program would be forfeited.

  In head-worn protectors, pressure of the head band and size of the cup around the ear should be checked. A seal pressing against an edge of the external ear can cause a great deal of pain.

  Liquid or grease-filled seals may harden when used in extremely cold work areas. A plastic foam filled seal would be a better choice in this type of environment.

The seal material itself may in some employees cause a dermatitis where it contacts the skin. "Socks" made of soft paper, cotton, or wool are available to place over the plastic seal but it should be remembered that these reduce attenuation by as much as 10 dB.

In some cases poor sanitation techniques may be the cause of the infection. Not cleaning the device frequently enough, using caustic cleansing agents, and insufficient rinsing to remove all residues of the cleansing material are common causes of skin inflammations. These factors hold true for insert protectors also.

16. Where inserts are worn what does irritated ear canals indicate as far as the sizing of the devices?

   A. Surprising as it may seem to some, irritated ear canals in the presence of insert protectors generally indicates that the employee has been undersized. Normal movement of the jaw will easily push the insert out of the canal. Frequently reseating by the wearer will quickly macerate the thin and tender lining of the canal.

17. What are some of the tricks employees will do to their protectors that ruins the attenuation of the device?

   A. In an effort to overcome some of the discomfort related to wearing ear protection, and even to beat "the system" ingenious counter-maneuvers are employed by some workers; Head band pressure is decreased by straightening the band so that the whole device flops crazily about on the head. Holes have been drilled in the cups and cushion seals removed or deflated in the case of air, liquid, or grease filled seals. Head protectors are sometimes worn as a necklace and see the ears only when the nurse, safetyman, or supervisor is in the area. Insert protectors are sometimes cut down or cut off so that only the tab and base remain. Unless the nurse or safety man actually inspects the whole device a "90 percent protection" announcement will have some red faces behind it. Nurses who insist on seeing the protection devices the man has in his ears can give an on the spot lecture if there has been any tampering and get good compliance. Pin-holes burned through the protector should be checked for also.

18. Will *high* or *low* frequencies be less attenuated if small leaks develop in the ear protector?

A. Small air leaks around the seal of the protector (head or insert type) will reduce the low frequency attenuation ability of the devices.

19. What precautions should be taken if hard molded ear plugs are used?

A. It is generally recognized that inserts made of hard plastics or which contain metal cores are unsafe for many industrial purposes. Blows to the ear caused by accidents or interemployee disagreements can drive these devices deep into the canal causing trauma.

20. Does dry cotton make a good ear protector?

A. Plain, dry absorbent cotton is insufficient as an ear protector.

21. Should insert type protectors be re-issued?

A. For hygienic and esthetic reasons, insert type protectors should not be re-issued after being worn by an employee. Head worn protectors have replaceable parts and are more easily sanitized for redistribution.

22. What four fillers are commonly used in seal cushions of head-worn protectors?

A. Cushion seals are filled with either air, liquid, grease, or plastic foam; the latter being in more common usage.

23. What factors will cause an originally well fitted insert plug to lose its effectiveness?

A. The initial fitting of ear inserts on a particular employee may not be his sizing for the rest of his employment tenure. Size changes may be needed due to changes in the dimensions of the canal, or in the insert itself due to aging, chemical reaction to the ear excretions, breaking off of parts of the sealing flange, surgery of the ear canal, and doctoring of the device by the employee.

24. What factor should be kept in mind when reading attenuation curves published by the ear protector manufacturer?

    A. Most ear protection manufacturers supply attenuation curves with their product. The methods they are required to use by the Standards Institute have some shortcomings and for this reason the Z-137 of ANSI is investigating better methods of evaluating and classifying ear protection devices. At present attenuation is evaluated on at least 10 normal hearing listeners, on at least three separate occasions at each test frequency. Some manufacturers published the "best" of the results, others provide mean readings along with standard deviations at each test frequency.

    The "missing 6 dB" found in measuring sensation of loudness under earphones as compared to listening to a loudspeaker in a free field (6-10 dB higher in the low frequencies with earphones) is sometimes misleadingly added to the low frequency attenuation findings.

    Also, attenuation tests are conducted at relatively low sound levels and the published results may have no relationship under actual usage in high noise areas.

    Finally, the ear protectors are not used under laboratory conditions. The way the worker "wears" his protection may be highly dissimilar from paid laboratory subjects who become highly sophisticated as testing progresses.

25. At what noise level does ear protection become mandatory according to the OSHA for long time exposure?

    A. Chapters 16 and 17.

26. Machine operators and repairmen know their equipment by their sound. Does wearing protection upset these references?

    A. Chapters 16 and 17.

27. How is the ear protection program monitored to check its effectiveness?

    A. Chapters 16 and 17.

28. Why should wearing of ear protection apply to *all* personnel entering a designated noisy area?

    A. Chapters 16 and 17.

REFERENCES

1. References Chapters X and XI and the American Industrial Hygiene Noise Manual.
2. Ibid.
3. Ibid.
4. Ibid.
5. Ibid.
6. Ibid.
7. Ibid.
8. Ibid.
9. Ibid.
10. Ibid.
11. Ibid.
12. Beranek, L. L.: *Acoustics,* McGraw-Hill, 1956, p. 364.
13. Ibid.
14. Ibid.
15. Chapter X and XI and the American Industrial Hygiene Noise Manual.
16. Ibid.
17. Ibid.

INDEX